الطب النبوي

The Prophetic Medicine

Ibn Qay'em El-Jozeyah

Qadeem Press

Qadeem Press

Qadeem Press Edition
Breathing Life into Forgotten Pages
www.qadeempress.com

Find our titles on your favourite online bookstore using the keyword 'Qadeem Press'

In the name of Allah the Most beneficent the Most Merciful

Verily, the all praise is to Allah, we have recourse to Him and we ask forgiveness from Him. We ask refuge of Allah, The Glorious, from the evils of ourselves and the sins of our works. Whom does Allah guide, there is no one can misguide him, and whom Allah misguides, no one will guide him. I witness that there is no God but Allah, He is alone and I witness that Mohammed is His slave and his messenger. This book which I have got the honor to translate, it is one of the best books which saved us from treatment of chemicals and poisons that may have got bad sides effects.. I ask Allah The All Mighty The All Great to make my work in this book is pure for his Holy Face. The translators; Abd El Qader and Dr. Enjey R.K

Kinds of Diseases

There are two types of diseases that attack the heart, one doubt and error, and the second lust and desire, both are mentioned in the Qura'an, Allah says about the disease of doubt:

﴿ فِي قُلُوبِهِم مَّرَضٌ فَزَادَهُمُ ٱللَّهُ مَرَضًا ۖ وَلَهُمْ عَذَابٌ أَلِيمٌۢ بِمَا كَانُوا۟ يَكْذِبُونَ ﴾ (١٠) البقرة .

"In their hearts is a disease (of doubt and hypocrisy) and Allah has increased their disease." (2:10)

In addition, He said:

﴿ وَلِيَقُولَ ٱلَّذِينَ فِي قُلُوبِهِم مَّرَضٌ وَٱلْكَٰفِرُونَ مَاذَآ أَرَادَ ٱللَّهُ بِهَٰذَا
مَثَلًا ۚ كَذَٰلِكَ يُضِلُّ ٱللَّهُ مَن يَشَآءُ وَيَهْدِي مَن يَشَآءُ ۚ وَمَا يَعْلَمُ
جُنُودَ رَبِّكَ إِلَّا هُوَ ۚ وَمَا هِيَ إِلَّا ذِكْرَىٰ لِلْبَشَرِ ﴿٣١﴾ ﴾ (٣١) المدثر

"... and that those in whose hearts is a disease (of hypocrisy) and the disbelievers may say: 'What Allah intends by this (curious) example?'" (74:31)

Allah says concerning those who refuse to make the Qura'an and Sun'ah the basis of their judgements:

﴿ وَإِذَا دُعُوٓا۟ إِلَى ٱللَّهِ وَرَسُولِهِۦ لِيَحْكُمَ بَيْنَهُمْ إِذَا فَرِيقٌ مِّنْهُم
مُّعْرِضُونَ ﴿٤٨﴾ وَإِن يَكُن لَّهُمُ ٱلْحَقُّ يَأْتُوٓا۟ إِلَيْهِ مُذْعِنِينَ ﴿٤٩﴾ أَفِي
قُلُوبِهِم مَّرَضٌ أَمِ ٱرْتَابُوٓا۟ أَمْ يَخَافُونَ أَن يَحِيفَ ٱللَّهُ عَلَيْهِمْ
وَرَسُولُهُۥ ۚ بَلْ أُو۟لَٰٓئِكَ هُمُ ٱلظَّٰلِمُونَ ﴿٥٠﴾ ﴾

(٤٨ : ٥٠) النور

"And when they are called to Allah (i.e.. His Words, the Qur'an) and His Messenger ﷺ, to judge between them, lo! a party of them refuses (to come) and turns away. However, if the truth is on their side, they come to him willingly with submission. Is there a disease in their hearts? Alternatively, do they doubt or fear lest Allah and His Messenger ﷺ should wrong them in judgement. Nay, it is they themselves who ore the Zalimun (polytheists, hypocrites and wrongdoers). "(24:48-5O)

This is the disease of doubt and error. In addition, Allah says about desire and lust, adultery in this case:

﴿ يَٰنِسَآءَ ٱلنَّبِيِّ لَسۡتُنَّ كَأَحَدٖ مِّنَ ٱلنِّسَآءِ ۚ إِنِ ٱتَّقَيۡتُنَّ فَلَا تَخۡضَعۡنَ بِٱلۡقَوۡلِ فَيَطۡمَعَ ٱلَّذِي فِي قَلۡبِهِۦ مَرَضٞ وَقُلۡنَ قَوۡلٗا مَّعۡرُوفٗا ﴿٣٢﴾ ﴾ (٣٢) الأحزاب

"O wives of the Prophet! You are not like any other women. If you keep your duty (to Allah), then be not soft in speech, lest he in whose heart is a disease (of hypocrisy, or evil desire for adultery) should be moved with desire..." (33:32)

Physical diseases that attack the body

Allah says:

﴿ لَّيْسَ عَلَى ٱلْأَعْمَىٰ حَرَجٌ وَلَا عَلَى ٱلْأَعْرَجِ حَرَجٌ وَلَا عَلَى ٱلْمَرِيضِ حَرَجٌ ۗ وَمَن يُطِعِ ٱللَّهَ وَرَسُولَهُۥ يُدْخِلْهُ جَنَّٰتٍ تَجْرِى مِن تَحْتِهَا ٱلْأَنْهَٰرُ ۖ وَمَن يَتَوَلَّ يُعَذِّبْهُ عَذَابًا أَلِيمًا ﴿١٧﴾ ﴾

(١٧) الفتح

"There is no restriction on the blind, nor any restriction on the lame, nor any restriction on the sick..." (48:17)

These Verses refer to ailments that might attack a person while performing the Hoy, while fasting or making ablution. They contain c tremendous secret and wisdom, indicating the greatness and divine wisdom of the Qura'an and its sufficiency for those who have sound understanding and comprehension.

The science of medicine consists of three basic rules preserving good health, avoiding what might cause harm (i.e. establishing immunity) an(ridding the body of harmful substances. Allah has mentioned these three basic principles in connection with the performance of Hajj,

Fasting, and ablution mentioned above,

﴿ فَمَن كَانَ مِنكُم مَّرِيضًا أَوْ عَلَىٰ سَفَرٍ فَعِدَّةٌ مِّنْ أَيَّامٍ أُخَرَ ۚ وَعَلَى ٱلَّذِينَ يُطِيقُونَهُۥ فِدْيَةٌ طَعَامُ مِسْكِينٍ ۖ فَمَن تَطَوَّعَ خَيْرًا فَهُوَ خَيْرٌ لَّهُۥ ۚ وَأَن تَصُومُوا۟ خَيْرٌ لَّكُمْ ۖ إِن كُنتُمْ تَعْلَمُونَ ﴿١٨٤﴾ ﴾

(١٨٤) البقرة

"But if any of you is ill or on a journey, the same number (should be made up) from other days." (2:184)

Allah has allowed the sick to break their Fast because of their illness. Allah has In addition permitted the traveler to break their fast in order to protect and preserve their health and strength while traveling. Traveling uses tremendous physical effort that requires nourishment to sustain the body's energy. This is why the traveler is given an exemption from fasting so his body can be supplied with the required nourishment Further, Allah said:

﴿ فَمَن كَانَ مِنكُم مَّرِيضًا أَوْ بِهِۦٓ أَذًى مِّن رَّأْسِهِۦ فَفِدْيَةٌ مِّن صِيَامٍ أَوْ صَدَقَةٍ أَوْ نُسُكٍ ﴾ (١٩٦) البقرة

And whosoever of you is ill or has an ailment in

his scalp (necessitating shaving), he must pay a Fidiah (ransom) of either observing Sawm (fasts) (three days) or giving Sadaqah (charity - feeding six poor persons) or offering sacrifice (one sheep)." (2:196)

Allah has allowed the sick and those suffering from lice or sensitive scalp, to shave their head, which is normally prohibited, while wearing Ihram. Shaving the head and exposing the scalp in these cases removes the harmful substances and thus allows the sick person to get rid of whatever caused his illness and to recover from the condition that was aggravated because of the hair. This is an example of ridding the body of harmful substances, which had a higher priority (thus the exemption) than the general rule, no shaving of the head while in the state of Ihram. There are ten things that might cause harm to the body when congested, unless the body eliminates them: blood when it is irritated, sperm when it is excessive, urine, excrement, air, vomit, the need to sneeze, sleep, hunger and thirst. When any of these ten things are not properly dealt with or satisfied, as in the case of sleep, they will cause a particular type of illness. When Allah permitted shaving the head to remove harmful substances on the scalp, His statement inspired His slaves to use the same practice in removing harmful substances caused by other ailments.

As for observing a certain precautionary measure

(i.e, diet, or other type of abstention), Allah said:

﴿ وَإِن كُنتُم مَّرْضَىٰٓ أَوْ عَلَىٰ سَفَرٍ أَوْ جَآءَ أَحَدٌ مِّنكُم مِّنَ ٱلْغَآئِطِ أَوْ لَـٰمَسْتُمُ ٱلنِّسَآءَ فَلَمْ تَجِدُوا۟ مَآءً فَتَيَمَّمُوا۟ صَعِيدًا طَيِّبًا فَٱمْسَحُوا۟ بِوُجُوهِكُمْ وَأَيْدِيكُمْ ۗ إِنَّ ٱللَّهَ كَانَ عَفُوًّا غَفُورًا ﴿٤٣﴾ ﴾

(٤٣) النساء

"And if you are ill. or on a journey, or one of you comes after answering the call of nature, or you have been in contact with women (by sexual relations) and you find no water, perform Tayammum with clean earth and rub therewith your faces and bands (Tayammum)." (4:43)

Allah has allowed the sick person to use clean earth instead of water to perform his ablution for prayer; this spares his body from the repercussions of using water while ill. This Ayah sets the precedent for every type of precautionary or preventive measure (diet etc.) that protects the body from harmful substances that one consumes or his body produces.

Allah, all praise is due to Him, has emphasized the three basic rules of the science of medicine that we mentioned above.

We will now give several instances and examples that prove Prophetic medicine is superior and more comprehensive than any other method.

Providing proper remedies for ailments of the heart (referring to spiritual or emotional ailments) only occurs at the hands of Prophets عليهم السلام and Messengers of Allah. The heart becomes well when it acquires knowledge of its Lord and Creator and in His Names, Attributes, Actions and Commandments. The heart In addition becomes well when it prefers acquiring Allah's Pleasure and prefers what He likes, all the while avoiding His prohibitions and what might lead to His displeasure. There is no life, health, or wellbeing for the heart except by this method, which only the Messengers can provide. It is wrong to think that one can ever attain the heart's wellbeing through any other way than through the guidance of the Messengers of Allah, These errors result from confusing the heart's true wellbeing with satisfying and strengthening its lower animal lusts and desires. By this way, the heart will be far from acquiring its true wellbeing, strength and even its very existence will be in danger. Those who do not distinguish between these two paths should grieve for their heart's life and health, or in fact for the lack of it. Let such people In addition grieve because of their lacking the light of true guidance and because they are completely submerged in an ocean of darkness.

Remedies for physical illnesses are divided into two categories

One depends on instinct, which all species have. There is no need for the doctor to cure this type of illness, which entails responding to hunger, thirst, cold and fatigue.

The second, requires deep thought and analysis and entails subduing and resisting the ailment, and moderating the patients condition (temperament), which can result from fever, heat, coldness, dryness, or a combination of these symptoms. These ailments have two types of causes: physical and one that relates to temperament. These ailments are the result of a physical cause or are due to changes that affect the mood and the temper (of the body). The difference between the two types is that the ailments of the temperament occur after the physical causes are eliminated. Their effects remain and alter the temperament. The ailments that are caused by physical elements have their causes with them. In these cases of physical disease we should look at the cause first, the ailment second and the cure third.

Further, deep thought and careful analysis are In addition required concerning repelling and removing the ailments that affect the various organs and cause some alterations in the organs whether in the shape, cavity, vessel, roughness, touch, number, bone, and so forth.

When these organs, which collectively constitute the body, are working properly, they are described as being connected. Otherwise, they are described as having lost their proper connectivity.

These ailments that affect and alter the organs are included in the general ailments that affect the body.

As we have stated, these same ailments negatively affect the mood and temperament. The changes that accompany such ailments come in eight types, four simple types and four compound types. The simple types include coldness, hotness, wetness and dryness. The compound types include being hot and wet, hot and dry, cold and wet or cold and dry. The causes of these ailments are either physical or due to changes in the mood or temperament as we have stated.

In addition, there are three states that the body can be in normal, abnormal and in the middle (between normal and abnormal). When the state of the body is normal, the body is healthy. The second state occurs when the body is ill, while the third is in the middle, as one extreme does not become the opposite extreme except after passing through a middle stage.

There are internal reasons for the abnormal state the body passes through, for the body consists of coldness, hotness, wetness and dryness. In addition, there are external reasons for the abnormal state, which could find the body susceptible and affect it.

The potential harm inflicted on the body could result from bad temperament, that was not moderated, an ailment that attacks an organ, or a general weakness in the overall power of the body, or even the soul, which sustains such power, The ailment could be caused by an increase in what should not be increased, or a decrease in what should not be decreased. In addition, a break in the connection could be the cause, where the connection is essential, or due to a connection between that which should not be connected. The ailment could In addition occur due to an extension of what should not be extended or an alteration and change in the shape or place of some of the body organs.

The doctor is able to distinguish between what might harm the body when connected and what should be connected. The doctor In addition distinguishes between what might cause harm if increased and what might cause harm if decreased. The doctor helps bring about good health or what preserves good health, and helps fend off the ailment with its antidote (opposite) or by using a corrective diet. You will see that all these guidelines are met by the guidance and advice of the Prophet **b** **by** Allah's Will, Power and Support.

The Prophet b used medicine himself and prescribed medicine for his family and Companions

Yet, the type of medicines that the Prophet **b** and his companions used to take was nothing like the chemical mixtures that are called, "Aqrabathayn (Pharmacopoeia)". Rather, the majority of their medicine consisted of only one ingredient. Sometimes, they would take another substance to assist the medicine or make it taste better. This was, and still is, the case with most of the medicine used by many cultures such as Arabs, Turks, Indians and nomads. The Romans and the Greeks, on the other hand, use a mixture of substances or remedies in their medicine.

The medical authorities agree that whenever an illness could be fought with nourishment and diet, then medicine should be avoided. In addition, they agree that whenever it is possible to use only one substance or ingredient as a remedy, a compound remedy should not be used. They agree that the body will be harmed if doctors over prescribe medicine. This is because the remedy might not find an illness to cure, or might find an illness that it cannot cure, or might be suitable for the illness, but an excess dose may be given, thereby compromising the health of the body.

The most experienced doctors use medications that contain one ingredient, The medication should be similar or related to regular foods that the patient is used to eating. Cultures that consume one or only a few types of food in their regular diet, generally suffer from few illnesses, they should not use compound medicines. Those who live in cities and whose diets are complex need medicines that are a mixture of several substances or ingredients, as these are the types of medicines that most suit their illnesses. The ailments of the people who live in the deserts are usually simple and thus simple medications are suitable for them. These arguments entail facts that are known in the medical profession.

Prophetic medicine has a divine element to it. This element makes comparing Prophetic medicine to the medicines offered by regular doctors similar to comparing the medicine offered by doctors to folk medicine. The best medical authorities agree to this fact, since the science that they excel in is a result of comparisons, experimentation, inspiration, visions and hypothesis. Some of them state that their knowledge is acquired through the animal kingdom, for example they observe cats swallowing a venomous creature and then observe it lick the oil in the lamp, thus neutralizing the effect of the venom. They In addition observe a snake that has something wrong with its eyes. The snake then wipes its eyes on fennel leaves and cures its condition. In addition, they observe some birds that sip seawater when constipated. There are many similar examples that doctors mention concerning their observations of nature.

This type of knowledge cannot be compared to revelation from Allah to His Messenger and which informs him of what is good for him and what is not. Comparing scientific knowledge to revelation is like comparing the rest of the sciences to what the Prophet b has been sent with. In fact, the Prophets provide us with a kind of medicine that the doctors can barley understand or reach by their experimentation, hypothesis and theories. The Prophets deliver remedies that cure the heart from whatever attacks it. These Prophetic remedies strengthen the heart and increase the reliance and dependence on Allah. It In addition aids in seeking refuge, being humble and showing meekness before Him, Egging Him, giving charity and supplicating to Him. It In addition includes repenting to Allah, seeking His forgiveness, practicing kindness towards His creation and aiding those in desperate need and those who have suffered a calamity. These cures have been tried by various nations who have indeed found them to carry the cure doctors can never prescribe on their own, whether by experimentation or scientific observations.

We have tried the Prophetic cures and found that they are more powerful than any type of regular medicine. Further, it is a fact that comparing the Prophetic medicines to the medicines that doctors prescribe is just like comparing regular medicine to folk medicine.

The hearts that are connected with the Lord of the Worlds - the Creator of the illness and its cure and He Who governs the affairs of everything and everyone - require special types of remedies that are nothing like those required for the hearts that are far away from their Lord. Furthermore, whenever the soul and the heart become stronger (spiritually), they will cooperate to defeat the illness. How can anyone deny that the most effective cure for the ailment that afflicts the heart and soul occurs by feeling delight and joy when drawing closer to the Lord, loving Him, remembering Him, being totally dedicated and attentive to Him, depending on Him and seeking His help? Only the most ignorant people deny these facts, especially those who have the dullest intellect, the worst comprehension and who are the farthest from Allah and from knowing the true reality of mankind. Soon after, Allah willing, we will mention the reason why reciting Al-Fatihah (the first chapter in the Qura'an) has removed the effects of a poisonous sting, enabling the poisoned person to stand up as if he never suffered pain.

We will mention two types of Prophetic medicine in as much detail as possible, according to the limited strength, knowledge and resources available to us. We rely only on Allah for every type of good and righteous matter, while seeking His Bounty, for He is the Cherished Who grants favors without limit.

Every sickness has got a cure

Muslim narrated in his Sahih that the Prophet **b** said:

"Every illness has a cure. and when the proper cure is applied to the disease, it ends it, Allah willing."

In addition, it is narrated in the Sahihan that the Messenger of Allah said:

"Allah has not sent down a disease except that He has In addition sent down its cure."

Further, Imam Ahmad narrated that Usamah bin Shuraik said:

" I was with the Prophet **b** when the Bedouins came to him and said, 'O Messenger of Allah, should we seek medicine?' He said, 'Yes, O slaves of Allah, seek medicine, for Allah has not created a disease except that he has In addition created its cure, except for one illness.' They said. 'And what is that?' He said, 'Old age."

In addition, it is related in the Al Mosn'ad (by Imam Ahmad) that the Prophet **b** said:

"Allah has not sent down a disease except that He In addition sent down its cure; whoever knows it (the cure), knows it, and whoever is unaware of it (the cure), he is unaware of it." (the medicine) while those who are ignorant of it are unaware of it." [An-Nasa'y, Ibn Majah, Al-Hakim and Ibn Hibban].

In addition, it is narrated in the Musnad (by Imam Ahmad) and the Sunon (of At-Termezey and Ibn Majah) that Abu Khuzamah said:

"I said, 'O Messenger of Allah ﷺ about the Ruqya (divine remedies - Islamic supplication formula) that we use, the medicine we take and the prevention we seek, does all this change Allah's appointed destiny?' He said, 'They are a part of Allah's appointed destiny."

These Ahadeeth indicate there are causes for whatever occurs in this world and removal of these causes.

The Prophet's statement that there is a cure for every disease might include both the curable and the humanly incurable diseases, for Allah may have hidden these types of cures from mankind and blocked their path to acquiring them. Allah knows best. The Prophet **b** said that the disease ends when the proper cure is applied to it, indicating that there is an opposite for every creation and thus there is an antidote for every disease. The Messenger of Allah **b** has stated that when the two opponents meet, meaning, the proper remedy and the disease, recovery from the illness occurs. When the medicine is given in a dosage higher than what is needed, or when it is not the required medicine, it might lead the body to another type of disease. When the dosage is less than what is needed, it will not be sufficient to cure the disease. When the sick person and the disease are not treated with the suitable medicine, cure and recovery does not occur. In addition, when the time is not suitable for the cure, or when the body is unable or unsuitable for the prescribed medicine, the cure will not be effective. When all circumstances are favorable, the cure will surely be effective. This is the best explanation available for these Ahadeeth.

On the other hand, these Ahadeeth might be specific, in that Allah has not created a disease that can be humanly cured but has sent down a cure for it. This is similar to what Allah said:

﴿ تُدَمِّرُ كُلَّ شَيْءٍ بِأَمْرِ رَبِّهَا فَأَصْبَحُوا لَا يُرَىٰ إِلَّا مَسَاكِنُهُمْ ۚ كَذَٰلِكَ
نَجْزِي الْقَوْمَ الْمُجْرِمِينَ ﴿٢٥﴾ ﴾ (٢٥) الأحقاف

"Destroying everything by the Command of its Lord!" (46:25)

This Ayah means that everything prone to be

destroyed was destroyed by the wind. In this case, the Ahadeeth do not include incurable diseases.

Those who observe various substances and their opposites in this world, and analyze the pacifying effect, opposing nature and resistance in relation to each other, would appreciate Allah's perfect power, eternal wisdom and perfect creation and His Oneness in the Lordship and in His Actions. Everything else except Allah has an opponent or an antidote, but Allah Alone is the Self Sufficient and Irresistible, while everything and everyone stands in need of Him.

These authentic Ahadeeth command Muslims to seek and take the appropriate medicine, while indicating that this action does not contradict dependence on Allah Alone for everything. Just as one satisfying his hunger, thirst or reacts to being hot or cold does not contradict the dependence on Allah. On the contrary, the belief in Tawheed (Oneness of Allah) can only be complete by pacifying and responding to the various harmful elements in the manner and method that Allah has commanded and that which will help in such cases. Furthermore, refraining from using these cures or antidotes is, in fact, contradictory to total dependence on Allah, along with contradicting the Commandments and the Wisdom (of Allah). Not using these cures will In addition weaken our Tawakkul (reliance and dependence on Allah) even though the person might be thinking that he is strengthening his reliance and dependence by abandoning seeking the cure. Abandoning the cure is in fact contradictory to the true reliance and dependence, in that, reliance and dependence in essence includes the heart of the slave relying on Allah in acquiring what benefits him in his life and his religious affairs, while fending off what harms his life and religion. The correct method of reliance and dependence includes seeking these benefits for the slave; otherwise one will not be implementing the Commandments and the Wisdom. The slave should not call his inability, dependence on Allah, nor consider his true reliance and dependence as an inability.

These Ahadeeth In addition contradict those who do not seek medicine, saying:

"If the cure has been written or is destined to occur, then the medicine will be of no use. If the cure was not destined, then the medicine will not be useful."

In addition, one might say:

"The disease has occurred by Allah's will, and no one and nothing can resist Allah's will."

The last statement is similar to the question that the Bedouins asked the Messenger of Allah. As for his close companions, who had more knowledge of Allah,

His Wisdom and His Attributes, they did not think the way the Bedouins did.

The Prophet b gave the Bedouins an answer that comforted their heart, saying that these Ruqya (Islamic prayer formulas), medicines and preventative measures, are all part of Allah's Appointed Destiny. Therefore, nothing escapes Allah's Destiny, except by Allah's Destiny, Taking medicine is a part of Allah's Destiny and it repels a part of Allah's Destiny. In short, there is no way that the creation can escape Allah's Destiny no matter what they do. This is the exact same case with ending the hunger, thirst, warm or cold conditions with what satisfies or pacifies them. In addition, it is similar to repelling the enemy, which is a part of Allah's Destiny, with Jihad, which is In addition Allah's Commandment and appointed Destiny. Thus, the cause, its removal and those who remove it are all a part of Allah's appointed destiny.

Another way of answering those who ask similar questions (concerning taking medicine) is that this logic requires them to refrain from seeking their benefit or fending off harm. Following their logic, if the benefit or harm was destined to occur, then it would surely occur, and if it were not destined, then it would never occur! This method, if implemented, would bring utter destruction to life, religion and the entire world. Furthermore, this rhetoric only comes from those who arrogantly deny the truth and reject it, and this is why they mention destiny concerning this subject so as to refute the truth when it is offered to them. This is the exact case with the polytheists, who said:

﴿ سَيَقُولُ ٱلَّذِينَ أَشْرَكُوا۟ لَوْ شَآءَ ٱللَّهُ مَآ أَشْرَكْنَا وَلَآ ءَابَآؤُنَا وَلَا
حَرَّمْنَا مِن شَىْءٍ ۚ كَذَٰلِكَ كَذَّبَ ٱلَّذِينَ مِن قَبْلِهِمْ حَتَّىٰ
ذَاقُوا۟ بَأْسَنَا ۗ قُلْ هَلْ عِندَكُم مِّنْ عِلْمٍ فَتُخْرِجُوهُ لَنَآ ۖ إِن
تَتَّبِعُونَ إِلَّا ٱلظَّنَّ وَإِنْ أَنتُمْ إِلَّا تَخْرُصُونَ ﴿١٤٨﴾ ﴾ (١٤٨) الأنعام

"If Allah had willed, we would not have taken partners (in worship) with Him, nor would our fathers..." (6:148)

And:

﴿ وَقَالَ ٱلَّذِينَ أَشْرَكُوا۟ لَوْ شَآءَ ٱللَّهُ مَا عَبَدْنَا مِن دُونِهِۦ
مِن شَىْءٍ نَّحْنُ وَلَآ ءَابَآؤُنَا وَلَا حَرَّمْنَا مِن دُونِهِۦ مِن شَىْءٍ ۚ
كَذَٰلِكَ فَعَلَ ٱلَّذِينَ مِن قَبْلِهِمْ ۚ فَهَلْ عَلَى ٱلرُّسُلِ إِلَّا ٱلْبَلَٰغُ
ٱلْمُبِينُ ﴿٣٥﴾ ﴾ (٣٥) النحل

"If Allah had so willed, neither we nor our fathers

would have worshipped aught but Him." (16:35)

The polytheists issued these statements to refute Allah's proof against them when He sent the Messengers to them.

In addition, those who utter this question, concerning destiny, medicine and true reliance and dependence should know that there is an argument that they did not mention. Allah has decided that such and such matters will occur when such and such causes occur. Thus, if the cause is implemented or practiced, what was destined would In addition occur.

If one asks, "If I was destined to practice the cause, I would practice it. Otherwise, I would not be able to bring it into existence." We answer this claim by saying, "Would you accept such reasoning from your servant, children or workers if they deny what you have ordered them to do or commit an act that you have forbidden for them? Because if you accept such reasoning, then you have no right to blame those who disobey you, steal your property, question your honor, or transgress against your rights. If you chastise such persons for these acts, then how can you use the same logic to deny Allah's rights and Commandments on you?"

Jewish tradition states that Ibraheem عليه السلام once asked Allah, "O my Lord! Where does the disease come from?" He said, "From Me." Ibraheem عليه السلام said, "Where does the cure come from?" He said, "From Me." Ibraheem عليه السلام said, "What is the role of the doctor then?" He said, "A man in whose hands I send and cause the cure."

The Prophet's statement that there is a cure for every illness should strengthen the resolve of the sick person and the doctor, encouraging them to seek medicine. When the sick person feels that there is a cure for his illness, his heart will be full of hope, rather than despair, and thus the doors of positive anticipation will be wide open before him. When the resolve of the ailing person is strengthened, the various powers that exists within the person, the instinctive energy (or heat as Ibn Al-Qayyim puts it), the soul and the psyche, will In addition be strengthened. These powers will in turn strengthen that part of the body affected and the disease will be more easily dissipated and defeated.

In addition, when the doctor knows that there is a cure for that illness, he actively and energetically pursues that cure.

The diseases that attack the body are similar to diseases that attack the heart. Just as Allah has sent down a cure for every disease that strikes the heart, He has sent down a cure for every disease that attacks the body. If the person acquires knowledge of this cure and applies it in the proper manner, his heart will regain its health by Allah's Leave.

The Prophet's guidance concerning food and drink

Including observing diets, refraining from excessive eating and the general guidelines that should be observed regarding eating and drinking.

Al-Musnad (by Imam Ahmad) narrated that the Prophet b said:

"The son of Adam never fills a vessel worse than his stomach. The son of Adam only needs a few bites that would sustain him, but if he insists, one third should be reserved for his food, another third for his drink and the last third for his breathing."

Physical aliments

Physical aliments attack and harm the body and alter its normal functions, because of an excess amount of a substance. This type constitutes the majority of diseases and occurs, because of overeating or consuming more than what the body needs, that which brings about little benefit or is not digested easily, or due to complex meals, When the son of Adam habitually fills his stomach with these types of foods, he will end up with various types of illnesses, some of which take a long time to remedy. On the other hand, when one consumes moderate amounts of food and eats sensibly, the body will get the maximum benefit from this diet, as opposed to when one overeats.

The foods we eat are for necessity, sufficiency or excessiveness. The Prophet **b** told us that one only needs a few bites to sustain him, so that his strength does not fail him. When one wishes to exceed what is barely enough, he should reserve a third of his stomach for his food, another third for the water or drink and the last third for breathing. This is the best method of eating, both for the body and for the heart. When the stomach is full of food, there will not be enough space for drinking. When one consumes something to drink on a full stomach, one's breathing will be difficult, thus bringing about laziness and fatigue. One will feel heavy, as if carrying a load on his stomach. Consequently, one will be lazy fulfilling his obligations and will seek other desires now that his stomach is full!

Eating until one is full harms the body and the heart, when it becomes a habit. There is no harm if one occasionally eats his fill. For example, Abu Hurayrah ONCE drank some milk in the presence of the Prophet **b** until he said, "By He Who has sent you with the Truth! I do not find a place for it." The Companions at times used to eat their fill in the presence of the Prophet **b** . Eating until full as a matter of habit weakens the strength and the body, even as one becomes fatter. The body will be strong when it gets the nourishment it needs and can utilize, not from the quantity of food one eats.

The human body consists of three basic elements: water, solids and air (whereas the fourth basic element is fire, according to the Greeks), This is why the Prophet **b** gave each of these elements its due share in the body (the stomach being part of the body - editor). If someone asks about the share of fire in the body, we say that doctors confirm that heat is used in reactions that occur in the body. Other people disagree with this opinion and state that there is no fire part in the body. They reached these conclusions based on the following assumptions.

First, the firey part could either descend from the air and be mixed with the watery and solid parts (of the human body), or it could exist within the watery and solid matter.

The first assumption is not plausible, because fire naturally ascends and does not descend, otherwise it would depart from its center and descend to the earth. In addition, if in fact fire descends, it would have to pass through spheres of bitter cold that exist on earth and it would still have to remain intact. However, what we in fact observe in this world is that a great fire is extinguished with a little amount of water. Thus if the fire were to descend from its center, it would certainly be extinguished due to the bitterly cold spheres it would pass through.

The second assumption is that fire is formed inside the solid and watery bodies. This is even less plausible, because the body that has turned to fire must have been watery, earthly, or composed of air beforehand, along with being surrounded by such elements. In this case, the element that is surrounded and interconnected with the watery or solid elements would not turn to fire on its own, because it is not produces heat, the body would be cold. If the nature of the body is susceptible to coldness and the surrounding environment does not have the opposite effect, the body will reach the coldest degree there is. In this state, the body would not feel the coldness because it would have reached such coldness that it would be in fact frozen. Therefore, the state of coldness and the body would be in the same cool degree and thus the body would not feel the cold nor would it feel any pain because of the extreme cold. The same argument can be said when the body is in a lower temperature than the cold substance itself. Thus, if the body did not have any fiery part, it would not normally feel the cold nor be affected by it.

They In addition say that, "Your proofs only serve to refute the opinion that the fiery parts remain as fire within the bodies. We do not support this statement. Rather, we say that fire changes when it is mixed with the body."

Those who oppose this idea reply, "Why not say that the heat of the sun blends the earth, water and air? Then, when the resulting mixture reaches maturity, it would be ready to take new shapes whether these shapes are plants, animals or minerals, with the heat as the medium. Why not say that the inner heat and warmth that exist in the body are the result of certain qualities and powers that Allah brings into existence upon blending the mixture, not that they actually contain fiery parts? You have no way of denying this possibility, as some of the best medical authorities agree."

In addition, the fact that the body feels the cold only indicates that there is an inner heat in body. Who denies this fact anyway? But, what is the evidence that this heat is only produced by fire? Yes, the fire radiates heats, but not every type of heat is the result of fire. Rather, the correct statement in this regard is that some types of heat are produced by fire.

In addition, the statement that the fire's essence changes when it mixes with the body is not supported by the opinions of the best doctors, or by fact. In addition, some of your (those who say that the body is part fire) best supporters (i.e. Ibn Sina, the misguided philosopher) has admitted in his book Ash-Shifaa (The Cure) that the four essential elements (water, fire, earth and air) retain their essential qualities when blended in a compound.

The Prophet b used three types of remedies for various ailments: natural, divine and a combination of both natural and divine

We will mention the three types of remedies that the Prophet bprescribed and used, starting with the natural medicines, then the divine remedies and lastly those composed of the two types.

The Prophet s& was sent as a guide and a caller to Allah and to His Paradise. He acquainted the people with Allah. He In addition informed them of what pleases Him and commanded them to implement these actions, and informed them of what angers Allah and ordered them to avoid these actions. He told them stories of the Prophets and Messengers b and what occurred between them and their nations. He In addition acquainted the people with the creation of the world, its beginning, Resurrection and how and the reasons why souls will either acquire misery or happiness.

As for the remedies of the bodies, this is a part of the Prophet's Law that completes it and makes it whole. The remedies of the body should be used when needed. Other than that. it is better to spend the time and energy curing the ills of the heart and soul, preserving their health, and preventing any harm from touching them. This is the ultimate goal that the Prophet's mission seeks to achieve. It is a fact that curing the ills of the body without curing the heart does not work or benefit anyone. However, curing the heart while the body is ill does not cause extensive harm since soon after, this harm will be removed and will be replaced with the ultimate, eternal benefit. All success comes from Allah.

Curing fever

It has been narrated in the Sahihan that the Prophet said:

'Verily Fever- or severe fever- is a breath of the Hell Fire, so cool it using water."

This Hadith has caused confusion for many ignorant doctors as they thought it contradicts the common method of treating fever. We will explain this Hadith in detail, Allah willing.

When the Prophet sg issues a statement, it is either general for all people or for specific people and conditions. The majority of the Prophet's statements are of the first type. As for the second type, it is similar to the Prophet's statement:

"Do not face the Qiblah with urine or feces, nor leave it directly behind you. Rather, face either the East or the West."

This statement (facing the East or the West) is not for those who reside in the East, the West or Iraq, but for those residing in Al-Medina and Ash-Sham (Syria). It is the same case with the Prophet's statement:

"What is between the East and the West is a Qibl'ah."

Understanding this fact, we can realize that what the Prophet s, said regarding fever is particularly for the people of Hijaz (Western Arabia), for the people in this area are susceptible to a type of fever that results from sunstroke. This type of fever requires cold water, either by drinking it or taking a bath. Fever causes rising temperatures in the body that emanates from the heart and which spreads throughout the entire body via the blood vessels and the soul, which disrupts the proper functioning of the body.

There are two types of fever, accidental that is a result of tumors, sunstroke, movements, or intense heat and another type that results from an ailment that usually starts at a particular organ and then heats up the entire body. When the fever is of the first type, it ends in one to three days. If the fever is a result of harmful mixtures, it is called septic (or toxic) fever, which is divided into four types: bilious, melancholic, phlegm and sanguinary. If the fever originated in the basic organs of the body, it is called hectic fever, which has many types In addition.

The body benefits from the fever more so than it benefits from taking medicine. This is because; the fever heats up and matures harmful substances, which it could not have done without the fever. In addition, the fever causes various blockages to open especially those that medicines can not reach.

As for simple and chronic conjunctivitis, fever helps cure most of its types quickly, as well as, helping against facial paralysis, hemiplegia, paralysis affecting only one side of the body, spasms and many other ailments that result from thick substances or excesses.

Some of the best doctors feel a bit relieved when fever breaks out in an ailing body, just as the sick person rejoices upon recovering from illness. This is because fever is more efficient than medication in some cases, since it matures the spoiled and septic substances that harm the body. When such substances reach maturity, the medicine will reach it, as the substances are ready to be discarded out of the body, concluding this process. Thus, the fever becomes a part of the cure.

Based on these facts, it appears that the Hadith is talking about the accidental type of fevers that are relieved by being submerged into cold water or by drinking cold water. In this case, the sick person does not need any other medicine, because this type of fever is composed of heat that is connected to the soul. When a cold substance is introduced, the heat produced by the fever will be eliminated without having to get rid of any mixtures of substances or to wait for these substances to mature.

Galinus, one of the renowned doctors, admitted that cold water helps relieve this type of fever. He stated in the tenth article in his book, Healing Methods, "If a young, healthy man, who does not suffer from an internal tumor, took a bath in the heat of the day or swam in it, he will gain a benefit," He In addition stated that he used to prescribe this remedy on a regular basis.

In addition, Ar-Razi said in his book, Al-Kabir:

"If the strength is normal, but the fever is very intense and the maturity (of the harmful substances) is apparent, while not suffering from any internal tumors or any type of ruptures, then drinking cold water becomes beneficial. If the ailing person is fat, the weather is hot and the person is used to taking cold showers, let him do just that."

In the Prophet's statement: "The fever is a breath inferno's fire." There are two possible meanings.

First, the fever is a breath that was released from Hell so that the slaves are aware of it and thus learn a lesson from this fact. Therefore, Allah has created reasons and causes for the fever to appear and breakout. Similarly, comfort, joy, enjoyment and elation are a part of Paradise's joys that Allah has allowed to appear in this world as an example and a lesson, and He has allowed such feelings to be connected to reasons and causes behind their appearance.

Secondly, the Hadith equated fever and the heat of day, to the intense heat of Hellfire, so that our hearts could imagine the intense torment of the Fire and the heat that emits from it.

The Prophet's statement, 'Cool it off with water might entail all types of water, and this is the correct opinion. Another opinion states that the water here means Zamzam water. Supporters of this opinion used as evidence what Al-Bokhary narrated in his Sahih that Abu Jamrah, Nasr bin 'Imran Adh-Dhuba'i said, "I used to be in the presence of Ibn Ab'ass in Mecca until one day, I was struck by fever. He said to, 'Cool it off with Zamzam water, for the Messenger of Allah said:

"Fever is a breath of Hell's fire." therefore, cool it with water, or said with Zamzam water.'"

The narrator of the Hadith was in doubt as to the

exact words of the Prophet b . Otherwise, it would be established that the Prophet meant Zamzam water for the people of Mecca, because it is available. All others can use whatever water is available to them.

There is a difference of opinion concerning if the Prophet ^ meant by this Hadith to encourage giving away some water as a charity, or to actually use it. The correct opinion is that the Hadith means using it. I believe that those who thought the Hadith means giving away some water as a charity did not understand the goal behind using cold water for fever. Yet, there is a good explanation for the Prophet's statement, for the reward is of a type compa.able to the deed. Since thirsty people drink cold water to quench their thirst, Allah dissipates the fever with cold water, as well. Yet, this is an implication of the Hadith, as for the ruling contained in it, it simply means to use the water (not give it away in charity).

Abu Nu'aym said, Anas narrated that the Prophet said:

"If any of you comes down with fever, let him sprinkle cold water on himself for three consecutive nights before daybreak."

Ibn Majah narrated that Abu Hurayrah related from the Prophet b that he said:

"Fever is a bellow of Hell's heat. So remove it from you with cold water."

It is In addition narrated in the Sunon that Abu Hurayrah said:

"Fever was mentioned in the presence of the Messenger of Allah b and a man cursed it. The Messenger of Allah said:

'Do not curse it, for it removes the sins, just as fire removes the impurity of the iron." [In addition refer to Sahib Muslim].

Fever is usually followed by a diet avoiding improper foods and requires consuming beneficial foods and medicines. The sick person's body will be cleansed from all impurities and septic elements and materials, having a similar purifying effect as the fire has when it removes the impurity of the iron. The benefits that fever has are already known to the medical authorities.

As for cleansing the heart from its ills and impurities, only doctors of the heart (this does not refer to cardiologists-Editor) have access to this type of knowledge. Such experts will find that whatever the Prophet s^ stated in this regard is the plain truth. However, when the heart's ills become chronic, hope diminishes that it will ever be cured!

Fever thus helps the body and the heart. Therefore, cursing such a beneficial matter would be an act of injustice and transgression.

Abu Hurayrah said:

"No ailment that I might suffer from is dearer to me than fever, because it enters every organ of my body, and Allah gives each organ its due share of-the reward."

Therefore, using cold water to relieve fever during summer and in hot areas is beneficial, because the water would be the furthest from the rays of the sun just before daybreak (at its coolest). In addition, just before daybreak the body is at its strongest, for the ailing person would have taken his due share of sleep and relaxation In addition they would have less polluted air to breathe. The strength of the body will be added to the strength of the medicine - water in this case - and they will both relieve the fever that is not a result of malignant tumors or septic substances or conditions. Allah will then extinguish the heat of the fever by His will.

The Prophet's guidance on curing diarrhea

It is narrated in the Sahihan that Abu Sa'id Al-Khudri said:

"A man came to the Prophet s& and said, 'My

brother is complaining about stomach, or he is complaining about diarrhea.' The Prophet **b** said, 'Give him some honey.' The man went and came back later, saying, 'I have given him some honey, but it did not help,' or he said, 'It made his diarrhea worse.' He repeated this twice or three times, all the while the Prophet **b** continued saying to him, 'Give him some honey.' In the third or fourth time, the Prophet ^ said, 'Allah has said the truth while your brother's stomach has lied.'"

Honey has tremendous medicinal value, because it washes away the harmful substances that might be collected in the veins and the intestines. Honey In addition dissolves excess moisture, is beneficial as a drink and as an ointment, it is of great value for the elderly, and those suffering from phlegm and cold moods or condition (chills). Honey is nutritious, softens one's bowel movement and is a good preserving agent. In addition, honey reduces the bitter taste of other medicines, cleanses the liver and the chest, aids in producing urine, and dissolves the phlegm that is accompanied by coughing. When honey is consumed hot and mixed with rose oil, it cures animal bites and the effects of opium. Taking honey mixed with water helps against the bite of a rabid dog and the effects of eating poisonous mushrooms. If fresh meat is kept in honey, it preserves its freshness for three months. Likewise if gourds, cucumbers and eggplants are kept in honey, they too will be preserved.

Further, honey will keep some types of fruit fresh for six months. It preserves dead corpses, thus deserving to be called, "The true preserver." When honey is applied to someone that is infected with lice, it will kill both the lice and the eggs. Honey will In addition add softness and beauty to the hair while allowing it to grow longer. When honey is applied to the eye as a Kuhl, it will strengthen weak eyesight. Honey In addition whitens the teeth, preserves their health and the health of the gums, opens the orifice of the veins along with causing the flow of menstruation. Furthermore, licking honey on an empty stomach will help the body get rid of mucus and phlegm. It cleanses the stomach and rids it of harmful substances or mixtures, heats the stomach mildly and opens up the pores. Honey has similar effects on the kidneys, the prostate and the liver. Furthermore, honey is the least harmful sweet substance for congesting the liver and kidneys.

Adding to all these benefits that we mentioned, honey does not have any side effects, nor harm except for those suffering from bile and who should take it with vinegar to neutralize its harm.

Honey is In addition a food, a drink, a sweet, a remedy, a type of refreshment and an ointment, along with its numerous medicinal values. Therefore, there is no other substance that is more beneficial than honey or that even rivals its value. This is why the people of old relied on honey, for most of the books of old do not mention sugar, as this was discovered in modern times.

The Prophet b used to drink some honey mixed with water on an empty stomach. There is a wonderful secret behind this practice regarding preserving the health. Only those who enjoy sound comprehension will be able to recognize such a secret. We will mention this subject again when we explain the Prophet's guidance regarding persevering good health.

A Hadith [narrated by Ibn Majah and others] stated that the Prophet b said:

"Make use of the two cures: honey and the Qura'an."

This Hadith joins the material and the divine cures, the medicine of the body and the soul, the earthly medicine and the heavenly cure.

Understanding these facts, let us go back to the man to whom the Prophet had prescribed honey to cure his diarrhea, which was caused by overeating. The Prophet ^ prescribed honey for him to rid his stomach and intestines from accumulating harmful substances or excretions that prevents the food in the stomach from being digested, because honey has a cleansing effect. The harmful, viscid substances were adhering to the stomach walls, which is similar to the material of a towel, polluting both the stomach and the food. Honey removes these substances that engulf the stomach, and it is the best cure for this condition. Honey is a potent cleanser and is effective in treating cases of diarrhea, especially when the honey is mixed with warm water.

The Prophet b repeated his command to the man to give some honey to his sick brother for a good reason. The prescribed medicine should be in sufficient doses; otherwise, the ailment will not be fully cured. When the prescribed medicine is in a larger than necessary dose, it will weaken the body and cause side effects. When the Prophet ^ first ordered the man to give his brother honey, he did not give him a sufficient amount to cure his condition. When the man said that his brother was not cured, the Prophet s& knew that the dose was not sufficient, so he told the man several times to give his brother more honey, so that the dose would reach a sufficient amount. When the sick person has several doses of honey in a sufficient amount to fight the disease, the cure occurs by Allah's permission. Giving the correct dose of the proper medicine is a major part of the science of medicine.

When the Prophet b said to the man:

"Allah has said the truth and your brother's

stomach has lied."

This indicates the sure effectiveness of the honey. It In addition indicates that the illness remained not because the prescribed medicine was not effective, but because the stomach had a large amount of spoiled substances in it. Therefore, the Prophet **b** . ordered the man to take more medicine because his stomach contained excessive amounts of spoiled substances.

Prophetic medicine is not similar to that offered by doctors and physicians. Prophetic medicine is indeed the effective treatment and cure provided by the revelation and the guidance of the Prophet **b** that is coupled with a sound and perfect mind. In comparison, the majority of remedies prescribed by other than a Prophet **b** are built on hypothesis, observation and experimentation.

It is a fact that many people do not benefit from Prophetic medicine, because it will help only those who acknowledge and have faith in it. Thus, they believe that it will help them and they then submit to it. If the Qura'an, which is a cure for whatever the heart conceals, is not acknowledged and accepted with faith, it will not provide a cure for the heart. In fact, the Qura'an will only add more evil and disease to the hearts of the hypocrites.

Prophetic medicine is only suitable for good and pure bodies, just as the Qura'an is only suitable for righteous souls and feeling hearts. Therefore, when the people ignore Prophetic medicine, it is like ignoring the help and guidance of the Qura'an, which is the most effective medicine. Again, when the medicine (the Qura'an and the Prophetic medicine) do not work, it is due to the negativity in the body and soul that are not suitable for accepting the medicine, not because the medicine does not work. All success comes from Allah, Wherein is healing for men

There is a conflict of opinion concerning what Allah said:

﴿ ثُمَّ كُلِي مِن كُلِّ ٱلثَّمَرَٰتِ فَٱسْلُكِي سُبُلَ رَبِّكِ ذُلُلًا ۚ يَخْرُجُ مِنۢ بُطُونِهَا شَرَابٌ مُّخْتَلِفٌ أَلْوَٰنُهُۥ فِيهِ شِفَآءٌ لِّلنَّاسِ ۗ إِنَّ فِى ذَٰلِكَ لَءَايَةً لِّقَوْمٍ يَتَفَكَّرُونَ ﴿٦٩﴾ ﴾ (٦٩) النحل

"There comes forth from their bellies, a drink of varying color wherein is healing for men." (16:69)

The disagreement revolves around the words "wherein is healing for men" if they refer to the drink or the Qura'an?. There are two opinions on this matter, the closest to the truth is what Ibn Mas'ud, Ibn Ab'ass, Al-Hasan, Qatadah, and the majority of the scholars stated, that these words refer to the drink. The Ayah, (Verse) is talking about the drink and not the Qura'an. Adding to this fact, the Prophet **b** said in the previous Hadith, "Allah has said the truth," as it is clear in determining that the verse is referring to the drink. Allah knows best.

The Prophet **b** commanded Muslims not to enter a plague-infested area

In the Sahihan it is narrated that Sa'd bin Abi Waqqas asked Usamah bin Zayd about what he heard the Prophet :ge say concerning the plague. Usamah said that the Messenger of Allah **b** said:

"The plague is a punishment that was sent down on some of the Children of Israel and on those who were before your time. So if you hear that it has struck a land do not enter that land. and if it breaks out in a land that you are residing in, do not go out of that area escaping from it."

Furthermore, in the Sahihan it is narrated that the Messenger of Allah **b** said:

"The plague is a martyrdom for every Muslim."

Linguistically, Taoon, the plague, is a type of disease. In medical terms, the plague is a fatal, vicious tumor that causes a very strong and painful infection, quickly turning the infected area into black, green or brown color. Soon afterwards, ulcers start to appear around the infected area. The plague usually strikes three areas, under the arms, behind the ear and the tip of the nose, and / or, the soft (flaccid) tissues of the body. A'esha narrated that she asked the Prophet b about the plague, and he said:

"A gland that is similar to the camel's gland and which appears in the tender parts of the abdomen and under the arms."

Doctors say that when a septic infection occurs in the soft flesh, such as under the arms or behind the ears, it is called the plague. The plague is caused by spoiled, septic blood [infected by a bug that carried the disease from infected rodents]. The infected blood spoils the part of the body that it strikes, sometimes causing blood hemorrhaging and pus. In this case, the inflicted organ sends the infected blood to the heart, thus causing vomit, unconsciousness and rapid heartbeat. Although the plague describes every infection that sends septic blood to the heart, becoming fatal sometimes, it particularity describes the infection that attacks the soft tissues of the body. Since the infected blood is septic, the various organs reject the blood, except those that have become weak. The worst types of the plague are those that strike behind ears and under the arms, because they are closer to the essential organs of the body. There is little chance to be cured from the black plague, while the red plague then the yellow plagues are the least dangerous. Since the plague breaks out in polluted areas, it is called a plague, although this word describes every epidemic, as we have stated, and as Al-Khalil has concurred.

The word epidemic is more general than the plague. Every plague is an epidemic while not every epidemic is a plague.

The plagues cause infections, ulcers and malignant growths in the areas of the body we described. It is my judgment that these are only the symptoms of the plague, since this is what doctors visibly observe, thus prompting the doctors to call them symptoms of the plague.

There are three meanings for the word plague. First: the symptoms of the disease that the doctors observe and record.

Second, the death that occurs to those inflicted by the plague, as the Prophet **b** said:

The plague is a martyrdom for every Muslim."

Third, the reason behind the outbreak of the plague, which is mentioned in the Hadith,

"The plague is the remnant of a punishment that was sent on the Children of Israel."

In addition, the plague was described in another Hadith that:

"It is a result of the Jinn's touch." Further, the Prophet **b** said that the plague is:

A Prophet's supplication.

The doctors cannot refute the reasons we have mentioned explaining why the plague breaks out, although they feel that there is no physical proof that supports them. The Messengers informed us of matters of the Unseen, while the doctors' expertise deals with the physical symptoms of the plague. However, the symptoms of the plague that doctors are familiar with do not provide them with any material evidence that the plague does not engage the soul in some manner, for there is a tremendous connection between the soul and what the body suffers due to disease and ultimately death. Only the most ignorant people will deny the effects of the soul on the body and on human nature as a whole. Allah gives the soul certain powers over the body of the sons of Adam, at such times when an epidemic breaks out or when the air is unhealthy. In addition, the soul has certain effects on the body when it experiences the ailments that are caused by septic substances, especially when blood, semen or black bile is irritated. Evil forces take control of the body when it experiences such emotions and ailments, unless the person repels it with an even stronger power, such as remembering Allah, supplicating to Him, invoking and pleading to Him giving in charity and reciting the Qura'an. In this case, angels will descend and will defeat and neutralize the evil effects of the devilish souls (evil forces). We have successfully tried this method many times, that which only Allah is Able to count, and we witnessed the wonderful effects of such positive forces (good souls) in strengthening one's resolve and ridding him of bad elements when in the early stages. This method almost never fails. When one feels that evil is close-by him, he should turn to good deeds as we have explained, so that they deter and fend off the evil forces (souls). This is the best medicine in such cases for those whom Allah leads to success. But when Allah decides that His appointed destiny takes over, He draws the slave's heart away from knowing and intending to perform these good deeds. In this case, the slave does not decide or intend to perform these good deeds, so that what Allah has decided takes over,

Allah willing, we will elaborate further on this subject when we discuss the divine remedies of Islamic prayer formulas (Ruqya literally: incantations), the Prophet's supplications, the various types of D"O"AA (supplications and prayers), specific forms of remembering Allah and performing righteously good deeds. We will In addition affirm that comparing Prophetic medicine to regular medicine is just like comparing folk medicine to that provided by doctors, as some of the best doctors have conceded. We will In addition elaborate on the fact that bodies are more affected by the soul and that Islamic prayer formulas and supplications are better and more powerful than the most powerful medicines; that they can even neutralize the effect of deadly poisons.

We must reemphasize the fact that unhealthy air plays a major role in causing the plague. Air becomes unhealthy when it becomes polluted because of septic materials or pollutants, no matter what time of year, although it usually happens in the latter part of the summer and in the autumn. This is because during these times of the year (and when the air is most polluted), acute bilious excretions will accumulate during the summer, yet would not have maturated by the end of the season. In autumn, the air is usually cold and thus the immature excretions that accumulated in the summer will heat up and start to get spoiled and decayed, thus causing putrid illnesses. This is especially the case when the body is ready to accept such ailments, being inactive and having abundant septic materials, both of which rarely spare the body from ailments.

We should state that the best season of the year is spring especially regarding the air. Hippocrates said, "Autumn carries the worst types of ailments and deadly sicknesses. Spring, on the other hand, is the best season and has the least occurrences of death," Pharmacists and those who prepare dead bodies for burial usually borrow money during spring and summer, rather than autumn. This is because to them, autumn is their spring that they are eager for its coming and feel happy when it starts (due to the increased number of deaths in the autumn).

It was reported in Hadith that:

"When the Najm (literally: star) appears, every epidemic is removed from every land."

The Najm is said to mean the star, or the plants that appear in spring.

"And the herbs (or stars) and the trees both prostrate themselves (to Allah)." (55:6)

Meaning during spring, because it is the season when the trees are at their prime and thus the epidemics are removed.

As for the Najm (North Star in this case), ailments intensify when it rises and then sets just about dawn. At-Tamimi said in his book, 'The Secret of the Existence', "The worst two times of the year and the most harmful for the body are: when the North star sets just before dawn, and when it appears from the east before the sun rises on the world. This is the time when spring is about to end. Yet, the harm that occurs when it appears is less than the harm caused by its setting." Further, Abu Muhammad bin Qutaibah said:

"Whenever the Pleiades (in astronomy, the star cluster was named by the ancient Greeks after the "Seven Sisters" of mythology, the Arabs called it Atharaiya) rises or sets, it brings about an epidemic for people and camels. Yet, its setting is worse than when it is rising."

There is a third opinion regarding the meaning of the Hadith, that is, the star means the Pleiades and the epidemic is that which attacks the plants and fruits during winter and in the beginning of spring. When the star rises, the plants will be safe from such epidemics during that time, This is why the Prophet **b** disallowed selling or buying fruit before it is apparent that they are good.

The Prophet **b** commanded Muslims not to enter a plague-infested area and to remain in the infected area

Once there was an outbreak of the plague where one happened to be. This is the best type of prevention, for when one enters a plague infested area, he exposes himself to the risk of infection and harm. Exposing oneself to such danger defies religion and a sound mind. Staying away from plague infested areas is a type of prevention that Allah has directed and guided the people to. In this case, one observes a form of diet or prophylactic by avoiding contaminated areas and air.

As for the Prophet's prohibiting the Muslims from escaping from the epidemic infested area, it has two possible meanings.

1. Encouraging the heart to depend and rely on Allah while observing patience and being content with what Allah has decided.

2. The best medical authorities say in order to avoid becoming sick during an epidemic requires helping the body to get rid of harmful fluids and moisture, observing a diet and preserving the body's dryness in general, they warn against sports activities and taking baths. The human body usually contains harmful substances that are idle and which sometimes become activated by sports and taking a bath. They would then mix with the beneficial substances in the body and cause several ailments. Therefore, when the plague strikes a land, the best thing one can do is to remain idle in that land, so that the harmful substances in his body are not aroused or irritated. Leaving the plague-infested area requires motion and physical effort, both of which are very harmful in this case.

These are the statements of the best medical authorities of old and present, helping to shed light on the correctness of the Prophet's commands that assure the wellbeing of the heart and body.

If someone asks, "When the Prophet **b** said: 'Do not abandon it and take flight,' Refutes the meaning that has been stated. Leaving the infested land for another purpose than escaping, such as travelling, is exempt from the prohibition."

We answer this question by stating that no person, whether a doctor or otherwise, said that all types of motion is prohibited when the plague strikes a land, for the people cannot act as if they were fixed objects. Rather, engaging in excessive physical movements and activities that are not necessary is discouraged during the outbreak of an epidemic. There is no reason behind abandoning the plague-infested land other than escaping from the plague, whereas being idle and calm are better for the people's hearts and bodies in this situation. In addition, staying inactive satisfies the required dependence and reliance on Allah and submitting to His decisions. As for those who need to move about, such as hired hands, manufacturers and travelers, they are not required to remain completely inactive, but to refrain from any unnecessary movements such as traveling to escape the plague.

There is a great wisdom behind commanding the

people to remain in the plague-infested area, as follows.

1. Avoiding harm and the paths that might lead to harm.

2. Preserving one's health, which is the vehicle that people rely on to acquire life's necessities and to fulfil the requirements of the Hereafter.

3. So that the people do not fall sick upon breathing polluted and contaminated air.

4. Avoiding close association with those afflicted with the plague, so as not to catch the plague themselves.

5. Preserving the body and soul from contamination and superstition, which only harms those who believe in it.*

In short, prohibiting entering plague-infested areas is a preventive measure and a type of diet (prophylactic) that leads away from the paths of harm. Prohibiting leaving the area where the plague has struck entails submitting to Allah's will and decisions. The first order teaches and trains, while the second order entails submission and referring all matters to Allah's will.

" Umar was on his way to Ash-Sham when he reached the area of Sargh where he met Abu Ubaydah bin

Al-Jarrah with some people. They told 'Umar that there was an outbreak of the plague in Ash-Sham. They disputed among each other about what to do. So 'Umar said to Ibn Ab'ass 'Summon the early Migrants.' Ibn Ab'ass said, 'I summoned them and they In addition disputed, as some of them said (to Umar) you went out for a certain purpose and we recommend that we do not go back until it is fulfilled.' Other Migrants said, 'You have the best of the people in your company and the remainder of the Companions of the Messenger of Allah **b** Therefore, we do not recommend that you send them towards the epidemic.' 'Umar said, 'Go away from here.' He then said, 'Summon Al-Ansar for me.' I (Ibn Ab'ass) summoned them and Umar asked for their opinions. The Ansar disputed just as the Migrants disputed and copied their behavior. 'Umar said, 'Go away from here.' 'Umar then said, 'Summon whoever is present from the leaders of Quraish from those who embraced Islam in the aftermath of the Fath (conquering of Mecca).Ibn Ab'ass summoned them and no two among them disputed, as they all said, 'We recommend that you go back with the people and do not expose them to the epidemic.' 'Umar then ordered the people to leave, saying, 'In the morning, I will be riding on my animal's back, and so you too should.' Abu 'Ubaydah bin Al-Jarrah said, O leader of the believers! Do you run away from Allah's appointed destiny?' Umar said, 'I wish that somebody else had uttered these words, O Abu 'Ubaydah! Yes, we run away from Allah's appointed destiny to Allah's appointed destiny. If you had a herd of camels that arrived at a valley that has two slopes, one fertile and the other barren and you let your camels graze on the fertile slope, you will do so by Allah's leave, will you not. And if you allow them to graze on the barren slope, you will do so by Allah's Leave, will you not?' Soon after, Abdur Rahman bin Awf came back from attending to some of his needs and said, 'I have knowledge regarding this matter. I heard the Messenger of Allah **b** said:

"If you bear about it (the plague) in a land that you are in, do not run away from it, and if you hear that it broke out in a certain land, do not enter that land." [Al-Bokhary, Muslim, Abu Dawood, At-Termezey, An-Nasal, Ibn Majah and Ahmad].

The Prophet's remedy for dropsy

In the Sahihan it is narrated that Anas bin Malik said:

"Some people of (the tribes of) 'Ukl and 'Uraynah tribe came to Al-Medina and its climate did not suit them. So the Prophet **b** ordered them to go to the herd of camels reserved for charity, and to drink their milk and urine (as a medicine). Therefore, they went as directed. After they became healthy they killed the shepherds of the Prophet's camels and drove away all the camels, thus becoming aggressors against Allah and His Messenger b The Prophet b sent (men) in their pursuit and they were captured. The Prophet b then ordered that their hands and feet to be cut off (and it was done), and their eyes were branded with heated pieces of iron. They were then kept in the sun until they died."

The proof that these people were complaining from dropsy, is from Imam Muslim who narrated in his Sahih from the same Hadith above that the Bedouins said, "We have not found Al-Medina suitable for us and our stomachs swelled, our organs became weak..." until the end of the Hadith.

Dropsy is a physical disease that occurs when a harmful cold substance penetrates the external organs of the body and in addition the body organs other than those that are used in digestion, causing them to swell. There are three types of dropsy: in body tissue (fleshy), which is the most serious of the three, in a body cavity, and in an organ (drum). The remedy required for this disease includes mild laxatives and diuretic medicines that help rid the body of fluids. These diuretic qualities exist in the milk and urine of camels and that is why the Prophet b ordered them to drink them. Camel milk is a mild laxative, diuretic, cleanses and opens that which is closed and removes the obstructions and soothes the body. This is especially the case when the camels graze on beneficial herbs, such as wormwood, lavender, chamomile, daisy and lemongrass. These herbs help against dropsy.

Dropsy is usually symptomatic of an ailment in the liver, especially due to congestion in the liver. The milk of the Arabian camels helps in this case, because of its many benefits as mentioned and which help open the clogged passages and the obstructions. Ar-Razi said, "The she-camel's milk soothes the liver and the effects of a spoiled constitution," Al-Israili In addition said, "The she-camel's milk is the softest, least concentrated and lightest milk. It is the best choice for moving the bowels, as a laxative and for opening the clogged passages and obstructions. What makes this evident is the fact that this type of milk is mildly salty, as a result of the animal's instinctively hot nature. Therefore, the she-camel's milk is the best remedy for the liver as it soothes it, opens its pores and veins and softens the hardness of fresh food. Fresh, warm camel's milk is beneficial against dropsy, especially when taken with fresh, warm camel urine, thus making the combination more salty and adding strength to its effectiveness in dissolving harmful fluids and as a laxative. If the [combination of milk and urine] did not purge the stomach, then one should take a stronger laxative.' The author of AI-Qonon In addition commented, "Do not listen to those who claim that milk does not provide cure from dropsy. Rather, know that camel's milk is an effective cure, because it cleanses gently and easily, due to its other qualities. This type of milk is so beneficial that if a person substituted water and food with camel's milk, he would be cured [from dropsy and other ailments], Some people tried this remedy and were soon cured. We should state that the best camel urine is that of the camels of Bedouin people."

The story that was mentioned in the last Hadith has several areas of interest, as follows. The Hadith encourages the use of medicines and cures. The Hadith In addition indicates the purity of the milk of the animals that Muslims are allowed to eat, for using what Allah has prohibited in medicine is disallowed. Further, the people mentioned in the Hadith were not commanded to rinse their mouths or their clothes for the prayer, although they were new Muslin ݫ [indicating that rinsing the mouth and the clothes in such cases is not necessary]. The Prophet **b** cannot delay the necessary details of a religious command when such elaboration is necessary. In addition, this story emphasizes the fact that the aggressor is punished by the same method he transgressed. The people mentioned in the Hadith killed the shepherd and branded his eyes, as evident in another narration of this Hadith by Imam Muslim. The Hadith In addition mentioned that the entire group was killed for killing one person. In addition, this story indicates that whereas the aggressor deserves to be punished for multiple crimes, one punishable according to the law of equality and the other for an act of aggression, then both laws are applied. The Prophet ordered that the hands and feet of the aggressors be cut off, as a punishment from Allah for their audacious raid and aggression. They were In addition killed because they had killed the shepherd. In addition, the Hadith indicates that when armed aggressors steal money and In addition commit murder, their hands and feet are cut off, and they are then executed. The Hadith In addition indicates that the punishment for multiple crimes is multiplied, because the people who were mentioned in the story reverted from Islam, killed a human being, disfigured the dead shepherd, stole other people's property and announced their armed aggression. In addition, the entire armed band mentioned in the story were executed, not only those who actually committed the murder, as the Prophet **b**, did not consider this fact, nor did he ask about who actually committed the murder. Furthermore, assassination warrants capital punishment and cannot be pardoned [by the relatives of the deceased] or compensated, according to the scholars of Al-Medina and the Mathhab of Imam Ahmad, which our Shaikh (Ibn Taymiyyah) has chosen.

The Prophet's guidance on treating wounds and cuts

In the Sahihan it is narrated that Sahl bin Sa'd was asked about how the Messenger's injuries in the battle of Uhud were treated. Sahl said, "The Prophet's face was injured, his tooth was broken and the helmet he was wearing was smashed on his head. Fatimah, the daughter of the Messenger of Allah **b**, was washing the blood off while 'Ali was pouring water on her hands with his shield. When Fatimah realized that the bleeding did not stop, she took a burned mat (of palm leaves) and inserted the ash in the wound of Allah's Messenger and the bleeding stopped." The ashes of burnt palm leaves are very effective in stopping bleeding, because it is a strong drying agent and because it has the least burning effect (on the exposed skin). Other strong drying remedies have a burning effect on the skin and cause the blood to be irritated and the bleeding to intensify. Further, when the ashes of palm leaves are applied alone or mixed with vinegar in a bleeding nose, it will stop the bleeding. The author of Al-Qonun said, "Al-Baradii (Papyrus) is effective in stopping bleeding and coating exposed flesh when it is placed on a wound. In old Egypt, paper was made of the Baradii, which has a cold, dry condition. Baradii ash is effective in treating oral fungus and infection, hemoptysis (spitting up blood) and In addition prevents malignant infections from spreading."

The Prophet's guidance using honey, cupping and cauterizing as remedies

Al-Bokhary narrated that the Prophet said:

"There is cure in three substances, a drink of honey, a slash with a knife used for cupping and cauterizing by fire. I forbid my Nation from cauterizing by fire."

Abu 'Abdullah Al-Maziri said, Plethoric (excessive substances) conditions are either sanguineous (bloody), bilious, phlegm, or melancholic. Curing sanguineous plethora entails extracting the blood. If plethora was from the other three types, its cure is in softening the stool as warranted for each disease. The Prophet Us has indicated that honey is used as a laxative and that cupping is used to extract [septic] blood. Some people said that when the slash by a cupping knife does not work, the last resort is branding by fire (cauterizing). The Prophet b mentioned branding by fire as a last resort when the body has a strong resistance against medicine, rendering it ineffective. The Prophet b then said: "I forbid my Ummah (Muslim Nation) from branding by fire (cauterizing)," and in another narration, "I do not like to be branded by fire." Cauterizing by fire should be the last resort and only used when warranted. The fire should not be the first choice because of the intense pain it causes and which will be used to remove a lesser pain!

Some doctors said that diseases related to the temperament are either material or non-material. The material types are either cold, hot, wet or dry or a combination of these conditions. The four conditions, hotness and coldness are effected, while the other two, wetness and dryness, are usually affected. When one of the two effective temperaments is stronger than the other, one of the affected temperaments usually accompanies it. Every type of temperament in the body has two parts, effective and affected.

Temperamental ailments are usually caused by whichever effective condition is stronger, hotness or coldness. The Prophet's statement directs us to the origin of ailments, hotness and coldness. If the ailment was hot, the cure entails extracting the blood by cupping or puncturing the veins, both of which help extract the septic matter, cooling the temperament. If the ailment is cold, we treat it with heat, such as by taking honey. If we In addition need to extract the cold material that has caused the ailment, honey In addition helps in this case because it leads the various substances to maturity along with its other qualities of cleansing, softening, soothing and purging the affected organs. In this case, the septic material will be gently extracted while saving the body the annoyance of using strong laxatives.

Physical ailments are either acute, not needing cauterization because they would soon be neutralized, or chronic ailments, for which cauterizing the proper organ is the best remedy after extracting the septic substances. Chronic diseases usually result from thick, cold septic substances residing in the affected organ, ailing it, spoiling its constitution and, thereby, inflaming the parts of the body that are directly connected to the affected organ. Therefore, cauterizing should be used to dissipate and extract the septic substances in the affected organ with fire.

The Hadith explains treatments for all type of physical ailments, just as we learned the treatment method for all simple ailments (accompanied by fever) from the Hadith,

"The heat of the fever is a breath of the Hell Fire; cool it with water."

Cupping continued

As for cupping, Ibn Majah narrated in his Sunan that the Messenger of Allah b said:

"During the night of Israa' (the overnight journey from Mecca to Jerusalem and then to the heavens), every company (of angels) that I passed by would say, 'O Muhammad! Order your nation to use cupping.'"

In addition, in the Sahihan it is narrated that the Prophet ate once had his blood cupped (medically) and paid the person who applied the cupping.

Further, in tne Sahihan it is narrated:

Abu Taybah cupped Allah's Messenger b who then ordered that Abu Taybah be paid one So" (a measure pertaining to food) of dates and ordered his masters to reduce his tax (as he was a slave and had to pay a tax to them). The Prophet a§ then said:

"Cupping is among your best remedies."

The benefits of cupping include cleansing the exterior parts of the body more than puncturing the veins, or puncturing the veins, is better when used to extract blood from the internal parts of the body. Cupping entails removing blood from the various parts of the skin.

Using either cupping or puncturing the veins depends on the time of year, the area, the age and state of the ailing person. For instance, cupping is more beneficial than puncturing the veins in warm areas, warm weather and hot-tempered people, whose blood is near maturity (concerning the septic substances in the blood). In this case, the septic, maturing blood will collect near the skin. Cupping extracts the septic blood more efficiently than puncturing the veins. This is why using cupping for children and those who cannot bear puncturing the veins is better and more useful.

Doctors affirm that cupping is better used in warm areas than puncturing the veins and that cupping is preferred in the middle of the month or soon after, especially in the last quarter in the month. In the beginning of the month, the blood will have already become irritated (thus carrying septic materials that need to be cupped). In the end of the month, the blood will be idle, unlike the case in the middle and last quarter of the month when the blood is agitated and sufficiently produced.

The author of Al-Qanun said, 'Cupping is not preferred in the beginning of the month, because the body's various conditions will not be agitated then, nor is it preferred in the end of the month, because by then the conditions would have decreased. Cupping is preferred in the middle of the month when the substances (of the constitution, or condition) accumulate and become agitated.' It was reported that the Prophet b said:

"Cupping and puncturing the veins are your best remedies."

This Hadith is directed at the people of Hijaz and warm areas in general, for their blood is delicate and circulates closer to the surface of the skin, while the pores on their skin are wide and their strength weakened (i.e., during summer). Puncturing the veins is harmful for them. Puncturing of each of the veins usually has a special benefit. For instance, puncturing of the basilica vein (the large vein running on the inner side of the upper arm) is useful against the heat of the liver and spleen and various blood-related tumors in these two organs. It is In addition useful for tumors of the lungs (emphysema), arterial pulsation, pleurisy and all blood-related diseases of veins in the lower part of the knee to the hip. Further, puncturing of the median vein helps against the various swellings that appear throughout the entire body, especially when the swelling is blood-related, and contains spoiled blood in general. In addition, puncturing of the arm's vein helps against the ailments in the head and neck that result from excessive amounts of blood or from septic blood. Puncturing of the jugular vein helps against the ailments of the spleen, asthma, thoracic cavity and forehead pain.

Cupping the upper section of the back helps against the aches of the shoulder and the throat. Further, cupping the two jugular veins helps against the ailments of the head, face, teeth, ears, eyes, nose and throat, if these ailments were caused by excessive presence of blood, soiled blood or both.

Anas said:

"The Messenger of Allah used to apply cupping on the two jugular veins and the upper part of the back." [Abu Dawood, At-Termezey, Ibn Majah, Ahmad and Al-Hakim].

"The Messenger of Allah b used to apply cupping

on three areas, his upper back area and the two jugular veins." [Al-Bokhary and Moslem].

It is In addition narrated in the Sahih that the Prophet b used cupping on his head when he was in a state of Ihram (for Hajj or omrah) due to a headache.

In addition, Abu Dawood narrated that Jabir said that the Prophet s& used cupping on his hip because of a debilitation he suffered from.

Doctors have conflicting opinions regarding cupping on the nape cavity

Some doctors approved of this form of cupping, saying that it helps against exophthalmoses, the abnormal protrusion of the eyeballs, the heaviness in the eyebrows and the eyelids and against eyelid mange. A Hadith states:

"Use cupping on the nape cavity, for it cures seventy two kinds of ailments."

Further, it was narrated that when Ahmad bin Hanbal needed cupping on the nape cavity, he did it on the two sides of the nape but not on the cavity itself.

The author of the Qonun In addition disliked cupping the cavity of the nape saying that, "It causes forgetfulness just as our Prophet Muhammad b has stated. This is because the back of the brain is the location of the memory power and cupping it affects that power."

Other people did not approve of his opinion though, saying that the Hadith that he referred to is not authentic. They said that even if the Hadith is authentic, cupping weakens the brain if cupping occurs without a necessity that warrants it. When warranted, cupping the nape cavity is medically and religiously useful against the pressure of the blood on the cavity. Authentic narrations have stated that the Prophet ^ used cupping in many areas on the back of his neck and in other areas of his body as much as was needed.

Cupping under the chin helps against toothache, face ailments and throat infections when used at the proper time

Cupping under the chin In addition cleanses and purifies the head and the jaws. Further, cupping on top of the foot substitutes for the puncturing of the saphena, which is a vein on the heel. This kind of cupping In addition helps against the ulcers that occur on the thighs and legs, the interruption of monthly periods and skin irritation on the testicles.

Cupping on the lower part of the chest helps against spots, sores and mange on the thigh. It In addition helps against gout, hemorrhoids, elephantiasis and itchiness on the back.

When is cupping preferred

Anas related from the Prophet b that he said:

"The Messenger of Allah b used to have cupping on the jugular veins and the upper part of the back on the seventeenth, nineteenth or twenty-first (day of the month)." (At-Termezey)

Anas related from the Prophet b that he said:

"Those who intend to have cupping let them do that on the seventeenth, nineteenth or twenty-first (of the month), to prevent the septic blood from causing death to one of you." (Ibn Majah)

In addition, Abu Dawood narrated that Abu Hurayrah related from the Prophet b that he said:

"Those who have cupping on the seventeenth, nineteenth or twenty-first will be cured from every disease."

"Every disease" mentioned in the Hadith means the blood-related" diseases. [Both of the last two Ahadeeth are weak].

These Ahadeeth conform to the position taken by doctors that cupping is preferred in the latter half of the month and the third quarter, rather than the beginning or the end of the month. However, if cupping is necessary, it will be useful during any part of the month including the beginning and the end. It was reported that Imam Ahmad Ibn Hanbal used to practice cupping during any part of the month when the spoiled blood became agitated,

The author of Al-Qanun said, "Cupping is preferred during the day, the second or the third hour and after one takes a bath. When warranted, one should take a bath then rest for an hour or so and then use cupping." Cupping is not preferred when the stomach is full, for it might cause various ailments, especially after taking a heavy meal.

It was said that cupping on an empty stomach is a cure, and when one's stomach is full is a disease, and when it is done on the seventeenth [of the month] it becomes a remedy. Choosing the best time for cupping preserves good health and helps prevent harm from occurring to the body. However, when the illness intensifies, cupping becomes warranted and needed whatever the circumstances, for the Prophet **b** said:

"So that the septic blood does not cause death to one of you."

We stated before that Imam Ahmad used to use cupping during any time of the month if cupping was medically warranted.

As for the best days of the week to have cupping, Al-Khallal said that Imam Ahmad was asked about the days when cupping is not preferred, and he said, "Wednesday and Saturday." In addition Al-Khallal narrated that Imam Ahmad was once asked about the days when cupping is disliked and Imam Ahmad answered, "Saturday and Wednesday, and In addition Friday as was reported." [However, all the Ahadeeth that state the time when the cupping is either preferred or disliked are weak, according to the scholars of Hadith].

The previous Ahadeeth we mentioned state that seeking the cure, including cupping, is preferred. In addition, cupping is done in the part of the body that most needs it. In addition, those who have assumed ihram are allowed to use cupping, even if it involves cutting some hair and they do not have to pay a penalty. Further, it is allowed for those who are fasting to use cupping as Al-Bokhary narrated that the Messenger of Allah **b** used cupping while he was fasting.

There are several Ahadeeth that state that cupping breaks the Fast. The only Hadith that appears to contradict this ruling is the Hadith that the Prophet ^ had cupping while fasting. In this case, for the Hadith to mean that cupping does not break the Fast, it should satisfy one of the following four conditions.

First, Fasting should have been obligated by the

time the incident in the Hadith [narrated by Al-Kukhah above] occurred. Second, it should be proven that the Prophet b was not traveling [when he had cupping]. Third, that the Prophet b was not suffering from an illness that warranted cupping. Fourth, that this Hadith came after the Prophet g§ said, "Those having cupping and those who do it have both broken their Fast." If these four conditions are satisfied, only then can we say that cupping does not break the fast relying on the Hadith [that the Prophet b had cupping when he was fasting]. Otherwise, the Fast mentioned in the Hadith might have been a voluntary fast that one is allowed to break when cupping is warranted. Or it could have occurred during Ramadan but while the Prophet a& was traveling. Or, the Hadith could be talking about a compulsory Fast during Ramadan but that it was necessary to have cupping due to an illness. Or, cupping could have been done during Ramadan and without a necessity that warrants it, but before the Prophet b issued his statement that cupping breaks the Fast of those involved in it. There is no proof that any of the four conditions we mentioned above were satisfied, so how about all four of them? [That is why Ibn Al-Qayyim asserts that cupping breaks the Fast of those who are doing it and those who are having it done].

In addition, the Hadith proves that one is allowed to hire a doctor for a certain purpose and then pay him for his services without a service contract.

The Hadith [that the Prophet b paid the person who performed cupping for him] In addition indicates that some people are allowed to make cupping their profession. The Prophet b gave the man who performed cupping some money and that person spent that money on his necessities. Furthermore, cupping is similar to garlic and onion in that they are described as being impure. But we are still allowed to use them.

Finally, the Hadith proves that one is allowed to collect reasonable taxes from his slave and that the slave is allowed to use whatever is left after paying the tax. Otherwise, if the master is going to take all the money anyway, it will not be called a tax any more! Therefore, whatever is left with the slave beyond the required tax is his property and he can do whatever he wishes with it.

The Prophet's guidance regarding cauterization and puncturing of the veins

"Jabir bin 'Abdullah narrated that the Prophet b once sent a doctor to Ubay bin Ka'b and that the doctor used puncturing on one of Ubay's veins and then cauterized the wound." (Al-Bokhary)

Further, when Sa'd bin Moa'az was injured in his medial arm vein, the Prophet b, had it cauterized and then cauterized again when the wound became swollen. In another narration of this Hadith, the Prophet cauterized

Sa'd bin Mu'adh in his medial arm vein using the tip of an arrow. Afterwards, Sa'd bin Mu'adh, or someone else, cauterized the wound again. Another narration states that one of the Ansar was injured in his medial arm vein and the Prophet ordered that he be cauterized. [These Ahadeeth are narrated by Muslim, Abu Dawood, and others].

Abu 'Ubayd In addition narrated that a man, who was prescribed cauterization, was brought to the Prophet b and the Prophet a| ordered that he be cauterized. Then hot stones were applied on the wound to close it. In addition, Jabir narrated that the Prophet sis, once cauterized him in his medial arm vein.

Al-Bokhary narrated that Anas said that he was once cauterized because he was complaining from pleurisy while the Prophet b was still alive. At-Termezey In addition narrated that Anas said, "The Prophet b cauterized As'ad bin Zurarah when he came down with a septic finger,"

We have mentioned that the Prophet ^ said in the Hadith narrated by Al-Bokhary and Moslem :

"I do not like to be cauterized."

Moreover, in another narration:

I forbid cauterizing for my Nation."

Further, [At-Termezey, Abu Dawood and Ahmad] narrated that one of the Companions said that the Prophet b has disallowed cauterizing, "But we were tested (i.e., with various ailments) and we did have cauterization, so we neither were successful nor did we acquire an advantage."

Al-Khattabi commented, "The Prophet b only cauterized Sa'd to stop the bleeding, because he feared that bleeding would not stop until Sa'd died. Cauterization is usually used in drastic cases, such as when a hand or a leg is amputated. As for prohibiting cauterizing, it might be specifically directed at whoever was seeking a cure with it (not to close an open wound). In early times, the people used to superstitiously believe that whoever did not have cauterization would certainly die and this is why the Prophet b disallowed it. It was In addition said that the Prophet b disallowed "Imran bin Husayn in particular from using cauterization because he was suffering from a sore in a delicate place. That is why the prohibition could be specific to cases where cauterizing is dangerous. Allah knows best.

Further Ibn Qutaybah said that cauterizing is of two types. The first type entails a healthy person using cauterization to fend off illness and it is this type that is referred to by the statement, 'Whoever reverts to cauterizing would not have practiced Tawakkul (depending on Allah).' as such people seek to fend off whatever is destined for them in the future. The second type entails cauterizing infected wounds and amputated limbs, and cauterization is effective in these cases. As for the type of cauterization that might or might not work, it is apparently disliked.

There is a Hadith narrated in the Shahihan [Al Bokhary and Moslem] about the seventy thousand Muslims who will enter Paradise without reckoning, describing them as:

"They are those who do not seek prayer formulas (Ruqyah literally incantations), nor cauterization, nor are they superstitious, and they depend on their Lord (for each and everything)." [In addition narrated by At-Termezey and Ahmad].

In short, the Ahadeeth that discussed the subject of cauterization fall under four categories: practicing it, disliking it, praising those who do not revert to it and disallowing it. There is no contradiction between these categories. When the Prophet s. had someone cauterized, he indicated that practicing it is allowed. Further, the Prophet's disliking cauterization for his Ummah (Muslim Nation) does not indicate that it is prohibited. In addition, the Prophet's praising those who avoid cauterization indicates that avoiding it is better. Finally, disallowing cauterization can be explained that in general, either cauterization is disliked, or that it is directed at those who revert to cauterizing to fend off a future illness. Allah knows best.*

There is another point that needs to be clarified and that concerns the word prayer. What we call prayer in English has two different words to describe it in Arabic. Sallat, the formal prayer with specific movements and D"O"AA, the informal prayer in which one asks the Creator for what they want in their own words or according to formulas set by the Prophet 8! or the Qura'an. One of the pillars of Islam is the five daily prayers. This is a formalized system of praying that has specific movements and times. In Arabic this is called Salatt. The other form of prayer, when we ask Allah for anything, in our own words or in prayer formulas set by the Prophet b or by the Qura'an, is called D'ouaa. This form of prayer is sometimes referred to as supplication in English, which is a very good word to describe this form of prayer. The only problem with translating D"O"AA as "supplication" is that the word "supplication" is very formal and rarely used in verbal communication. Supplication is used constantly throughout the day. Any English speaking person who is continuously calling on God, will describe what they are doing as praying, which is the simple common way to describe this act. When we call Ruqyah (literally incantations) Islamic prayer formulas, we are using the word prayer in its informal meaning (Doaa) and not the formal meaning (Salatt).

The Prophet's guidance on treating epilepsy and spiritual possession*

In the Sahihan it is narrated that 'Ata bin Raba'h said, "Ibn Ab'ass said to me, 'Should I tell you about a woman from among the people of Paradise?' I said, 'Yes.' He said, 'That black woman, who came to the Prophet **b** and said, 'I suffer epileptic fits during which I inadvertently take off my clothes. So invoke Allah on my behalf.' He said,

'If you wish, be patient and you will acquire Paradise; and if you wish, I will supplicate to Allah to cure you.'

She said, 'Rather, I will observe patience.' She then said, 'I keep taking off my clothes during these fits, so supplicate to Allah for me that I do not do so. The Prophet **b** supplicated (to Allah) on her behalf.'"

Epilepsy is two kinds, one that results from negative forces and the second type is physical that results from bad mixtures (chemical and material imbalance). The doctors often talk about the second type and explain its causes and how to cure it.

As for the epilepsy that results from negative forces, the best doctors and the wise ones among them affirm that it exists. They In addition confirm that curing this type of disease occurs by the support of the righteous, exalted souls so that they neutralize the effect of the evil and render its efforts harmless. When Hippocrates explained the cures for epilepsy he stated that, "These cures are effective in treating the epilepsy that results from chemical and material causes. As for the epilepsy that results from negative forces, these remedies (that he explained and detailed) do not cure it."

As for the most ignorant, unknowing and immoral doctors, and those who consider heresy a virtue, they deny the type that occurs by negative forces and deny that it has any effect on the body. They have only ignorance to support them, because the medical authorities cannot actually disprove the epilepsy that is caused by these negative forces. Fact and experience assert and prove the existence of this type of epilepsy. That is why when the doctors explain the reason behind epilepsy as being natural or physical, their statement is true regarding some types of epilepsy but not all of them.*

The doctors of old used to call epilepsy, The divine disease', stating that it is caused by negative forces. On the other hand, Galinus and other doctors misinterpreted the term divine ailment, saying, "They called it divine because it attacks the head and thus causes harm to the apparent divine organ where the brain resides." This explanation, however, resulted from their ignorance of the soul and its effects.

As for the heretical doctors, they only confirm the kind of epilepsy that results from physical causes. Whoever has a sound mind and good knowledge of the soul and its effect, will laugh at the ignorance shown by these doctors and at their weak minds.

Curing the type of epilepsy caused by negative forces has two parts, a part that involves the person afflicted with epilepsy and a part that involves those who treat them.

The part that the person afflicted with epilepsy plays in his treatment involves strengthening his heart and being sincere in repentance to the Creator from the negative forces and seeking sincere refuge with Him both by heart and tongue. This is a type of warfare that the person afflicted with epilepsy engages in against evil. To defeat the enemy, warfare requires the warrior to acquire beneficial, suitable weapons and to have a strong arm. When one of these two elements does not exist, the effort will not be very effective. The situation becomes more difficult when the person is missing both essential requirements, in this case, the heart will be lacking Towhid (Oneness of Allah), Tawakil (trusting in Allah),

Taqwa (righteousness), and Tawajhu (awareness of Allah's Presence), plus the person does not have sufficient material armament.

The second part of epilepsy treatment involves the person who is treating the ailment and who is In addition required to have the same necessary weapons mentioned above. When these weapons are ready, one sometimes merely needs to say (to the evil spirit), 'Get out of him,' or, 'In the Name of Allah,' or, 'There is no power nor strength except with Allah.'

The Prophet **b** used to say in such cases:

"O enemy of Allah, Depart! I am the Messenger of Allah."

I once witnessed our Shaikh (Ibn Taymiyyah, the renown Imam of Islam) send someone to speak to an evil spirit that had possessed a person, saying, "The Shaikh says this to you: get out of this body for you are not allowed therein." The person afflicted with epilepsy (possession) then woke up from his seizure. Sometimes, our Shaikh would even speak to the evil spirit directly, or would use physical punishment to repel the rebellious evil spirit. When the patient would wake up, he would not feel any pain, as we have ourselves witnessed on numerous occasions. The Shaikh would sometimes read the following Ayah, verse, in the ear of the person afflicted with epilepsy (possession),"Did not think that We had created you in play (without any purpose), and that you would not be brought back to Us?"

The Shaikh once told me that he read this Ayah, verse, in the ear of the person afflicted with epilepsy and that the evil spirit that possessed him answered by saying, 'Indeed,' extending her voice (mocking the Qura'an). So the Shaikh said, "So I took a stick and beat the sick person on his neck with it until my hands became tired. Those present did not doubt that the patient would die from this severe beating.

While beating the patient, the she-devil said 'I love this person.' I said, 'But he does not love you.' She said, "I want to accompany him to perform Hajj. I told her, 'He does not want to go to Hajj with you.' She said, 'I will leave him in your honor.' I said, "No, but as an obedience to Allah and His Messenger **b** She said, 'Then, I will leave him alone.' The patient then woke up and started looking around, saying, 'What brought me to the presence of the Shaikh?' They asked him, 'What about the beating you took?" He said, 'Why would the Shaikh beat me while I have not done anything wrong?' He had no idea that he had been beaten.'"

Further. the Shaikh used to recite Ayatil kors'ey[2:255] and would order those who suffer from and those who cure epilepsy (possession) to recite it along with the last two chapters of the Qura'an [113 and 114].

In general, no one can deny the type of epilepsy that is caused by negative forces except those who have little knowledge and comprehension. We should In addition state that the majority of those afflicted by the touch of evil spirits are themselves in error due to weak Faith and hearts and tongues that don't remember Allah, they fail to seek refuge with Him and they fail to use Prophetic guidance, (supplications and remedies). The evil spirits find the people that are vulnerable and take advantage of them.

If the truth was uncovered, we would discover that the majority of mankind is under the influence of negative forces which guides the people according to their evil wishes. The people are unable to set themselves free from this control or even oppose it. Most people suffer from this common type of possession (epilepsy), from which the afflicted person cannot wake up. And unless the veil that obstructs their sight is removed, they will not realize that it is they who are actually afflicted by epilepsy. We seek Allah Alone for His help.

Curing (epilepsy) possession that results from the touch of evil requires the cooperation of a sound mind and sincere faith in what has been sent down to the Prophets **b** Then one would act as if both Heaven and Hell are right in front of his eyes and heart. They would remember that the people of this earthly life suffer calamities and trials that come down on their homes just as the rain does, all the while being unaware of what is going on around them.

The epilepsy that evil causes is truly severe, but since it touches so many people and is so common, the people are no longer surprised by it. Since they are so many, it is strange to see someone who is not touched by it.

When Allah wills that a certain slave should acquire what is good for him, that slave will wake up from these fits of epilepsy and will realize that the children of this life are suffering from epilepsy. He will discover that some of them have surrendered to insanity and that some of them might briefly recover from a bout to fall back into another bout soon after. Some of them would be awake from a bout and would act like sane people, but when he falls into another bout, he would act confused. [This is the state of those who do not have the correct Faith.]

The epilepsy that results from physical causes

This type of epilepsy alters the constitution and is accompanied by spasms that prevent the limbs from functioning normally or from normal movements. The physical or constitution related epilepsy occurs due to the accumulation of thick, viscous substances near the brain that partially obstructs the cerebral cavities. In this case, the area of the brain responsible for the senses and the various movements are impeded, and accordingly, the organs (including limbs) of the body suffer from the same condition. There are other causes for this type of epilepsy, such as the accumulation of thick flatulence that impedes the soul in some manner, or a viscous vapor accumulates in an organ of the body and ascends to the brain, or from an acute ailment. The brain suffers from spasms due to fighting the harmful substances that are affecting the brain, and accordingly, the various organs of the body suffer from spasms. The person will not be able to stand up straight for very long he or she will fall down and foam accumulates in and around the mouth.

This type of epilepsy causes intense pain during seizures. It is In addition a chronic illness that is hard to cure and that remains for many years, especially if the person afflicted by it is more than twenty-five years old, who repeatedly falls into epileptic fits. Hippocrates said that epilepsy remains with such people until they die.

As for the woman mentioned in the Hadith who suffered from epilepsy and who used to take off her clothes because of epileptic fits, she might have been suffering from the physical type of epilepsy. That is why the Prophet promised her Paradise if she observes patience, or otherwise, the Prophet would have asked

Allah to cure her without guaranteeing her that she will be cured. She chose Paradise, but the Prophet asked Allah on her behalf not to take off" her clothes during these fits.

The Hadith indicates that it is allowed for Muslims to forgo the use of a remedy. Furthermore, the Hadith indicates that the cure of the soul is exclusively tied to invoking Allah and turning to Him sincerely and that this type of medicine has such profound effects on the human body that no regular medicine prepared by any doctor could ever compare to it. We have tried this medicine on numerous occasions [and witnessed its success].

The best medical authorities confirm the fact the psyche has an effective role in curing disease. The medical profession suffers from some ignorant, heretic doctors who do not do service to their profession.

As we have stated, it appears that the woman mentioned in the Hadith suffered from the epilepsy that is caused by a physical condition (chemical imbalances). Yet, she might have been suffering from the type that is caused by evil negative forces. We stated that the Messenger of Allah gave her the choice to observe patience and then acquire Paradise or that he would invoke Allah to cure her. She chose the first option but asked to be relieved from discarding her clothes because of the epileptic fits.

The Prophet's guidance on curing sciatica

Ibn Majah narrated in his Sunan (collection of Hadith) that Anas bin Malik said, I heard the Messenger of Allah **b** saying:

"Curing sciatica is accomplished by melting the fat from the tail of a nomad's ewe. Then, the fat is divided into three parts and one part per day is drunk on an empty stomach."

Sciatica is an ailment that starts from the hip's joint, then descends to the thigh from the backside of the body. Sometimes, sciatica reaches the ankles and the longer the ailment remains, the lower it descends and the weaker the legs and thighs become.

There are two beneficial understandings in the Hadith mentioned, medical and linguistic.

Linguistically, the Hadith proves that we are allowed to call this ailment a 'Irq (nerve) Nasa (sciatic nerve), to the contrary of the opinion of some people. They said that the Noso is the nerve itself and thus the two words together are redundant.

Answering this claim takes two forms. First, the word 'Irq (nerve) is more general than the word Noso (sciatic nerve). Hence the term 'Iraq An-Nasa gives the general and the specific meanings desired. Second, the Nasa is an ailment that attacks the nerve and thus the word Nasa should be included in the name given to the ailment [as it specifies the area where the nerve is causing pain]. It was reported that the name 'Irq Nasa is called as such because it makes the people forget (Nasa) any other pain. The sciatic nerve starts from the hips until the bottom of the foot from behind the ankles.

The Messenger of Allah ^, as we have noticed in previous Ahadeet'ı, may use two types of meanings in his expressions. One meaning may be general, for all conditions and people, while the other specific, its meaning and indications are specifically directed at some particular people or situation. The Hadith in this section is the specific type, it is directed at Arabs and the people of Hijaz in particular, including the Bedouins of those areas. The remedy mentioned in the Hadith is the best cure for the people of those areas as 'Irq An-Nasa is caused by dryness or thick, septic accumulations. The best treatment for this ailment is using a laxative. The fat on the ewe's tail has two qualities: bringing the septic substances to maturity and softening (the stool in this case), both are required to cure 'Irq An-Nasa.

In addition, the nomad's ewe has several qualities, such as being small in size, producing lesser excrements and having a soft essence. The nomad's ewe In addition grazes on beneficial wild plants, such as wormwood and lavender cotton, and so forth. When the ewe feeds on these wild plants, they will mix with and soften the ewe's flesh, especially the fatty tail. Although the ewe's milk carries in it the effective ingredients of the wild plants, the tail has two qualities that the milk does not have, being a laxative and leading the septic substances to maturity [making them ready to be extracted from the body].

We mentioned before that the regular medicines and remedies of different nations and peoples is based on the type of diet that the people are used to. Indians and Bedouins have a simple diet therefore the do not use complex medicines. As for the Romans and the Greek, they use compound medicines. They all agree, however, that the best treatment for an ailment is a specific diet. Otherwise, the doctors will first prescribe simple and then compound medications, when necessary.

If the diet is simple, simple medications are suitable for the simple ailments. The compound ailments, on the other hand, usually occur due to a complex diet and this is why compound medicines are suitable in those cases. Allah knows best.

The Prophet's guidance on treating constipation

At-Termezey and Ibn Majah narrated that the Messenger of Allah b asked Asma bint 'Umais,

"How do you deal with constipation?" She said, "By using Shubrum (euphorbia piteous)." The Prophet b said, it is hot and to strong laxative." She then said. "I In addition use Senna," and the Prophet replied, "If there is a cure that prevents death, it would be Senna."

Further, Ibn Majah narrated that Abudllah ibn Umm Haram said that he heard the Messenger of Allah b saying:

"Use Senno and Sanoot (cumin), because they cure every disease, except Saam." He was asked, "What is Saam?" He said, 'Death'. "

The Prophet m, asked the woman about what she uses to treat constipation, meaning what cure she uses to help soften the stool, so that the body is able to get rid of its harmful waste.

In another narration of the Hadith, the Prophet ^ asked Asma' about what she uses to cure constipation, and she mentioned the Shubrum (euphorb piteous), which is the bark of the root of the euphoric tree and which is dry and hot in the forth degree. The best type of Shubrum is the one reddish in color, which is soft and feels like wrapped skin.

Shubrum is among the medications that doctors do not advise people to use because it is a very strong laxative. In the Haditb, the Prophet sg described Shubrum as being hot and a strong laxative.

Senna is a plant that grows in Al-Hijaz (Western Arabia) and the best kind of it grows in Mecca, Senna is hot and dry in the first degree and it is a good, mild medication that does not cause any side effects. Senno helps against bile and black bile ailments and strengthens the heart, which is another good quality that this medication contains. Senno is useful against melancholic obsession and corporal incisions, relaxes the muscles and improves the hair. Senno In addition helps against lice, headache, mange, pustules, rashes and epilepsy. It is better to cook the Senno whole and drink three measures of its soup than cooking it crushed. In addition, it is better to cook the Senno mixed with violet flowers and red raisins, after removing the seeds,

Ar-Razi said, "Senna and fumitory help extract mature humors (bodily wastes) and helps against leprosy and rashes, when one takes four to seven measures of each remedy."

As for Sonoot (cumin), there is a difference of opinion concerning its nature. Umar bin Bakr As-Saksaki, for instance, said that Sonoot is either honey or butter extract. Another opinion suggests that Sonoot is a seed that resembles the Kammon (cumin), as Ibn Al-Arabi has asserted. The fourth and fifth opinions suggest that

Sonoot is the Persian cumin or fennel, according to Abu Hanifah Ad-Daynoori. The sixth opinion suggests that it is the Shibitt (dill), and the seventh opinion suggests that it is the date, according to Abu Bakr bin As-Sunni. The eighth opinion suggests that it is honey that exists in butter-skin, according to Abdul-Latif Al-Baghdadi. Some doctors In addition stated that the last meaning is the most probable. In this case, the Sanoot is prepared by blending Senno powder with some honey mixed with ghee, as this is better than taking the Senna by itself. Then one licks the mixture that contains the Senna, as in this case the Senna taste will be made milder, because of the honey and butter, which will In addition assist the laxative power of the Senna. Allah knows best.

The Prophet's guidance on treating skin rashes and scabies caused bv mites

In the Sahihan it is narrated that Anas said, "The Messenger of Allah **b** has allowed Abdur Rahman bin Awf and Az-Zubayr bin Al-'Awwam to wear silk garments because of a skin rash they had." In another narration, "Abdur Rahman bin Awf and Az-Zubayr bin Al-Awwam complained to the Prophet **b** during a battle that they had mites, and he allowed them to wear silk garments which I saw them wearing."

There are two areas of interest regarding this Hadith, one in the area of Fiqh (Islamic Jurisprudence) and another medical.

In the area of Fiqh (Islamic Jurisprudence), the Sunnah of the Messenger of Allah is that wearing silken garments is allowed for women and disallowed for men, except when there is a legitimate need. For instance, [men are allowed to wear silken garments] in cold weather, when one has only a silken garment to wear and when complaining from mange, rashes, mites or lice, as evident by the last Hadith.

According to Imam Ahmad and Shafi'i, wearing silken garments is allowed [for men if a necessity warrants it]. The permission given to some Muslims [such as wearing silken garments for men in this case] due to special circumstances applies to all those who face similar circumstances.

Several scholars said that the Ahadeeth that disallow silken garments for men apply in general. They said that the Hadith (narrated above) might entail a specific permission for only Abdur-Rahman bin 'Awf and Az-Zubayr. They say that it is possible, though, that this permission applies to other Muslims. When there is a probability, adhering to the general text is warranted. This is why some of the narrators of this Hadith commented, "I do not know if the permission applies to whoever comes after them (Abdur-Rahman bin Awf and Az-Zubayr)."

The correct opinion is that the permission is general in its indication and that there is no evidence that it is specific or restricted. Similarly, the Prophet st once said to Abu Burdah, "This permission applies to you and none else after you." In addition, Allah said to His Prophet ^ regarding the woman who offered herself in marriage to the Prophet **b**:

"A privilege for you only, not for the (rest of) the believers."

Since disallowing wearing silken garments for men is a precautionary measure, it is allowed in certain situations and for a benefit that warrants it. For instance, gazing at women is disallowed as a precautionary measure, but it is allowed when there is a real need. Such is the case with disallowing performing voluntary prayers at certain times [while the sun is rising or setting], to prevent even a hint of resemblance between Muslims and sun worshippers. Yet, in some cases, it is allowed for Muslims to offer voluntary prayers during these times for a real need and benefit. We have explained the cases when wearing silken garments is allowed in our book on this subject, At-Jabiri.

Medically, silk is produced by an animal and is a remedy. Silk has many benefits, such as soothing and strengthening the heart and helping relieve several of its ailments. Silk In addition helps against black bile and whatever ailments it might cause. Further, silk strengthens the eyesight when used as eyeliner. Raw silk, which is used in preparing medications and remedies, is hot and dry in the first degree. When silk is used in clothes, it is mild and heats the body. Sometimes it could chill the body.

Ar-Razi said, "Silk is hotter than linen, colder than cotton and develops the flesh. Every type of thick clothes weakens the body and hardens the skin."

There are three types of clothes, one that brings warmth and In addition heats the body. Another type of clothes brings warmth but no heat to the body. The third type does not bring warmth or heat. There is no type that brings heat but not warmth to those wearing it. For instance, clothes made of wool and animal hair elevate body temperature and bring warmth to the skin. On the other hand, silk, Kittan (linen) and cotton garments only bring warmth to the skin. Kittan clothes are cold and dry, wool clothes are hot and dry, while cotton garments are moderate. Silken garments are softer and less hot than wool. The author of Al-Minhaj stated that wearing silk, "Does not bring as much warmth as cotton, because it is milder."

Every type of soft, polished clothes heat the body less and is less effective in helping the decomposition process. That is why it is better that this type of clothes is worn during summer and in hot areas.

Since silken garments are neither dry nor thick as the other types of clothes, they help as a treatment for skin rashes that result from dry, thick material. Hence, the Prophet ^ allowed Az-Zubair and Abdur-Rahman to wear silken garments due to their skin rash. In addition, silken garments are the least hospitable to mites or lice, for it is not the best environment where mites live and thrive.

The types of body wear that neither elevates the body temperature nor brings warmth are made of iron, lead, wood, sand, and so forth.

If one asks, "Since silk provides the best type of clothes and the most suitable for the body, why was it prohibited for men) by the Islamic legislation, which is the mot honorable, perfect legislation and which allows the good and pure things and only disallows the impure things?" We should mention that this is a question that the Muslims differ regarding its answer.

Those who deny that there is wisdom behind the Islamic legislation do not even need to answer this question.

As for those who affirm that there is a wisdom behind the Islamic legislation, who are the majority, say that Islam disallowed silken garments for men so that they observe patience and abandon wearing them for Allah's Sake. In this case, they will be rewarded by Allah, especially since there are other types of clothes to wear.

Some people say that silk was created for the benefit of women, such as the case with gold. Hence, silk is prohibited for men so that they do not imitate women. Some Muslims say that silk was prohibited because it leads to arrogance and pride.

Others say that silk was disallowed because of its softness on the skin that leads to feminine behavior while weakening manhood and masculinity. Hence, you rarely see a man wearing silken garments who is not affected by its softness by inadvertently imitating feminine behavior and softness, even if he was among the most masculine men. Wearing silken garments will certainly diminish the manly qualities and masculinity, although these qualities will not disappear all together. As for those who do not comprehend these facts, let them submit to Allah's wise decisions. Finally, we should state that according to the correct opinion, young boys should not be allowed to wear silken garments, because they will acquire feminine behavior.

An-Nasa'y narrated that the Prophet b said:

"Allah has allowed silk and gold for the females of my Ummah (Muslim Nation) and disallowed them for the males of my Ummah (Muslim Nation)." In another narration, the Prophet **b** said:

"Wearing silk and gold is disallowed for the males of my Nation and allowed for the females."

Al-Bokhary In addition narrated that the Messenger of Allah **b** has disallowed wearing and sitting on silken garments and Dibaj (pure silken clothes), and then added, "It is for them (whoever wears them among men) in this life and for you in the Life Hereafter."

The Prophet's guidance on treating pleurisy

The doctors divide pleurisy into two types, real and unreal. The first type is an infected growth that appears in the pleura that coats the ribs. The second type causes a similar pain and attacks the pleura as a result of thick, congested flatulence between the peritoneum's (smooth transparent membrane that lines the abdominal cavity and part of the pelvic region). The pain caused by the unreal pleurisy is acute while the real pleurisy causes stinging pain.

The author of the Qonoon said, "Sometimes, the flank (of the body), the peritoneum, chest muscles and ribs and surrounding areas suffer from an extremely painful growth called pleurisy. Sometimes, there could be pain in these same areas of the body but not as a result of growth but of accumulating harmful gasses (flatulence), and thus, the people think that it is the first type when in fact it is not."

He In addition said, "Know that every type of disease that attacks the side or the flank is called 'Thatul janb (pleurisy), which is derived from the place where it appears (i.e., the Janb, the flank). That is why every type of pain on the side or flank is called Jhatul janb regardless of the cause of the ailment. This is the meaning of Hippocrates' statement that those suffering from That Al-janb will benefit from taking a bath. It is said that his statement includes those who suffer from pleurisy, as well as, lung disease (pulmonary) pains that result from a bad constitution, congested conditions without tumors or fever."

Some doctors said that in Greek, the term pleurisy means the warm growth that appears on the side and In addition the tumors of all internal organs. The tumor of any organ is called pleurisy when it is a warm tumor only. Further, there are five symptoms that accompany the real pleurisy: fever, coughing, stinging pain, hard breathing (dyspnea) and pneumonia.

Sea-costus (Indian costus) is used to treat the unreal pleurisy. When the Indian costus is ground to fine powder, blended with hot oil and then used as an ointment on the affected area, or when the ailing person licks it, it will be a good cure for that ailment. In this case, the costus decomposes the septic substances, strengthens the internal organs and opens the obstructions or clogs. Al-Masi'hi said, "Costus is hot and dry and constipates, strengthens the internal organs, dissipates the wind, opens the clogs, helps against pleurisy and dries out excess moistures. In addition, costus is good for the brain and might help against the real pleurisy, if a phlegmy substance had caused it, especially when the illness is weakening. Allah knows best."

Thotul janb is a dangerous disease. An authentic Hadith related by Umm Salamh reads, "The final ailment that the Messenger of Allah ^e suffered from started while he was in Maymunah's house. Whenever the Prophet b felt the pain had eased, he would go out and lead the people in prayer. Whenever the pain intensified, he would say, 'Order Abu Bakr ^ Ai ^ to lead the people in prayer,' The pain kept intensifying until the Prophet m, lost consciousness. When the pain intensified, his wives, his uncle Ab'ass, Umm Al-Fadhl bint Al-Harith and Asma' bint 'Umair discussed among each other about giving a medicine to the Prophet m,, and they did just that while he was unconscious. When he woke up, he said, 'Who did this to me. This is the work of some women who came from there, pointing to the direction of Ethiopia with his hand.' Umm Salamah and Asma were the ones who had administered the medicine to the Prophet b (they were among those who had migrated to Ethiopia), and they said, 'O Messenger of Allah! We were afraid that you were suffering from Thatul janb.' He said, 'What medicine did you give me?' They said, 'Some Indian costus, Wars and some drops of oil.' He said, 'Allah would never inflict this type of disease on me.' He then said, 'I order you that every person present in this house take some of the same medicine, except for my uncle Al-Ab'ass."

Further, in the Sahihan (Al-Bokhary and Muslim) it is narrated that

A'esha said:

"We administered some medicine to the Messenger of Allah b although he indicated that he did not want to be given medicine. But we attributed his refusal to what the sick usually feel about taking medicine. When he woke up, he said: "Did I not disallow you from giving me this medicine? Therefore, everyone present should take some of that medicine, except for my uncle Al-Ab'ass because he was not with you."

The last Hadith allows treating the aggressor in the same manner he treated others, as long as what the aggressor has committed is not prohibited by Allah, and there are more than ten proofs to this ruling that we elaborated on in another book. In addition, this ruling confirms the rulings of the Four Guided Caliphs and

Imam Ahmad. In addition, this Hadith indicates that reprisal for striking the face and hitting is of the same nature, as there are several Hadith on this subject that are unequivocal.

The Prophet's guidance on treating headaches and migraines

Headaches resemble a pain that appears in some part of the head or all of it, but when the headache attacks one side of the head, it is called migraine. The type that attacks the entire head is sometimes called a helmet, for it resembles the helmet that covers the head. Furthermore, headaches sometimes attack only the back or the front side of the head.

There are many types of headaches that result from various conditions. Headaches usually start when the head becomes hot due to the pressure of a septic vapor that accumulates near the head and which seeks a way out of the body but fails. Then, the pressure of the vapor intensifies, just as a pot when it is heated but the steam is not able to escape from it. It is a fact that when moisture heats up, it seeks more space to expand. Similarly, the vapor accumulates near the head and then causes a headache in the entire head because it is unable to expand or escape from the body as it heats up. This condition causes a type of dizziness.

There are various specific causes for headaches. First, when one of the four essential conditions (coldness, hotness, dryness and wetness) becomes predominant. Second, ulcers of the stomach cause headaches, because the cephalic (relating to the head) nerves and the stomach are connected, Third, thick flatulence might accumulate in the stomach then later ascend to the head and cause headaches. Fourth, headaches are sometimes caused by a tumor in the gastric veins that cause pain in the head, because the stomach and the head are connected. Fifth, when the stomach is full of food it sometimes provokes headaches, as some of the food remains undigested. Sixth, headaches sometimes occur after sexual intercourse because the body will then be weakened and thus exposed to the heat of the air. Seventh, headaches sometimes occur after vomiting due to excessive dryness, or to accumulating gaseous materials (flatulence) that ascend to the head from the stomach. Eighth, sometimes the hot weather and air provoke headaches. Ninth, headaches are sometimes caused by the cold weather and from the vapor that accumulates in the head and which is unable to decompose. Tenth, not having enough sleep In addition causes headaches. Headaches are sometimes caused due to the pressure exerted on the head, such as when one carries a heavy object on his head. Twelfth, excessive talking sometimes weakens the mind in a way that causes headaches. Thirteenth, excessive movements and sports activity can In addition provoke headaches. Fourteenth, sadness, depression, obsession and evil thoughts In addition provoke headaches. Fifteenth, excessive hunger provokes headaches, as in this case; the excess gaseous materials (flatulence) that accumulate in the stomach ascend to the brain and provoke headaches. Sixteenth, those who suffer from a tumor in the cerebral lining sometimes feel as if hammers are constantly pounding on their heads. Seventeenth, fever In addition provokes headaches because of the intense heat that the body suffers from them. Allah knows best.

Headaches result from changes in the system that affects the cerebral arteries

The weaker side of the brain will accept septic material and the migraine headache will be accompanied by pulsation in the arteries. The pain could be relieved in this case when one ties a bandage so that the pulsing of the arteries is stopped and thus the pain is lessened.

Abu Na'im said in his book on Prophetic medicine that the migraine type of headache used to attack the Prophet ss and that it would prevent him from going out of his house for one or two days at a time. In addition, Abu Na'im related from Ibn Ab'ass that he said, "Once, the Messenger of Allah ;ig delivered a speech while a cloth was tied around his head."

In addition, the Sahih states that the Prophet ^ said

during the illness that preceded his death: "O my head!" He used to tie a piece of cloth around his head.

Tying a piece of cloth around the head helps soothe the pain of headaches and migraines.

Treating headaches varies according to their type and causes

Hence, headaches could be relieved by vomiting, eating, being calm and idle, using cold rags, cooling the body, elevating the temperature, avoiding noise, etc.

Knowing these facts, we should mention that treating headaches with Henna is partial and that it treats some types of headache, If the headache is caused by high fever and not a spoiled substance that requires extraction, Henna helps soothe the headache somewhat. Crushed Henna blended with vinegar and applied to the forehead will relieve the headache. Henna In addition soothes the nerves when used as a bandage. Finally, Henna is not only favorable to relieve headaches, but In addition for the various organs of the body and for the hot tumors and inflammations when used as a bandage.

Henna is cold in the first degree and dry in the second degree

The Henna tree has two special qualities,

decomposing due to its warm watery essence, and constipating due to the cold earthly essence it contains.

Henna is useful in treating burns and soothes the nerves when used as a bandage, as we have stated. When chewed, Henna helps treat the cankers and thrush that appear in the mouth. Henna In addition heals stomatitis (inflammation of the mucous membranes of the mouth) that appear in the child's mouth. Using the Henna to bandage hot tumors In addition helps, as it has a similar effect on open sores as the dragon's blood tree has on them. When the Henna flower is blended with pure wax and rose oil, it will help against the aches of the side (Thatul janb).

When the symptoms of smallpox start to break out on children and Henna is then applied on the bottom of their feet, the eyes will be immune from the sores that accompany smallpox. In addition, when the flower of the Henna is placed between wool clothes, it will perfume it and will prevent mold or mite. Furthermore, when the leaves of the Henna are submerged in fresh water, then squeezed and drunk for forty days, twenty measures each day along with ten measures of sugar while eating the meat of a young ewe, it prevents leprosy with its amazing qualities.

We were told that a man once complained from fissuring in his fingers and that he offered monetary rewards to whoever could cure him, but to no avail. Later on, a woman prescribed for him a drink of Henna for ten days but he could not stand the idea of drinking it. Later on, he soaked Henna leaves in water and drank the water and his fingers were healed and regained their beauty.

Henna is In addition used as an ointment for the fingers, as it polishes and strengthens them. Henna is In addition useful when blended with butter and then used as a bandage for the hot tumors that drain yellow residue. Henna a so benefits against chronic mange, helps the hair grow, makes it stronger and In addition strengthens the head. Finally, Henna helps against the blisters and the pustules that appear on the legs and feet and the rest of the body in general.

The Prophet's guidance concerning feeding the sick with what they like and not forcing them to eat or drink

At-Termezey and Ibn Majah narrated that the Prophet ^ said:

"Do not force your patients to consume food or drink, for Allah, the Exalted and Most High, feeds them and gives them drink."

Some doctors commented, "How beneficial and true is this statement by the Prophet **b** that contains divine wisdom, especially for the doctors who treat patients. When the patient does not feel like eating or drinking, it is because the body is busy fighting the illness, or because the instinctive heat (or the appetite) becomes weaker. Either way, it is not allowed to give the patients food in this case."

The feeling of hunger results from the body's appetite for food so that it refuels itself with the needed energy replacing that which the body has spent. The various organs of the body will spend the available energy until it runs low on supply, the stomach will alert the person, who would then feel hungry. Food will then be distributed from the stomach to the rest of the organs of the body starting with the closest ones. When one is ill, the body will be busy maturating and getting rid of the alien, septic substances and does not require food or drink. When the sick person is forced to eat some food, the body's energy will be divided between digesting the food and concentrating on fending off the invading septic substances that caused the ailment. The patient will be harmed in this case, especially when one is suffering from acute ailments or lessening in the instinctive heat, as these conditions will only add strength to the ailment and bring about harm. The patient should only eat what is required to sustain his strength and should avoid what can aggravate his condition. The patient should consume light food and juices like nenuphar (similar to carrot), apples and tender rosewater drinks, etc. As for the types of foods the patient should consume, they should include aromatic chicken soup. In addition, the patient should refresh his body with good scents and listen to good news.

The doctor is the servant of nature not one who hinders it or obstructs its path.

We should state that fresh, healthy blood provides nutrition to the body. We should In addition know that phlegm is a type of blood that has not properly matured. Therefore, when the patient's body has excess phlegm on an empty stomach, the body will lead the phlegmy blood to maturity and then turn it into fresh blood that will supply energy to the organs of the body. The nature of the human body is the engine and vehicle that Allah has entrusted with preserving the body and its health and guarding it throughout its term.

Sometimes, compelling the patient to eat and drink becomes warranted when the ailments involve sanity.

The Hadith indicates that the patient could live without nourishment for longer than a healthy person could.

The Prophet's statement: "For Allah provides food and drink for them," entails more far-reaching implications than the doctors think. Only those who are experienced in knowledge of the heart and soul and in their effects on the nature of the body and vise versa will be able to uncover the implications of the Prophet's statement.

It is a fact that when the heart is busy with such feelings as joy, sadness or fear, it will be busy attending to these feelings, thus ignoring the need to eat or drink. In this condition, one does not feel hunger or thirst or even the cold or the heat. Rather, the body in this case will be busy attending whatever made it concerned and whatever caused it pain. Every person experiences such moods and thus would agree that when the heart is busy attending to a concern, it will not feel the need for food.

When the concern is a matter that brings joy, the feeling of elation will be a substitute for the food. Jubilation will fill the body and will energize it and the blood will be pumped to the various organs until it appears under the skin. In this case, the face will radiate with delight and life. Indeed, happy feelings relax the heart and fill the veins with blood. The organs do not require food in this case because they are busy dealing with what is even better for their nature than food. When human nature acquires what it likes, then it will disregard what is less favorable or important.

When the concern entails sadness, anguish or fear, the body will be busy attending to such concerns and will ignore seeking food in this case, because it is busy conducting its own war. When the body wins the war against such feelings, the feelings of joy will re-ignite the body's strength and will become a substitute for the-regular energy through food and drink. When the war against these concerns is lost, the body will feel as low and weak as the size of defeat it suffered. If the war against such concerns is sometimes won and sometimes lost the body will feel energetic at times and weak at other times. Certainly, this type of war resembles the actual war between two enemies, where the upper hand belongs to the victorious, while defeat entails suffering casualties, dead, wounded or captured.

The sick person receives supplies from Allah that provide nutrition for him, in addition to the nutrition that he receives through the blood which the doctors confirm. This divine help varies in amount according to the amount of submission and meekness that one shows before his Lord and which will earn him closeness to Him. The closest the slave will be to his Lord is when his heart submits to Allah and in return Allah's mercy will draw closer to the slave. When the slave is one of Allah's, loyal supporters, his heart will receive sufficient support and aid that will nourish his body and strength more than the nourishment that his body receives through material nourishment. The stronger the slave's love, happiness, certainty, eagerness and contentment with Allah becomes, the more divine strength he will feel. This cannot be described with words, nor can any doctor explain or attain knowledge of it on his own.

Those who do not have sound comprehension and thus are unable to understand the aforementioned facts, let them observe the miserable condition of whoever covets a part of the material existence, whether a picture, a position, money or knowledge. Many people have discovered amazing facts concerning their own selves and other people by deep observation.

In the Sahih it has been stated that the Prophet **b** used to continue fasting for days at a time, yet he would prohibit his Companions from imitating him, saying:

"I am not like any of you, my Lord provides me with food and drink."

The food and drink mentioned in the Hadith is not the type that people eat with the mouth. Otherwise, the Prophet ^e would not have been continuing the Fast. Rather, the Prophet sjg said: "My lord provides me with food and drink," thus drawing a difference between him and the Companions in that he is able to bear what they cannot bear. If the Prophet as were talking about the regular food and drink, he would not have said:

"I am not like any of you." Those who understand

regular food and drink from this Hadith do not have a significant supply from the true nutrition that the heart and soul require. Nor do they have knowledge of this divine nutrition's effect on the strength and revival of the body, along with providing it with the true sustenance that is much more powerful and sustaining than the material food.

The Prophet's guidance on treating tonsillitis and administering the medication orally

In the Sahihan it is narrated that the Prophet b said:

"Cupping and manne costus are among your best remedies; and do not torture your children by pressing their uvula to cure tonsillitis."

In addition in the Sunon and the Musnad (by Imam Ahmad) it is narrated that Jabir said, "The Messenger of Allah came to 'A'esha and saw a boy with a bleeding nose and said, 'What is this?' They said, "He is suffering from tonsillitis, or a headache.' He said:

"Woe unto you! Do not kill your children. Let the mother whose child is suffering from tonsillitis or headache scrub Indian costus (aloes) with water and then administer it to the child through the nose.'

When 'A'esha ordered that the prescription be followed, the boy was cured." [Ahmad, Al Hakim, Abu Ya'la and Al-Kazzar].

Abu 'Ubaidah said, "Tonsillitis, according to Abu 'Ubaidah, is a blood related throat irritation." It was In addition said that tonsillitis is an ulcer that appears between the ear and the throat that especially afflicts young boys.

Administering scrubbed aloes through the nose helps against tonsillitis, which is essentially composed of blood related phlegm that accumulates in the bodies of young boys. Costus or Aloes tighten the uvula and pulls it up to its proper place. Aloes In addition help against other hot ailments. The author of Al-Qanoon stated that costus, Yemeni alum and marjoram seeds help against tonsillitis.

The marine costus mentioned in the Hadith is the Indian aloes, particularly the one whitish in color, and it is sweet and has many benefits. Before, the people used to treat their children who suffered from tonsillitis by pressing the uvula and sometimes affixing an object to the uvula. The Prophet ^ disallowed this practice and guided the people to what is better, more beneficial and easier for the afflicted children.

Administering the medicine through the nose involves either simple or compound remedies that are ground and dried. Then, when warranted, the medication is administered through the nose of the afflicted person while he lay on his back and while his shoulders are elevated so that the head lay back. In this position, the medication would reach the head and extract the disease by sneezing.

The Prophet s, has praised using this method when there is a need that warrants it. Further, Abu Dawood mentioned in his Sunon that the Prophet sg used this method himself.

The Prophet's guidance on treating diseases of heart

Abu Dawood narrated that Sa'd said, "Once, I became ill and the Messenger of Allah b came to visit me and placed his hand on the center of my chest, until I felt its coldness on my heart. He then said:

"You ore complaining from your heart. Go to Al-Harith bin Kaladah, from (the tribe of) Thaqhif, for he knows about medicine. Let him take seven dates from Al-Medina, grind them with their seeds and then give them to you."

Dates in general and dried dates in particular, especially from Medina, posses tremendous qualities and are especially effective in treating heart aliments. Using seven dates is another quality that can only be known through the revelation.

In the Sahihan it is narrated that Sa'd bin Abu Waqqas said, "The Messenger of Allah **b** said:

"Whoever eats seven dates from the area of Al-Aliab when he gets up in the morning then no poison or magic would harm him that day."

In another narration, the Prophet **b** said:

"Whoever eats seven dotes produced between the two areas in Al-Medina that are covered with burned black stones in the morning, will not be harmed by poison until he reaches the night."

Dates are warm in the second degree and dry in the first degree. Dates constitute a good type of nutrition, especially for those whose regular diet contains dates, such as the people of Al-Medina. Dates are the best type of food for the residents of the hot and mildly warm countries, more so than for the residents of cold areas who have an elevated inner temperature, whereas those in warm areas have a colder inner temperature. This is why the people in Hijaz, Yemen and Tai'f, and similar areas, eat hot foods such as dates and honey. They In addition use pepper and ginger in their food more than other areas; sometimes ten fold as much. Some of them even eat Zanjabil (ginger) just as other people eat sweets. They even transport these types of foods with them when traveling. As we have stated, these types of food are suitable for the residents of warm areas and do not harm them because of the lower inner temperature of their bodies. On a similar note, we should mention that well-water becomes colder during summer and warmer during winter. Further, the stomach digests because thick (or complex) foods in winter more than during summer.

For the people of Medina, dried dates are their staple like wheat is to other people. In addition, dried dates from the area of Al-Aliyah in Medina are one of the best kinds of dates because they are firm, delicious and sweet.

Dates are a type of fruit that is In addition used for its nutritional and medicinal value, being favorable for most bodies and for their role in strengthening the natural heat. In addition, dates do not produce harmful wastes or excrements such as the other types of foods and fruits. Rather, dates preserve the bodily wastes from being spoiled and from rotting, especially for those used to eating dried dates.

The Hadith we mentioned about dried dates [in the beginning of the chapter] is specifically for the people of Al-Medina and surrounding areas. It is a fact that the medicinal value of the herbs and plants that grow in certain areas is closely related to the quality of the air and the type of soil in those areas. A certain medicinal herb might be useful in its natural habitat but not if it is grown elsewhere. The various lands differ in their nature and characteristics, just as people differ from each other. Sometimes, a certain type of plant might be a regular staple in the diet in a certain area, while it is poisonous in other areas. Sometimes, certain remedies that people use in a certain land might be a regular staple for other people in another area. Some types of medicine might provide a cure for some illnesses for some people while curing other kinds of diseases for other people. Furthermore, there might be a beneficial cure in some area that does not work in other areas.

Using seven dates has a spiritual and material significance. Allah has created seven heavens, seven earths, seven days in the week and made the creation of mankind pass through seven stages. In addition, Allah made the Tawaf seven circumambulations, and the Sa'i In addition seven trips between Safa and Marwah. In addition, the Jamrat are stoned with seven pebbles each and the Takbir during the 'Gd prayer is made seven times. In addition, the Prophet sag said about young children,

"Command him to pray upon reaching the age of seven."

In addition, when the child reaches the age of seven, he is given the choice between his father and mother, according to some opinions. When the Prophet m, was ill he ordered that water be poured on him from seven different water skins. Allah has In addition sent the destructive wind on the people of Ad for seven consecutive nights. The Prophet of Allah In addition asked Allah in supplication to test his people with a similar seven years of famine that the people of the Prophet Yusuf (Joseph) were tested with. Furthermore, when Allah gave the example of charity, He compared it to a grain (of corn); it grows seven ears, and each ear has a hundred grains. In addition, the ears of corn that the king saw during the time of Prophet Yusuf (Joseph) were seven and the number of the years during which the king's people would farm the land was In addition seven. In addition, charity is multiplied seven hundred times, to much more. Further, there are seventy thousand members of the Muslim Nation who will enter Paradise without questioning. The number seven has a special significance more than other numbers and only Allah has full knowledge of the wisdom behind choosing this number above other numbers.

The Hadith mentioned that eating seven dates from a certain area in Al-Medina prevents poisoning and magic, indicating the special qualities of this type of date. Had it been Hippocrates or Galinus who issued this statement rather than the Prophet m,, the doctors would quickly accept the statement without question, even though they would be issuing it based on guessing and not on fact. The statrments that come from the Prophet ^, whose words are certainly true and divinely revealed, deserve to be believed in more and submitted to, without any hesitation or denial.

The dried dates mentioned in Hadith, being useful against certain poisons and only in some areas Further, we should state here that it is a condition that the sick person should believe that the medicine will help him, so that his body accepts it and benefits from it. It is a fact that sometimes merely believing that the medicine will work helps cure some ailments, as many people have witnessed in this regard. When the heart accepts that a certain medicine carries the cure, the body will feel an elevation in its strength and in the instinctive heat that will help the body get rid of and extract harmful substances. On the other hand, sometimes an effective medicine fails to work because the patient does not believe that it will cure him, and consequently, his body neither accepts it, nor benefits from it.

Even the Qura'an, which is the best, most beneficial remedy ever, both in this life and in the Hereafter, and which is a cure for every disease, will not benefit the heart that does not believe in its value as a cure and a remedy. Rather, the Qura'an only adds more disease to such evil hearts.

There is not a more effective cure for the diseases of the heart than the Qura'an, for it completely eradicates the ills of the heart, preserves the heart's health and wellbeing and defends it against all that might bring harm to it. Yet, most of the hearts ignore the Qura'an and do not believe in it, and thus refrain from using it. Instead, such people refer to other types of medicine that were prepared by their like from among mankind, thus preventing their hearts from benefiting from the Qura'an. Consequently, the symptoms that attacked their hearts will persist and will expose their hearts to even more ailments. By the passage of time, both the doctors and the patients will get used to the medicines produced and prescribed by their like, leaders, or those whom they respect. In this case, disasters will accumulate and the diseases will become harder to cure. And the more they (those who ignore the Qura'an) use these medicines, the more strength they will add to the ailment!

The Prophet's guidance on neutralizing the harm of various foods and fruits

In the Sahihan it is narrated that 'Abudllah bin Ja'far 'a. AI ^3 said, "I saw the Messenger of Allah s&. eat ripe dates with cucumbers."

Ripe dates are hot in the second degree, increase sexual desire and add strength to the cold stomach. But, ripe dates rot quickly, bring thirst, harm the teeth, spoil the blood and cause headaches, various clogs and pain in the prostate. Cucumbers are cold and wet in the second degree and they prevent thirst, have a refreshing aroma and cool the stomach. When the seeds of the cucumbers are dried then crushed and are boiled with water, they produce a drink that will quench the thirst, help produce urine and soothe the pain in the prostate. When cucumber seeds are crushed and then sifted, it will whiten the teeth when brushed with it. Further, when cucumber plant leaves are crushed and blended with raisin jelly and used as a bandage, they will help against the bite of the hydrophobic dog.

In general, dates are hot while cucumbers are cool, and each is suitable for the other and In addition neutralizes each others harm. This is a type of balancing off the harm of one substance by combining it with its opposite or antidote, and these are the goals that preventive science seeks to achieve. In fact, these are the goals that the science of medicine as a whole seeks to achieve.

Combining the foods or medicines with their antidotes or opposites makes the product milder and rids it of any harmful side effects. Consequently, the body will preserve its health, strength and wellbeing.

'A'esha \^i AI ^.3 once said, "They tried to make me fatter using every type of food, but I did not get fatter.

But when they fed me ripe dates and cucumbers, I became fatter."

In short, neutralizing the effect of the hot substance with the cold, the cold with the hot, the dry with the wet and the wet with the dry produces a milder substance that is considered among the best remedies and preventive measures. We mentioned before the Prophet's guidance concerning blending Senna and Sanoot (honey and butter) and stated that this method will make the Senno milder. May Allah bestow His peace and blessings on he who was sent with all that brings life to the hearts and bodies and what brings about their benefit in this life and the Hereafter.

The Prophet's guidance on observing a diet as part of the cure

All types of cures and medicines contain either a certain diet or preventive measures. When one feels ill, he will need to rid the body from harmful substances and bodily wastes. These three elements are what medicine is all about.

There are two types of diet, a diet from what might bring an illness and a diet from what might intensify the illness. The first type of diet is for the healthy and the second type is for those with an illness. When the patient observes a certain diet, the illness will not progress and thus the powers contained in the body will cooperate and collaborate towards ridding the body of the ailment.

The most basic element regarding the diet is what Allah said:

﴿ يَٰٓأَيُّهَا ٱلَّذِينَ ءَامَنُواْ لَا تَقْرَبُواْ ٱلصَّلَوٰةَ وَأَنتُمْ سُكَٰرَىٰ حَتَّىٰ تَعْلَمُواْ مَا تَقُولُونَ وَلَا جُنُبًا إِلَّا عَابِرِى سَبِيلٍ حَتَّىٰ تَغْتَسِلُواْ ۚ وَإِن كُنتُم مَّرْضَىٰٓ أَوْ عَلَىٰ سَفَرٍ أَوْ جَآءَ أَحَدٌ مِّنكُم مِّنَ ٱلْغَآئِطِ أَوْ لَٰمَسْتُمُ ٱلنِّسَآءَ فَلَمْ تَجِدُواْ مَآءً فَتَيَمَّمُواْ صَعِيدًا طَيِّبًا فَٱمْسَحُواْ بِوُجُوهِكُمْ وَأَيْدِيكُمْ ۗ إِنَّ ٱللَّهَ كَانَ عَفُوًّا غَفُورًا ﴿٤٣﴾ ﴾

(٤٣) النساء

"***And if you are ill, or on a journey, or one of you comes after answering the call of nature, or you have been in contact with women (by sexual relations) and you find no water, perform Tayammum with clean earth***." (4:43)

Allah has saved the sick person from using water when there is a chance that it might harm him.

Ibn Majah narrated that Umm Al-Munthir bint

Qays said, "The Messenger of Allah b came along with Ali ^ AI ^3 who was then recovering from an illness. At that time, we had some hanging clusters of dates. The Messenger of Allah a& started eating from them and then 'Ali ^ AI ^3 joined him. The Messenger of Allah kept saying to Ali Ai ^.3 &: You are still recovering, 'until Ali ^ -mi ^.3 Stopped eating.' I then made some barley and chard (similar to spinach) and brought it to them. The Prophet s& said, to Ali, 'Eat from this food, it is more beneficial for you." In another narration, the Prophet ^ said, "Eat from this food for it is more suitable in your condition." [Abu Dawood, Ahmod and Al-Hakim].

In addition, Ibn Majah narrated that Suhayb said, "I came by the Messenger of Allah ag and found that there were some dates and bread in front of him. The Prophet b said, 'Come closer and eat.' I picked up some dates and started eating from them. Then the Prophet ste said, 'Do you eat dates while you are suffering from conjunctivitis (an inflammation of the covering membrane of the eye)?' I said, 'O Messenger of Allah, I am chewing on the other side.' The Messenger of Allah then smiled.'" [At-Termezey and Al-Hoki'mJ.

In another Hadith, the Prophet s& said:

"When Allah loves a slave. He helps him observe a diet from the life of this world, just as one of you puts bis patient on a diet from food and drink. Allah puts His believing slave on a diet from the life of this world."

The famous statement that: "Diet is the top medicine; and the stomach is the home of disease; give each person what he is used to [of food and medicine]," this is not a Hadith, according to the scholars of Hadith. Rather, it is the words of Al-Harith bin Kaladah, the renowned Arab doctor.

Al-Harith stated that, "Diet is the head of medicine." To doctors, observing a diet by healthy people is as harmful as unhealthy eating habits for patients. Consequently, the best type of diet is that observed by those recovering from an illness, because until then, their body organs would not have regained their normal strength and wellbeing. In this condition, the digestion process would not be at its normal efficiency while the various organs of the body would still be prone to sickness. At this time unhealthy eating habits might cause the disease to come back stronger than it was before.

Know that the Prophet's disallowing Ali from eating the hanging clusters of dates while still recuperating from an illness is one of the best preventive measures. Fruits are not beneficial for sick or recovering patients as they get digested quickly at a time when the body is still fighting the ailment and is not strong enough to deal with an excess amount of food. Ripe dates in particular are heavy on the stomach at a time when the body is still resisting the ailment and removing its effects. Whatever part of the ailment that remains would either dissipate or re-intensify, depending on the condition of the body.

Therefore, when cooked barley and chard were brought to the Prophet **b** he ordered Ali to eat from it. Cooked barley and chard represent one of the best types of foods for the recovering patients and those with weak stomachs. It does not produce any harmful substances or bodily wastes. The water of cooked barley is cool and nourishing, along with its other qualities of soothing, relaxing the bowels and strengthening the body in general, especially when it is cooked with chard.

Zaid bin Aslam once said, "Umar once made a patient observe such a strict diet that he used to suck on date stones." In short, diet is one of the most beneficial preventive measures before and after the disease strikes, in which case diet will prevent the disease from spreading or progressing.

We should know that when healthy, recovering or sick people have a taste for a type of food or drink, it would not harm if one consumes little amounts of it. Rather, the food might even help and benefit the body, as the stomach will accept and easily digest the food, more so than when one takes a medicine that it detests. This is why the Prophet **b** allowed Suhaib to eat a few dates when he was suffering from conjunctivitis, since it was just a little and would not harm him.

It was reported that Ali said that he once came by the Prophet **b**, when he, (Ali), was complaining from conjunctivitis, and found the Prophet **b** eating dates. The Prophet ^ asked him, "O Ali, do you have a taste for dates?" He then threw a date and then another date to Ali, until he threw seven. The Prophet ^ then said, "That is enough, O Ali." [Abu Na'im in his book on the Prophetic medicine].

In addition, Ibn Majah narrated that Ibn Ab'ass said:

"Once, the Prophet **b** ate visited a sick person and asked him, "What do you have a taste for?" The man said, "I have a taste for wheat bread, or I have a taste for a cake." The Prophet ^ then said: "Whoever has wheat bread, let him send some to his

brother." He In addition said, "When yours sick have a taste for something, give them some of it."

The last Hadith contains a secret, because when the sick person eats what he has a taste for while In addition hungry, it will be less harmful than what he does not have a taste for. If what he has a taste for is not beneficial in his condition, then his preference for it will prevent its harm. In addition, eating what one does not like will cause harm to the patient even if the substance is beneficial itself. In general, the type of food that is tasty and that the person likes will be accepted by the body and will be digested in the best way, especially when the appetite for it is strong.

The Prophet's guidance on treating conjunctivitis with rest and observing a special diet

We mentioned that the Prophet b required Suhaib to observe a diet from eating dates when he was suffering from conjunctivitis, and did the same with 'Ali when he was suffering from the same condition. Furthermore, Abu Na'im narrated in his book, the Prophetic Medicine, "Whenever any of the Prophet's wives would come down with conjunctivitis, he would not touch her until her eyes were cured."

Conjunctivitis is an infection that attacks the conjunctiva, that is the white part of the eye. The disease is caused by one of the four conditions [hotness, coldness, dryness and wetness], or by the accumulation of hot flatulence in the head and body, that later reaches the eye and cause conjunctivitis. In addition, when the eye receives a hit, the blood and the soul will rush to the aid of the affected eye, which then becomes swollen.

We should know that there are two types of

moistures that ascend to the air. One is hot and dry and the other hot and wet. These moistures form the clouds that shade the sky from our eyes. Likewise, gaseous substances and moistures ascend from the stomach to the upper parts of the body and cause many ailments, such as conjunctivitis. When the body's resistance is strong, it will push these gaseous substances to the nose and cause a congestion that usually accompanies colds. When these substances are pushed up through the uvula and the nostrils, they cause angina. When these moistures are pushed towards the side, they cause causes pleurisy, and when they reach the chest they causes pneumonia. When the moistures reach the heart they cause rapid pulse, and when they reach the eyes they cause conjunctivitis. When they reach the intestinal cavity, they cause diarrhea and when they reach the brain they cause forgetfulness. If the brain receives excessive amounts of these gaseous moistures, they might cause heavy sleeping. This is why sleep is wet while being awake is dry. When the septic gases unsuccessfully seek to depart from the body through the head, they will cause headaches and less sleep. When these gases attack one side of the brain, they cause migraines. If these gases reach the cerebral divider and cause it coldness, hotness or wetness, it will cause sneezing. If the gases cause the accumulation of phlegm in the cerebral divider, so that its hot nature becomes weak, they cause unconsciousness and stroke. If the gases excite the black bile, they will cause obsession, and if they reach the nerves, they will cause real epilepsy. When the cerebral nerves receive these gases they will suffer from facial paralysis. If these gases were caused by inflamed yellow bile that heats the brain, they will cause cerebral tumors, and when the chest receives a part of these gases, they will cause pleurisy.

In short, the condition of the head and body will be irritated because of conjunctivitis, and having sex in this state will only aggravate the condition even more. Sex entails a movement that is shared by the entire body, the heart and the soul. As for the body, it heats up due to the intense movements during sex, while the heart will seek to acquire its lust and pleasures. The soul will follow the lead of the body and the heart, as the first part that is connected to the soul is the heart, which in turn affects the rest of the body. As for the body, it sends the semen that is needed to bring the sexual intercourse to conclusion. Thus, sexual activity involves a movement by the entire body, the heart and the soul, and every move excites the various conditions and causes them to move to the weaker parts of the body, such as the eye when suffering from conjunctivitis.

We should state that the body benefits from conjunctivitis in that it helps the body extract harmful substances and cleanses the body and the head from septic elements. In addition, conjunctivitis compels the affected person to observe a diet and avoid sadness, grief, strong movements and hard work. Further, one of our righteous predecessors said, "Do not hate conjunctivitis, because it prevents blindness."

In addition, conjunctivitis requires rest and avoiding touching the eye to prevent more harmful substances from accumulating in it. Some of the Salaf once said, "The example of the Companions of Muhammad y& is the example of the eye: its cure is in avoiding touching it."

A Hadith that we are not sure about its authenticity states that sprinkling cold water on the eye helps cure conjunctivitis. The remedy mentioned in the Hadith is beneficial for hot conjunctivitis, since water is cold and thus cools down the heat that accompanies conjunctivitis. This is why when the wife of "Abdullah bin Mas'ud complained about her eyes, he said to her, "If you had done what the Prophet **b** used to do, it would have been better for you and would have brought fast healing to your eyes. Splash water on your eyes and then say, 'Cure the ailment, O Lord of the people! Bring about the cure, for You Alone bring the cure and there is no cure except that which you bring about. Bring a type of healing that eradicates every ailment,"

We mentioned before that these types of remedies are suitable for certain areas and for some ailments that attack the eye. Do not understand the Prophet's statements that are specific to be general nor vise versa. Otherwise, mistakes will certainly occur.

The Prophet's guidance on treating narcolepsy

Abu Ubaid said in his book on the unusual words used in some Ahadeeth that some people passed by a tree that they ate from and they were soon immobilized, just as if a wind had swept through by them and froze them. The Prophet b said:

"Cool some water in water skins and then pour the water on them between the two Azanayn (the Fajr call to the prayer and the Iqamah)."

The Prophet a| mentioned the water skins because they cool the water more than clay containers. He In addition called the Iqamah an Azan in this Hadith.

Some doctors stated that the remedy that the Prophet $& prescribed in the Hadith is the one of the most effective against narcolepsy if it occurs in the area of Hijaz, which is a hot dry land. The inhabitants of that area have a weak instinctive heat. Pouring cold water on the people afflicted by narcolepsy during the above mentioned time, which is the coolest time of the night, will cause the instinctive heat that is scattered throughout the body to be energized and accumulate in the inner parts of the body where the ailment resides. The powers of the body will then concentrate on expelling and resisting the ailment by Allah's will.

If it were Galinus or Hippocrates who had prescribed this remedy, the doctors would have been amazed by its perfect effectiveness!

The Prophet's guidance on food and drink contaminated by flies

In the Sahihain [actually, only Al-Bokhary narrated it in his Sohih] it is narrated that the Messenger of Allah b said:

"If a housefly falls in the drink of anyone of you, he should dip it (in the drink), for one of its wings has a disease and the other has the cure for the disease."

In addition, Ibn Majah narrated that the Messenger of Allah said:

"One of the fly's wings carries poison while the other carries a cure. When it falls in the food, dip it, for the sake of Allah, for verily He (Allah) makes the poison (take affect) first and He makes the cure come last."

This Hadith contains two areas of interest, Fiqh (Islamic Jurisprudence) and medicinal. As for the Fiqh part, the Hadith states that when a fly falls in water or fluids, it does not make it impure, according to the majority of the scholars. None among the early generations contradicted this ruling.

The Prophet b ordered the fly that falls on the food be dipped ir. :t, thus killing the fly, especially if the food is hot. If the fly's death inside the food would make the food impure, the Prophet ^s would have ordered us to discard the food. On the contrary, the Prophet sought to salvage the food.

Bees, hornets, spiders and all similar insects are treated in the same manner as houseflies, because the ruling that we derived from the Prophet's commandment in this Hadith is general. Since the reason why dead animals are impure is that their blood remains trapped in their bodies, therefore the insects, which do not have blood are pure. The first person to use the words "What does not have a soul (meaning blood)" was Ibrahim An-Nukha'i and then the scholars used these terms after him,

As for the medicinal value contained in the Hadith, Abu 'Ubaidah said that the purpose behind dipping the fly [in the drink] is to extract the cure from [its other wing] just as the poison was extracted from [the wing that fell on the food].

Houseflies carry poisonous materials as evidenced by the effect of their bite, such as rash and infection, and this poison is the fly's weapon of defense. When the fly falls into what harms it, it tries to defend itself with the available weapons. The Prophet b ordered that we neutralize the poisonous substances produced by the fly with the cure that Allah has kept on its other wing. The fly should then be submerged in the water or the food so that the cure could neutralize the effect of the poison. This is a remedy that the best medical minds would never be able to discover on their own, because it is coming from Prophetic knowledge. The doctors who have good knowledge and comprehension submit to this Prophetic remedy and admit that he who was sent with it, is indeed the perfect human being who is supported by divine revelation that is beyond human power.

Several doctors have stated that when one anoints the inflammation caused by scorpion and hornet bites with the housefly, it would calm down the pain due to the cure that the fly carries in its wing. When the head of the housefly is amputated and the body is used to scrub the tumor that appears in the eyelid, it will cure it, Allah willing.

The Prophet's guidance on treating pimples

Ibn As-Sunni said in his book that one of the Prophet's wives said, "Once, the Messenger of Allah b came by when I had a pimple on my finger. He said:

"Do you have a Tharirah (arum)?' I said, 'Yes.' He said. Place it on the pimple. He then said, 'Say, O Allah who transforms the big to small and the small to big, make what I am suffering from small." [Al-Hakem In addition narrated the Hadith],

The Tharirah (Arum) is an Indian remedy made of arum cane. Arum is hot and dry and helps against stomach and liver tumors and dropsy and In addition strengthens the heart.

In the Sahihain it is narrated that 'A'esha said, "I perfumed the Messenger of Allah SB with my hand using Tharirah (Arum) during the Farewell Hajj during the state of Ihram and otherwise."

The pimple is a growth that results from hot harmful, septic substances that push towards the skin so as to find a way out of the body. The pimple needs to mature and to then be opened and extracted, such as by using the Tharirah, which helps extract the septic matter from the pimple, along with giving a good aroma. In addition, the Tharirah soothes the hotness of the pimple. This is why the author of ' the Al-Qonoon said, "There is no better remedy for fire burns than the Tharirah, when it is blended with rose essence and vinegar.

The Prophet's guidance in treating tumors and abscesses with surgery

Abu Hurayrah narrated that the Prophet **b** ordered a doctor to incise an abscess on the abdomen of a man. He was asked, 'Does medicine help, O Messenger of Allah **b** He said:

"He Who has sent down the disease has In addition sent down whatever He wills of the cure."

The tumor, which accompanies most ailments, is a growth in the organ due to the accumulation of unnatural, septic materials engineered by the four conditions hotness, coldness, dryness and wetness, plus water and wind. When the tumor swells with septic material, it is called an abscess. Every hot tumor ends up decomposing, or becoming pus, or hardening. If the body is strong enough, it dissolves the tumor, and this is the best end of tumors. If the body is not strong, it turns the tumor into a white substance, pus, and opens an exit for the pus to go out of the body. If the body is weak, the tumor will be full of immature pus and the body will not be able to open an exit to discard the pus. In this case, it is possible the tumor will spoil the affected organ. The doctor's help is then sought to incise the tip of the tumor to extract the septic substance.

Puncturing or incising the tumor has two benefits,

extracting the harmful substance and preventing more harmful substances from accumulating around the tumor making it even worse.

The Hadith stated that the Prophet b ordered a doctor to incise a tumor on a man's abdomen that was filled with putrid or rotten liquid.

The scholars have conflicting opinions regarding incising tumors, some of them did not allow it because it is dangerous in their opinion. Other doctors said that there is no cure for dropsy except incision. As we have stated, dropsy is of three types: drum dropsy, which causes the stomach to swell with accumulated gases, that if one pounds on the stomach it will produce a similar sound as the drum.

In addition, there is the fleshy dropsy that causes the flesh to swell accompanied by phlegm that spreads throughout the body through the blood. This type is worse than the first one.

Third, there is the dropsy that causes the accumulation of toxic materials in the lower part of the stomach. When one moves in this case, his stomach will produce a sound similar to the shaking of a water skin. Most doctors consider this type of dropsy the worst, while others consider the fleshy dropsy the worst of the three types.

Curing the third type of dropsy requires extracting the accumulating water by incision, which is similar to extracting spoiled blood by puncturing the veins. Yet, this procedure is dangerous, although the Hadith, if proven authentic, allows using this method. Allah has the best knowledge.*

The Prophet's guidance on treating the sick by encouraging them and strengthening their resolve

Ibn Majah narrated that Abu Sa'id Al-Khudri said, The Messenger of Allah **b** said:

"When you visit a sick person, say good words to him, for the sake of Allah for although that does not prevent any harm, it still brings relief to the patient's heart." At-Termezey In addition narrated the Hadith].

This Hadith contains one of the most honorable remedies, that is, relieving the anxiety of the sick with some good words that will enhance his resolve and strength. In this case, the inner energy would be elevated and would help the body against the disease, which is the best the doctor could wish for.

Relieving the anxiety of the sick person and bringing relief to his heart has a surprisingly good effect in curing the body and lessening the effects of an ailment. It will In addition bring strength to the heart and the soul of the sick person, further encouraging the body to fight the disease. People have witnessed that the sick feel refreshed and energized in the company of those they like and respect when they visit them. This is one of the benefits gained from visiting the sick, which carries four types of benefits: for the sick person, the visitor, the sick person's family and the general public.

We mentioned before that the Prophet $& used to ask the sick about what they complain from and how they felt. He would In addition ask them about what they had a taste for and would place his hand on the forehead, or even on the chest, asking Allah to bring about whatever benefits them in their condition. Sometimes, the Prophet as would perform ablution and then pour the water he used on the sick person. Sometimes, the Prophet **b** would say to the sick person:

"It is alright. You will be purified (cured). Allah willing."

This, indeed, is the kindest way to treat the sick when visiting them.

The Prophet's guidance on treating various illnesses with food and medicine the body is used to

This is In addition one of the major pillars and the most beneficial parts of the science of medicine. When

Al-Harith stated that the stomach is the residence of the disease. The stomach is a curved organ that looks like a gourd and consists of three layers of delicate and neural components called fibers and surrounded by flesh. The fibers of one layer are arranged longitudinally, while the second layer's fibers are horizontal and the third slanting. The tip of the stomach has more nerves, while the bottom has more flesh and its interior is coated and fuzzy. The stomach is located in the middle of the abdomen, leaning more to the right side, created in this shape by the wisdom of the All-Wise Creator. The stomach is indeed the residence of the ailment, it is the center of the digestion and maturing process of all food and drink. After that, the digested food descends to the liver and the intestines. Meanwhile, excess amounts of partially digested substances that the stomach was not able to completely digest remain, either because the amount of nourishment was excessive, spoiled, or was not consumed in the proper order, or all of these reasons. Some of this excrement remains in the stomach and the body is not be able to completely discard them, and this is why the stomach is the residence of ailments, Al-Harith indicates the importance of eating less food and preventing the heart from fulfilling its desires.

As for one's being accustomed [to certain things and foods] it is a part of the human nature. Habit has such a great influence on the person and on his body, that if we conduct an experiment on several people who have the same characteristics, the result will vary considerably. For instance, three young, hot-tempered men, one of them is used to eating hot foods, the second is used to cold foods, while the third man is accustomed to mild foods. When the first person eats honey, it would not harm him, unlike the second person, while the third person would be slightly bothered. Habit, therefore, is an important basis on which preserving the health and healing ailments relies. That is why the Prophet **b** said that each person should be treated according to what he is accustomed to of medicine and food.

The Prophet's guidance on treating the sick with the simplest types of food

In the Sahihain it is narrated that A'esha said that when a relative of hers would die the women would gather on that occasion and then would depart except for her family members and close associates. She would then order that milk soup be prepared. Then, Tharid would be made and she would pour the milk soup on it. A'esha would then ask them to eat saying, "I heard the Messenger of Allah **b** saying:

"Milk soup brings relief to the heart of the sick and takes away some of the anguish.'"

Milk soup, means the kind of soup that is similar

to milk in consistency. This is a beneficial food suitable for the sick, especially when well cooked until acquiring a soft consistency. The milk like soups, are as beneficial as barley soup, even better. Barely soup is made of whole barley grains, while the milk like soup is made of ground barley flour with its bran.

We mentioned that observing the habits and customs of a certain sick person benefits them with a favorable cure and nourishment. The people in Al-Medina were accustomed to eating barley soup ground not whole, thus making it more nutritious and beneficial for them. The doctors in cities recommend the use of whole barley grains, because the soup in this case is lighter and easier for the ailing person to digest. The people who live in cities are used to comfort and easy life and that is why ground barley grain is heavy on their stomachs.

Whole grain barley soup digests quickly, provides good nutrition, and cleanses the stomach, especially when taken while it is still hot. In this case, it's cleansing and digestive qualities are stronger and the soup will In addition develop its instinctive heat quicker and will soften the outer layers of the stomach.

The Prophet's statement that the Milk like soup takes away some of the sadness refers to the effect of sadness on the mood and in weakening the instinctive well being, which in turn affects the soul and the heart.

Milk like soup brings strength to one's inner energy and thus the body will be able to rid itself of the sadness and grief that took it over.

We could In addition say that some foods bring relief to the heart, such as the type of soup mentioned above, because they posses a special quality that effect people's mood and brings them relief and comfort. Allah knows best.

We might In addition say that the sick person's strength becomes weaker because of his grief and sadness that will translate to dryness in the body and the stomach due to the scarcity of food. The milk like soup brings wetness and strength to the stomach, which will In addition bring relief to the heart. In addition, the sick person may complain from an accumulation of harmful flatulence or phlegm in his stomach. The milk like soup will dissolve these harmful substances or dilute them, so that the pain and harm they cause are diminished, especially for those accustomed to eating barley bread, such as the people of Al-Medina. During that time, barley bread was the staple diet for the people of Al-Medina as wheat was scarce at that time.

The Prophet's guidance on treating poisoning

Abdul Razzaq narrated that, "A Jewish woman brought to the Prophet b a roasted sheep that she had poisoned, while he was in Khaybar. The Prophet an asked, 'What is this,' She said, A gift,' being careful not to say that it was from charity so that he would not eat it. The Prophet ^ ar J his Companions ate from the sheep, then the Prophet ^ said, 'Stop eating.' He said to the woman, 'Did you poison this sheep?' She said, 'Who told you that?' He said, 'This bone,' meaning the ewe's leg that he had in his hand. She said, 'Yes.' He said, 'Why?' She said, 'I thought that if you were a liar, the people would be relived from you. However, if you were a true Prophet ate, it would not harm you.' The Prophet **b** then used cupping thrice on the upper part of his back and commanded that his Companions do the same. Yet, several of them died.'"

In another narration narrated by Musa bin 'Uqbah, "The Messenger of Allah **b** used cupping on his back because of what he ate of the poisoned sheep. Abu Hind, a servant for Bani Bayadhah, used a knife to cup him. Three years later, when the Prophet **b** was suffering from the illness that he died from, he said:

"I still feel the effects of the poisoned sheep I ate from during the Day of Khaybar, until now, when it is the time the aorta is cut off (meaning when death is near)".

Therefore the Messenger of Allah **b** died as a martyr.

Poisons are treated by extracting the poison and by using the proper antidotes to neutralize their effect. Whoever does not have access to the medicine, or the antidote, should use complete disgorging, the best method of which is cupping especially in warm areas and during hot weather. The poison passes through the veins and the blood vessels to the heart and then to the rest of the body, bringing certain death. Since the blood is the means that transports the poison to the heart and -the organs, when the infected blood is extracted by cupping, the body will get rid of the poison. In addition, when one resorts to complete disgorging, the poison does not cause any further harm, the body gets enough strength to fight it and then weakens or even completely dissipates the poison.

When the Prophet ;a& used cupping, he did it in the upper part of the back, which is the most direct route to the heart, and so the poison was extracted with the blood, in this case only partially. A part of the poison remained in the Prophet's system, in order to fulfill what Allah had decided for His Prophet so he would acquire every type of good and righteous reward there is.

When Allah decided that it was time for His Prophet $& to die as a martyr, the effect of the poison reappeared, so that Allah's decision was fulfilled. Therefore the meaning of the following Ayah, becomes apparent where Allah says,

﴿ وَلَقَدْ ءَاتَيْنَا مُوسَى ٱلْكِتَـٰبَ وَقَفَّيْنَا مِنۢ بَعْدِهِۦ بِٱلرُّسُلِ ۖ وَءَاتَيْنَا عِيسَى ٱبْنَ مَرْيَمَ ٱلْبَيِّنَـٰتِ وَأَيَّدْنَـٰهُ بِرُوحِ ٱلْقُدُسِ ۗ أَفَكُلَّمَا جَآءَكُمْ رَسُولٌۢ بِمَا لَا تَهْوَىٰٓ أَنفُسُكُمُ ٱسْتَكْبَرْتُمْ فَفَرِيقًا كَذَّبْتُمْ وَفَرِيقًا تَقْتُلُونَ ﴿٨٧﴾ ﴾ (٨٧) البقرة .

"It is that whenever there came to you a Messenger with what you yourselves desired not, you grew arrogant? Some you disbelieved and some you killed." (2:87)

This Ayah uses the word disbelieve in the past tense and the word kill in the future tense, indicating an uncompleted action that would continue to occur [meaning the Jews would kill the Prophet]. Allah knows best.

The Prophet's guidance on treating sorcery

Some people have erroneously denied that sorcery could effect the Prophet, they believed that it was not befitting his grade and status. Actually, being effected by sorcery illustrates the human side of the Prophet, just like he suffered from various other illnesses, and sorcery is an ailment just like poison.

In the Sahihain it is narrated that 'A'esha said:

"The Messenger of Allah was effected by sorcery until he thought that he had slept with his wives, while in fact he did not."

This is the worst type of magic spell.

Qadi 'lyadh said, "Sorcery is just like any other ailment that the Prophet ate suffered from, and this fact by no means affects his status as a Prophet ate. Further, the fact that the Prophet ate imagined something which he did not do, does not detract from his truthfulness regarding religion, there is a consensus that he is immune from error in this regard. Sorcery is just like any other matter of this life, which has nothing to do with the reason why he was sent and preferred above mankind. The Prophet was subject to come down with all types of ailments that would touch other people. Therefore, it is not surprising that he would imagine doing something which in fact he did not do, and that he was soon cured."

The Prophet **b**. used two methods to treat sorcery, first by finding the spell and neutralizing it. The Prophet **b** supplicated to his Lord and Allah showed him that the evil spell was hidden in a well. The Prophet **b** removed the evil spell, which consisted of a comb, combed material (hair) and a dry male spathe. When he discarded these objects, he was immediately cured, as if he was restrained and then suddenly released. This is the best cure from sorcery and is similar to removing septic materials by complete disgorging.

The second type, extracting harmful substances from the organ most touched by magic works. Evil spells aggravate nature, produce harmful substances and adversely affect the mood. Disgorging the alien substance that affected a certain organ as a result of evil spells becomes necessary.

. The effect of the sorcery reached the Prophet's head and affected one of his senses, he imagined he did something while in fact he had not. The sorcerer, therefore, affects some of the natural powers of the body so that it does not function normally.

Sorcery is a combination of the powers of evil spirits and the adverse effects they have on the normal functions of the body. The worst type of magic is that which affects the senses of the affected organ. Drawing blood from the organ most affected by magic is the most beneficial cure, if used in the proper manner. Hippocrates said that, "Cupping (or disgorging) should be used on the part most affected using the most favorable means available."

Some people a so said that when the Messenger of Allah b suffered from this condition, he first thought that it was caused by spoiled blood that reached the brain and affected the senses. In such cases, cupping is the best medicine, and this is what the Prophet **b** did. Then, when Allah revealed to him that it was the effect of magic that caused his condition, he asked Allah to show him where the evil spell was hidden and then he retrieved and discarded it. When he did so, he was cured as if released after being restrained. Further, the magic spell only affected the Prophet's senses not his sanity or heart. This is why he did not believe what he imagined of sleeping with his wives because he knew that this sensation was not real.

Divine cures are the best remedies against sorcery. Since sorcery is the work of evil spirits, then its best cure is that which neutralizes it, such as certain prayers and recitations of the Qura'an. The more powerful the defending army, the more powerful the adversary it will be able to remove and neutralize. This case is similar to two opposing armies, each of which carries its weapons and armaments. The army that has more weaponry and supplies, is the army that will prevail in the war. When the heart is full of Allah's remembrance and invokes Him often for its needs, and when the heart is joined by the tongue and righteous deeds, these acts will be the best medicine there is against sorcery and magic spells. The sorcerers and magicians admit that their magic is most effective against those who have weak hearts that are busy satisfying the desires and lusts of the life of this world. That is why magic usually affects women, children, nomads, ignorant people, those who have weak Faith, lack trust in Allah (Tawakkul) and lack the fundamentals of Unity (Tawheed), and those who neither remember Allah often nor use the various Prophetic supplications and Islamic prayer formulas (Ruqyah). In general, the effect of sorcery and magic is more powerful against weak hearts that lean towards the lower desires of this world.

When the heart leans towards this earthly life, sorcery and magic becomes most effective against it, because evil spirits only search for evil in the soul that is prone to submit to their power. Surely, evil in the heart deprives one of divine power that is necessary to provide it with sufficient weapons of defense against these evil spirits. That is why these evil spirits, which seek evil, find the hearts weakened by evil unarmed and prone to submit to evil and this is when sorcery and magic spells are most effective. Allah knows best,

The Prophet's guidance on vomiting as a remedy

At-Termezey reported that a person narrated that Abu Ad-Dardaa said, "The Prophet sss, once performed ablution after he vomited. I met Thawban in the mosque of Damascus and mentioned what Abu Ad-Dardaa narrated to him and he said, 'True'. I poured water for him (the Prophet ^ then." At-Termezey then commented that this Hadith is the most authentic on this subject. [In addition, Ahmad, AI-Hakim, Ibn Al-jarud, Ad-Daraqutni, AI-Bayhaqi and At-Tahawi}.

Vomiting is one of the five methods used to disgorge septic substances from the body. They are diarrhea, vomiting, cupping, the passing of air or wind and sweating. The Sunnah has mentioned these five types. As for diarrhea, we mentioned the Hadith that states, "Diarrhea is the best of your remedies." We In addition mentioned the Hadith about Senna.

We mentioned cupping when we narrated the Ahadeeth about this subject,As for getting rid of septic gasses and steams, we will elaborate on this subject later on in this book.

As for getting rid of septic substances by sweating, it does not usually involve puncturing of the veins. The body naturally rids itself of these substances through the skin when sweat leaves the body through the open pores.

Vomiting involves throwing up the harmful substances through the upper part of the stomach. An enema and medicines that instigate disgorging artificially through the lower parts of the stomach are of two types, one that occurs naturally and one artificially instigated.

The naturally instigated vomit should not be prevented, except when it becomes excessive and becomes unsafe. In this case one should take the medicines that stops vomiting. The second type of vomiting is used for medicinal purposes, in the proper time and under proper conditions.

There are ten reasons for vomiting, the first, excessive amounts of bile that float in the stomach and seek an exit out of the body.

Second, excessive amounts of phlegm in the stomach that In addition seek a way out of the body.

Third, when the stomach is weak and unable to completely digest the food and the partially digested food seeks an exit out of the body.

Fourth, vomiting occurs when a harmful substance enters the stomach and causes a disruption in the digestion process.

Fifth, when one eats excessive amounts of food or drink, more than the stomach can bear. In this case, the stomach will not be able to tolerate these excessive amounts of nourishment and will seek to throw them out.

Sixth, vomiting occurs when the food or drink consumed is not suitable for the stomach, which then throws them out.

Seventh, when the stomach suffers from a condition that spoils the food and drink which then seeks an exit.

Eighth, nausea might In addition cause vomiting.

Ninth, depression, sadness and anguish cause disregard for the needs of the body and its necessities of food, including the need to mature and digest the food. The stomach gets rid of this undigested food. In addition, vomiting may occur under the pressure of various physiological conditions, because the body and the psyche both effect each other profoundly, Tenth, one might feel nauseous and then vomit upon seeing other people vomit.

Once, a doctor informed me that he had a nephew who was good at applying Ku'hl (antimony, a black powder used for the eyes) and when his nephew would apply Ku'hl to a person who was suffering form conjunctivitis, he himself would later catch conjunctivitis. When this was repeated several times, his nephew stopped this profession. I asked the doctor about the cause of his nephew's condition and he said that his nephew's body reacted to the condition of the men he was treating by catching the same ailment they suffered from. h-le In addition said that he knows of a man who saw a benign growth, an-abscess, on someone's body and that he started to scratch the same part on his body. Later on, he In addition had a growth in the same area.

I say that this proves that the psyche affects the body in such a way that when certain powers in the body are idle, it suddenly becomes active without a reason.

Vomiting is suitable as a remedy in hot weather and hot climates

In hot areas and hot weather, certain harmful substances are light and thus prone to float, and this is why vomiting becomes a proficient way to discard these mixtures. On the other hand, certain harmful substances in cold areas and in cold weather become thicker and are harder to extract from above. In this case, getting rid of these harmful mixtures is better done by diarrhea.

Getting rid of harmful mixtures is done by pulling them from the farthest exit or by extracting them from the nearest exit. For instance, there are various mixtures that are not stable and seek to either ascend or descend. If the mixture tends to ascend, then discarding it from below is better. If the mixture tends to descend, then pulling it from above is better. When the mixture becomes stable, then discarding it from the nearest exit is better. When the mixture starts to harm the upper organs, it should be pulled down through the lower parts, and vise versa. When these r-mixtures become stable, they should be discarded from the nearest exit.

This is why the Prophet ate had cupping sometimes in his arm vein, sometimes in his head and sometimes on the top of his foot, so that the spoiled blood is discarded from the nearest possible exit.

Vomiting cleanses the stomach from harmful substances

Vomiting strengthens the stomach, sharpens the sight, relieves headaches, ulcers, and infections in the kidneys and the prostate. Vomiting In addition relieves and soothes chronic illnesses, such as leprosy, dropsy, partial paralysis, or trembling.

A healthy person should instigate vomiting once or twice a month each time vomiting two times, so that the second vomit rids the body of the substances that remained after the first one. Excessive vomiting harms the stomach and weakens its protective layers. It a so harms the teeth, the sight and hearing along with causing headaches. In addition, those suffering from swelling in the throat, weak chests, those who have small windpipes, or those who find it difficult to vomit intentionally or those prone to spitting up blood should not vomit intentionally.

Those who have the bad habit of filling their

stomachs with food and then instigate vomit will find that this method accelerates old age and leads to many harmful diseases, along with making vomiting habitual.

In addition, instigating vomiting while suffering from dehydration, weak or defective intestines, senility, or general weakness in the body is dangerous for the health. The best time to instigate vomit is during summer and spring, not winter or autumn. When vomıtıng intentionally, one should cover his eyes, wash the face with cold water when finished and should then drink apple juice with some mastic and rosewater if possible. Vomit should be expelled through the mouth or pulled from below in the form of diarrhea. Hippocrates said, "Vomit during the summer should be (naturally) expelled from above more than by using Medicine, while in winter it should be pulled from below using medications."

The Prophet's guidance on seeking the best doctors

Imam Malik narrated in his Muwatta that Zaid bin Aslam said:

"During the time of the Prophet **b** a man was injured and the blood was congested in the wound. The man then called two doctors from Bani Amir to examine him. The man then claimed that the Messenger of Allah **b**asked them, 'Who is the best doctor among you?' They asked, 'Is there prefer ability in the medicine, O

Messenger of Allah **b** He said, 'The One Who has sent down the disease also sent down the cure.'"

This Hadith indicates that Muslims should seek the best authority in each and every matter and field, because such expertise will ensure that the job is done with excellence. For instance, those inquiring about a matter of religion should seek the most knowledgeable scholar to answer their questions. Further, those who are unsure about the direction of the prayer should imitate the most knowledgeable person available. This is the way Allah has created His slaves. For instance, those traveling on land or sea should seek the best guides because their hearts will feel safer following their lead and in their presence. The religion, the mind and the way Allah created mankind all emphasize this fact mentioned in the Hadith.

The Prophet's statement:

"He Who has sent down the disease also sent down the cure."

Like this has been mentioned in several other Ahadeeth. For example, Hilal bin Yasaf said:

"The Messenger of Allah **b** once visited a sick man and said, 'Send for a doctor.' A man said, 'Do you say that, O Messenger of Allah **b**' He said, 'Yes. Allah has not sent down a disease but In addition sent down a cure for it." (Ahmad)

In the Sahihain it is In addition narrated that the Prophet b said:

"Allah has not sent down a disease except that He sent down its cure."

There is a conflict of opinion on the meaning of sending down the disease and the cure. Some people say that sending the cure down means the slaves become aware of it. This opinion is not valid, although Allah has informed us about the fact that for every disease there is a cure still the Prophet b said:

"Those who know it ore aware of it, and those who do not know it are ignorant of it."

Some people say that the Prophet's statement indicates that Allah has created these cures on the earth, like another Hadith, "Allah does not create a disease but would create its cure." Although this opinion is better than the first one, it is still not valid because "sending down" is more precise and specific than creating.

Another group says that the statement means that Allah sends down the cure with the angels who are responsible for the affairs of mankind including the diseases and their cures. Indeed, the angels are responsible for the daily affairs of this world, especially the affairs of mankind from the time he or she is a fetus until they die. This opinion that the angels are sent down with the cure is more plausible.

Other people say that the majority of the medicine comes down with the rain, as the rain causes the growth of the vegetation and food, meaning the various sources for cure. In addition, rain washes down various minerals from the mountaintops which are used in remedies. In addition, various types of fruits, plants and even spring water are used in cures and remedies. This opinion is better than the previous three opinions, but Allah knows best.

This is the perfect wisdom of Allah, that He tests His slaves with the disease and yet helps them find the cure. He In addition tests His slaves with sins, but helps them erase these sins by repenting to Him, by performing good deeds and by their enduring different calamities and disasters. Allah In addition tests His slaves with evil, yet helps His slaves with angels. Allah In addition tests His slaves with desires, but has allowed them to satisfy their desires by taking from the good, pure substances that are In addition desirable. Allah has not tested His saves with anything but would In addition provide them with what helps them sustain themselves against that trial and test.

The difference between the slaves of Allah in this state is in their knowing and acquiring such aids. Allah is sought for help regarding each and every matter.

The Prophet's guidance on requiring compensation from those unqualified to practice medicine

Abu Dawood, An-Nasay and Ibn Majah said that the Messenger of Allah **b** said:

"Those who practice Tibb, but are not knowledgeable in this profession are responsible for their actions." [In addition Al-Hobm narrated this Hadith],

There are three types of benefits in this Hadith: linguistic, religious and medicinal.

Linguistically, Tibb entails preparing a thing. It In addition entails excellence and thus entails other than the profession of doctors. A person might be called Tabib (Usually means doctor) when they are proficient in anything. In addition, a proficiency might be called Tibb sometimes even magic.

In the Sahih it is narrated that 'A'esha said, "When the Jews worked magic on the Messenger of Allah **b**, two angels sat next to him one at his head and the other at his feet, one of them asked, 'What is the matter with the man?' The other angel said, 'He is Matbub (touched by magic).' The first angel asked, 'Who did Tibb (sorcery) on him?' The second angel said, 'Such and such Jewish fellow.'

Abu 'Ubaid said that those touched by magic are called Matbub, touched by magic. In addition, the medicine is called Tibb.

The word Tabib describes a knowledgeable person including doctors.

The religious benefit from this Hadith requires the ignorant doctor to pay for his mistakes, because he has practiced a profession although he was unqualified in it and then caused harm to the people, whom he in fact has cheated and deceived. Therefore, unqualified doctors are held responsible for any health risks they cause, according to the consensus of the scholars.

Al-Khattabi said, "There is no difference concerning the ruling that when one treats a sick person and causes him harm that he is financially responsible for his acts. Those who indulge in a profession that they are not proficient in are aggressors. Therefore, when their actions lead to harm, the aggressors ought to pay for their action, financially not physically since the sick person actually allows such ignorant people to treat him.

There are five types of doctors: a proficient doctor

who gives the profession its due right and who acts responsibly. When such a person treats a sick person, an act that is allowed both by the religion and the sick person, and then commits a mistake he is not liable for this mistake. For instance, when a doctor who is proficient in his job performs circumcision for a boy under favorable circumstances, but the organ suffers some type of damage, the doctor will not be liable for this mistake. In addition, if a swelling was cupped by a proficient person in the proper time and manner, but a certain damage occurred, the doctor is not liable for that mistake.

The second type is an ignorant doctor who treats a sick person and causes him harm. If the sick person had knowledge beforehand that this doctor was ignorant and yet allowed him to treat him, then there is no compensation required in this case. This ruling does not contradict the Hadith we mentioned in the beginning of the chapter. The wording of the Hadith indicates that those who have to pay for their mistakes have cheated the sick person and caused the illusion that they were proficient doctors.

If the sick person thinks that a certain person is a proficient doctor and thus allows him to treat him, the ignorant doctor is required to compensate the sick person for whatever damage he might cause. In addition, when such a so-called doctor prescribes a medicine for the sick person who takes the medicine thinking that the doctor prescribed the medicine to him with knowledge, and if the medicine causes any harm, compensation would be required in this case. The Hadith is clear in its indication regarding this type.

The third type is a proficient doctor who was given permission to treat a person but made a mistake and caused harm to a healthy organ (meaning not the organ he was treating), then in this case compensation is required because it is an aggression by mistake. Does this person pay the compensation from his own money or from the Muslim Treasury? There are two opinions on this subject. If the doctor is not Muslim, compensation is paid from his own money and if the doctor is Muslim there is a difference of opinion as we mentioned earlier. The fourth type is the proficient doctor who prescribes the wrong medicine for the sick person who dies as a consequence. There are two opinions on this subject, one of them requires the compensation from the Muslim Treasury while the other requires it from the doctor's resources. Both of these opinions were attributed to Imam Ahmad.

The fifth type is a proficient doctor who amputated an organ form an insane person or a child without permission, or who circumcised a boy without his parent's permission and the organ was harmed. Some scholars say that the doctor is required to pay compensation in this case because he was not given permission to operate. However, if the guardian or the parent allows the doctor to operate then the doctor is not required to pay for his mistake.

It is possible that the doctor who operates without permission may not have to pay compensation because he intended to do good and is therefore not liable for the damage he causes. The Hadith in the beginning of this chapter entails such medicinal professions as remedy prescription, applying Ku'hl, physicians, performing circumcision, cupping and incisions, splintering broken bones, cauterization and administering injections, veterinarians, and so forth. It is a recent practice to restrict the word doctor to mean a specific part of the profession.

The proficient doctor takes the following steps when treating any type of disease.

1. First diagnose the type of disease.

2. Search for the cause behind the disease.

3. Examine the sick person to decide if his body is able to fend off the disease or if it is weaker than the disease. If the patient is strong enough to resist the disease, the doctor should not prescribe medicine.

4. Examine the patient and his mood and condition.

5. Examine the changes in the state of the patient.

6. Examine the sick person's age,

7. Examine his habits and what he is accustomed to,

8. Remember seasonal effects.

9. Consider the sick person's place of origin.

10. Consider the atmospheric conditions at the time he caught the disease.

11. Search for the correct and suitable medicine.

12. Examine the effectiveness of the medicine and the correct dosage.

13. The doctor not only intends to cure the ailment, but In addition to prevent what is even more serious. For instance, if curing a certain disease leads the way to an even more serious disease, the doctor allows the current illness to remain and tries to make it milder. For instance, the orifice of the veins, which is treated by incision or cutting, might aggravate other acute ailments.

14. Choosing and prescribing the simplest medicine

for treatment is warranted. For instance, the doctor does not prescribe medicine unless he investigates his options of food and diet. In addition, the doctor should not prescribe multiple or complex medications until he investigates his options regarding simpler medications. It is a sign that the doctor is truly professional that he prescribes food when he can substitute it for medicine, and simple rather than complex medications.

15. The doctor examines if the illness is treatable or not. If the doctor finds out that he is unable to treat the disease, let him preserve his energy and reputation and avoid falling prey to his own greed so that he pretends to cure the incurable.

If the illness is curable, the doctor examines if it can be totally cured, or at least made milder. If the doctor discovers that he cannot cure the diseases or decrease its intensity, he should examine the ways to stop it from being aggravated. In this case, the medication should be administered for that purpose, to increase the body strength and stop the disease from increasing.

16. The doctor should not revert to excreting the septic substances before they become stable and mature.

17. The doctor should In addition be knowledgeable of the sicknesses of the heart and soul and the methods of treating such ailments. This, indeed, is a major aspect of medicinal science, for the effect of the heart's moods and feelings is apparent in the physical body. This is why we state that if a medical doctor is In addition proficient in the ills of the hearts, he will be the prefect doctor. On the other hand, the doctor who does not have knowledge of the ills of the heart while knowledgeable in the ills of the body, he will be only half of a doctor. He is not a doctor who does not examine the righteousness of the sick person's heart and encourages him to strengthen his soul and body by performing righteous, good deeds, such as charity and being interested in drawing closer to Allah and acquiring the good of the Hereafter. Rather, he is a fake doctor. In fact, the best cures are in performing righteous good deeds, charity, remembering Allah, supplicating to Him, seeking His help, invoking Him and repenting to Him, Such good deeds have a truly profound effect in curing illnesses, more so than the usual medications, providing that the ailing person has faith in such divine remedies.

18. Being lenient and forbearing with the sick

person, just as one is easy going and lenient with a child.

19. The doctor should use the various types of medicinal and spiritual cures, along with using his imagination.

20. The doctor should make his treatment revolve around the six major principles, which are the cornerstone of his profession. First, the doctor should preserve the health. Second he should try and bring back the lost health. Third, the doctor should cure the disease. Fourth, at least lessen the intensity of the disease. Fifth, the doctor should ignore the lesser evil and treat the bigger evil. Sixth, the doctor should ignore the lesser good to acquire the greater good. The science of medicine revolves around these six basics, and the doctor who does not rely on them is not a doctor. Allah knows best.

The sick person passes through four stages:

1. The beginning.

2. The intense stage.

3. fading.

4. the end of the illness.

Since the sick person passes through four stages the doctor has to examine each of these stages carefully and treat them in the proper manner. For instance, if the doctor feels the body needs to remove and excrete harmful substances, if they are mature, he should do so. If this is not possible in the beginning of the ailment, especially if the disease has already progressed, or because the body is weak, the weather is cold, or by mistake, the doctor should not resort to excretion in these cases. If the doctor ignores this warning, the body will be busy dealing with the medication and will not concentrate on resisting the disease. This is similar to requiring a soldier who is busy defending his post to do something else. Rather, the doctor's concern should be concentrated on preserving the strength of the body as much as possible at this stage.

When the disease has stopped progressing, the doctor should then use excretion and treating the causes of the disease. It is even better when the disease has started to subside and end. This case is similar to an enemy whose strength has started to depart and his ammunition nears its end, so capturing him in this case becomes easier. When the enemy starts to give flight, it is even easier to capture him. It is a fact that the strength of the enemy will be at a maximum in the beginning of his aggression. This is the exact case with medicine as regards the ailing body.

The skilled doctor uses the easiest treatment and cure first, then the more difficult or powerful medications. Therefore, the doctor moves from the less powerful to the more powerful, unless he fears that the strength of the body will be drained if he does not use the most powerful medicine first. In addition, the skilled doctor does not keep using the same medications in a way that will allow the body to get used to the medicine and thus it looses its effectiveness. We In addition mentioned that the doctor should first consider prescribing a diet before using medications. If the doctor is unsure about the nature of the disease, he should not prescribe medication before being sure of the correctness of his diagnosis. There is no harm if the doctor administers a medication that does not cause side effects or negative repercussions.

When several diseases attack the body, the doctor starts with the medicine that satisfies three condition: treating the disease that might lead to curing the other diseases, such as when confronted with a swelling and an ulcer, he starts with the swelling.

The second condition, the doctor starts with the disease that has caused the other. For example, if the doctor is confronted with an embolism (the obstruction of an artery by an embolus, usually a piece of clotted blood which breaks away from one part of the circulatory system and travels to another) and septic-related fever, he starts with the cause of the first disease.

Third, when one of the two diseases is more serious than the other disease, then the doctor should start with the acute ailment. Yet, the doctor should In addi..ion examine the progress of the other disease.

In addition, when a disease and a symptomatic ailment both attack the body, the doctor starts with the disease, unless the symptomatic condition is stronger, such as in the case of painful constipation. The doctor first treats the pai..ı then treats the embolism. If the doctor can substitute excretion or extraction (of the septic substances) with hunger, fasting, sleep, then he should do so.

The Prophet's guidance on preventing contagious diseases and enforcing quarantine

Muslim narrated that Jabir bin Abdullah said:

"Thaqifs delegation included a man with leprosy. The Prophet **b** sent to him, 'Go back, for we have accepted your pledge of allegiance." [Ibn Majah, Ahmad, Ibn Khuzaymah and ibn jarir}.

Al-Bokhary narrated that the Prophet if said:

"Do not keep looking at the person afflicted by leprosy." [Ahmad. At-Tayalisi, At-Tabarani and Al-

Kayhaqi].

Further, in the Sahihain it is narrated that the Prophet s& said:

"A healthy man should not be brought near a sick person." [Abu Dawood, Ahmad, Ibn Majah, Ahmad and Al-Bayhaqy]

Leprosy is an especially harmful disease that occurs due to the accumulation of black bile in the entire body, altering the condition or temperament and shape of the organs. In the final stages, leprosy might cause such bad corrosion that the affected limbs would start to fall off and disintegrate. Leprosy is In addition called the diseases of the lion, for three reasons. First, this disease usually attacks lions (or wild beasts). Second, because this disease causes the face to frown, like the lion's face. The third, leprosy is contagious and will devour its victim just as the lion devours its prey.

Leprosy is a contagious disease, and those who come near the person afflicted with leprosy will be bothered by the foul odor, just like those suffering from tuberculosis.

The Prophet, who was full of mercy and pity for his nation, commanded them not to expose themselves to what might bring harm to their bodies and hearts. There is no doubt that certain bodies are disease prone and are easily affected by the surrounding environment, and as we have stated, leprosy is a contagious disease. Sometimes, someone's fear of the disease might actually help the disease attack the body, because fear prepares the organs of the body for the possibility of catching the disease. Sometimes, when one even smells the foul odor emitted by persons inflicted by certain diseases, they in turn catch the same disease, if their body is susceptible to catch the disease. Some people stated that the Ahadeeth we mentioned in this chapter are overruled by some other Ahadeeth. They brought as evidence what the Prophet m, said: "There is no contagion nor evil omen." [Al-Bokhary, Moslem and Abu Dawood].

We should state that there is no contradiction between the authentic Ahadeeth. When there is an appearance of contradiction, one of the Ahadeeth might not be an authentic Hadith, sometimes, the narrators of Ahadeeth might have made mistakes, although they are truthful themselves. Or, one of the seemingly contradicted Ahadeeth might be overruling the other. Further, there are no two authentic Ahadeeth that are direct in meaning which contradict each other in every respect. Allah forbids that his truthful Messenger should ever contradict himself, and therefore, everything the Prophet **b** uttered is the ultimate truth, no doubt. Problems and errors sometime arise from the narrators of the Hadith, the shortcoming in comprehending the true meaning of some Ahadeeth or the inability to distinguish between authentic and forged Ahadeeth.

Ibn Qutaibah said in his book, Al-Hadith, while talking about the enemies of Hadith, They say, "These are Ahadeeth that contradict each other. You narrated that the Prophet said, There is neither contagiousness nor evil omen.' And that the Prophet **b** was told, 'Wet mange attacks the camel's lip and then the camels catch leprosy,' and that he said, 'What has transferred the ailment to the first camel?' You In addition narrated, 'No healthy person should be brought near a sick person, and avoid the one with leprosy just as you avoid the lion.' You In addition reported that a man with leprosy came to give his allegiance to the Prophet as on Islam and that he said to him that his pledge is accepted, ordering him to return without meeting him. He In addition said, "Evil omen is in three things: the woman, the animal and the house,' and all these statements contradict each other."

Abu Muhammad (Ibn Qutaibah) then commented, "We say that there is no contradiction, because each statement has its own meaning and timeframe. When the Hadith is used in its proper context, the appearance of contradiction will not be substantiated. There are two types of contagion, one of them is leprosy like contagion. For instance, when the odor of the person afflicted with leprosy is felt by those who talk and sit near to the leper for a long time, they might fall victim to the same disease. Such is the case with the wife of the person with leprosy who remains under the same roof with him and thus catches the disease. In addition, the children of the person afflicted with leprosy might catch the disease later on in their life (hereditary). Such is the case with those suffering from tuberculosis, hectic fever and mange. The doctors order that those suffering from tuberculosis and leprosy should be avoided, not because they fear that such cases are contagious but because the bad odor that emits from such people might affect the healthy persons when exposed to it for a long time. The doctors are the farthest people from believing in evil or good omens. The same argument is true in the case with the Nuqbah, which is a wet type of leprosy or mange that attacks camels. When the infected camel mixes or mingles with other healthy camels, the infection will be transferred through the water [open sores] or the mucus that the camel produces. This is the meaning that the Prophet **b** intended when he said:

'No sick person should be brought near a healthy person.'

He disliked that the sick people associated with healthy people, so that the healthy are not exposed to any substances or rashes that the body of the sick person produces. The second type of contagion, is the plague, for instance, that appears in a land and the person thus seeks to flee that land for fear of catching the disease. The Prophet s& said, 'If it (the Plague) appears in a land where you are residing, do not depart that land. If it appears in a land, do not enter it,' The Prophet gs ordered the people not to depart the land afflicted by the plague, as they might be thinking that by fleeing they would be avoiding Allah's appointed destiny. In addition, the Prophet ^ ordered the people not to enter a land afflicted by the plague, for remaining in the healthy land brings calmness to their hearts and tranquility in their livelihood. In addition, this type includes the husband who suffers an affliction and attributes it to the bad omen of his wife or the house as is common. This is the type that the Prophet **b** meant when he said, "There is neither contagion...' "

Some other people said the Prophet safe only recommended that leprosy patients be avoided and that it is still allowed to eat with them, as the Prophet himself did.

Some other people said that these Ahadeeth contain specific commands for different types of people. For instance, some people have such a strong faith and reliance on Allah that the strength of their faith would save them from contagious diseases, just as the natural powers that exist in the body sometimes fend off the harm of the disease. Some people, on the other hand, do not have a strong faith, so the Prophet ^ commanded them to be cautious, The Prophet **b** implemented his own commands in both cases, so that the strong imitate his acts, depending on their trust in Allah. On the other hand, the weak would imitate the Prophet **b** (when he avoided leprous patients, for instance) to be cautions. Both ways are correct, but one is suitable for those who have strong faith while the other is suitable for those who have weak faith. Consequently, both groups of the believers will have their own method that is suitable for their own situation. As another example, the Prophet s has used fire for medicinal purposes, cauterization. Yet, he praised whoever refrains from using cauterization and mentioned avoiding it with the good deeds of shunning the bad omen and having total dependence on Allah. There are many other examples on this subject. The Prophet's method is always very gentle, and those who comprehend it in the correct manner will get rid of many suspicions that the authentic Sunnah contradicts itself.

Some other people stated that ordering the people to run away from the one with leprosy prevents the transfer of the disease by mingling with the sick or by smelling their odor when such mingling and associations are extensive. As for short visitations with such people for a good purpose, there is no harm in it and catching the disease will not be plausible during these brief contacts. The Prophet **b** prohibited long exposures to sick people to preserve health and allowed brief contacts that would not cause harm. Therefore, where is the contradiction here?

Another group of people said it is plausible that the person who suffered from leprosy with whom the Prophet as sat and ate was suffering from mild leprosy. There are several types of leprosy that vary in their seriousness and the degree of their contagion. In such cases, it is possible to mingle with some people suffering from mild leprosy that has not progressed and avoid catching the disease. When the illness is unable to progress in the sick person's body, it will be even less able to attack another person's body.

Another group of people said that the people before Islam believed that diseases themselves are contagious, without referring this matter to the power and will of Allah in the beginning and the end. The Prophet refuted their belief and ate with a person with leprosy to prove that Allah is the One Who causes the disease to come and Who brings about the cure. The Prophet In addition prohibited the Muslims from mingling with the sick to teach them that sickness and diseases are made by Allah to have a certain effect on people. The prohibition affirms these effects while his action teaches us that such effects are totally controlled by Allah, and that if He wills, these effects will not have any power. In addition, if He wills, these effects will cause the harm that He has decided and willed,

Finally, some other people say that these Ahadeeth might be overruled by other Ahadeeth, and that in case we are unable to produce the latter Hadith that overrules the previous Hadith, we should refrain from discussing this matter further.*

The Prophet's guidance on prohibiting using what Allah has forbidden for medicinal purposes

Abu Dawood narrated that Abu Ad-Dardaa said that the Messenger of Allah **b** said:

"Allah has sent down the disease and the cure and has created a cure for every disease. Seek the cure, but do not use what has been prohibited for medicinal purposes." [At-Tabarani].

Al-Bokhary In addition narrated that Ibn Mas'ud said:

"Verily Allah has not made your cure in that which has been forbidden for you".

In addition in the Sunan [Abu Dawood and At-Termezey] it is narrated that Abu Hurayrah said:

"The Messenger of Allah **b** has disallowed using impure (prohibited) substances for medicinal purposes."

In addition, Imam Muslim narrated that Tariq Ibn Suwayd Al-Ju'fi said that he asked the Prophet s& about alcohol and that he has disallowed it or hated that he makes it. He said, "I only make it for medicinal purposes." The Prophet b said:

"It is not a cure. Rather, it is a disease."

In addition in the Sunan it is narrated that the Prophet b was asked about Al-Khamr [alcohol] for medicinal purposes. The Prophet ^ said:

"Verily that is not a cure, rather it is a disease.." [Abu Dawood and At-Termezey].

In addition, Muslim narrated that Tariq bin Suwayd Al-Hadhrami said, "I said, 'O Messenger of Allah !. There are some vines in our land that we squeeze (for alcohol) and that we drink from.' He said, 'Do not do it.' So I went back to him and said, 'We use it for medicinal purposes.' He said:

"It is not a cure. Rather, it is a disease.'" [Abu Dawood and At- Termezey].

An-Nasa'y narrated that a doctor mentioned using frogs to make medicine and the Prophet b prohibited killing the frog for that purpose. [Abu Dawood, Ahmad]

Using what Allah has prohibited in medicines is

an evil act according to the religion and the mind. As for the religion, we mentioned several Ahadeeth on this subject.

As for the mind, Allah has prohibited whatever substances He has prohibited because they are impure. Further, Allah has never disallowed a good, beneficial matter for the Muslims, as He has decided in the case of the Children of Israel:

"For the wrong-doing of the Jews, we made unlawful for them certain good foods which had been lawful for them, and for their hindering many from Allah's Way".

Allah has prohibited some matters and substances because of the harm that they carry and to save His slaves from such harm. It is not suitable that the slaves seek these harmful substances for medicinal purposes. Even if such substances appear to have an affect on the disease, they bring about a more serious illness in the heart because they are impure and unclean. In this case, the sick person who uses what Allah has disallowed for medicinal purposes might be able to remove the physical illness but would cause himself a more serious disease in the heart.

Further, the Muslims are required to avoid what Allah has disallowed, while using them in medicine means that one will not avoid them, as the religion requires. This is the opposite of what the prohibitions seek to achieve.

In addition, what Allah has prohibited is a disease as the religion states by the tongue of the Messenger. Therefore, Muslims are not allowed to use it as a medicine.

Furthermore, prohibited substances affect the heart and soul and make them impure, since the various substances that the body consumes affect the body. When a substance causes an evil outcome in the body, the nature of the body will acquire this evil temperament, What about if the substance is impure and evil itself? In this case, when the substance is impure, the body becomes impure, as well. This is why Allah has prohibited the impure types of foods, drinks and clothes because of the evil effects that such substances have on the body and soul.

In addition, allowing using prohibited substances for medicinal purposes will later on encourage taking these substances to satisfy desire and the lust, especially when the heart likes such substances. This is especially the case when the heart thinks that such substances cure the illnesses of the body, thus making them even more desirable and likable. The religion, on the other hand, has closed the door to consuming or using prohibited substances. There is a contradiction if the religion closes the door to using prohibited substances on one hand and opens the door to using them in other instances on the other hand.

In addition, prohibited substances that people might use in medicine carry more types of harm than the harm that they might remove. For instance, the mother of all evil substances, alcohol, which Allah has not made a cure or a remedy, is very harmful to the brain, which controls the body, according to the doctors and many scholars of Fiqh (Islamic Jurisprudence). Hippocrates, for example, said while discussing serious illnesses, "Alcohol has a serious harmful effect on the brain, because it reaches the brain quickly along with some other harmful substances that the body contains, thus causing harm to the brain." The author of Al-Kamil In addition said, "Drinking [alcohol] brings harm to the brain and the nervous system."

There are two other types of disallowed medicines, one that the heart does not like, such as snake meat and poisons. Such substances are heavy on the heart and the stomach [let alone being dangerous] and are thus a disease not a cure. There are In addition some other medicines that are not disliked themselves, such as some drinks that pregnant women take.

These substances carry more harm than benefit, and consequently, the mind and the religion corroborate on disliking them.

There is another wisdom behind disallowing taking prohibited substances as medicine. That is that a condition that the medicine works is one's belief that it would work and bring the cure by Allah's blessing. Indeed, whatever is beneficial is In addition blessed, and the more benefit it carries, the more blessing it will bring about. In addition, what the people consider the most blessed is the substance that they think carries the most benefit. The Muslim, on the other hand, believes that what Allah has disallowed is not beneficial or blessed. Consequently, he will not have a good idea about the disallowed substance and his system will not accept it. Rather, the stronger the slave's faith is, the more he hates the disallowed substances and believes that it is impure. In this case, if the save takes such a substance it will indeed be a disease not a cure for him, unless he believes that it is pure and thus his dislike for it subsides. Therefore, the believer will not accept the disallowed substance and will consider it a disease, otherwise he will be contradicting the Faith.

The Prophet's guidance on treating and removing lice from the head

In the Sahihain it is narrated that Ka'b bin 'Ujrah said, "I was suffering from lice and I was carried to the Messenger of Allah b while lice were falling off on my face, the Prophet b, said:

"I did not realize that your trouble had reached the condition that I see (you in). The Prophet b then ordered him to have his head shaved and either fast three days or feed six poor persons or slaughter one sheep as a sacrifice." [In addition, narrated by Ahmad]

Lice appear on the head and body for two reasons, external and internal. The external cause occurs due to uncleanness and impure substances that the skin might carry. The internal reason is caused by rotted substances that the body expels through the skin and then rots due to the wetness in the skin's pores. The lice appear then (and feed on these rotted substances). Many times, lice appear after one suffers from various illnesses and diseases, because in this case cleanliness is ignored. In addition, children are the typical victims of lice because they usually play in and deal with wet things and because of their careless nature. This is why the Prophet ^ ordered that the heads of the sons of Ja'far be shaved, as shaving is one the best cures for lice because it exposes the skin to the sun and allows the harmful moistures under the skin to evaporate. Then, the head should be anointed with the cures that prevent lice from reproducing and kill them.

Shaving occurs for three reasons, as a legal ritual, as an act of innovation and polytheism, and as a cure. The first type is performed during Hajj and Umrah. The second type occurs for other than Allah,

Shaving the head is an act of humility and worship, and this is why it is a ritual that completes the Hajj acts. Imam Shafi'e even considers shaving the head a cornerstone of Hajj since it entails lowering the sides of the head in humility before the Lord and since it is In addition an honored act of worship. Furthermore, when the Arabs wanted to humiliate a captured warrior and then set him free, they would first shave his head. Later on, the teachers of false guidance and evil who seek to acquire the rights of lordship for themselves and whose ministry concentrates on polytheism and innovations came along. Such evil teachers wanted their students to perform the acts of worship for their sake. Consequently, they encouraged their students to shave their heads for their sake, just as they lured them to prostrate before them, calling this act by other than its true name and claiming that it is not prostrating, but merely lowering the head before the teacher. By Allah! What is prostrating for the sake of Allah, if it is not lowering the head before Him?

The evil teachers In addition lured their students to vow to them, repent to them and swear by their names! This is taking such teachers as gods beside Allah. Allah said:

"It is not (possible) for any human being to whom Allah has given the Book and Al-Hukm (the knowledge and understanding of the laws of religion) and Prophet hood to say to the people: "Be my worshippers rather than Allah's." On the contrary (he would say):

"Be you Rabbaniyyin (learned men of religion who practise what they know and In addition preach others), because you are teaching the

Book, and you are studying it. "Nor would he order you to take angels and Prophets for lords (gods) Would he order you to

disbelieve after you have submitted to Allah's Will?" (3:79,8O)

The prayer is the highest act of worship. Yet the teachers of false guidance, the so-called scholars and tyrants have divided the acts of prayer between themselves. For instance, the teachers of false guidance chose the highest act in the prayer, prostrating, for themselves. Some so-called scholars have In addition acquired bowing down for themselves. When they meet each other, some of them bow down before the others just as one does while praying to Allah! As for the tyrants, they acquired standing up for themselves! Free and slave men stand up before the tyrants while the tyrants are sitting down.

The Messenger of Allah **b** has prohibited these three acts for other than Allah. Therefore, committing these prohibited acts is a clear violation of the Prophet's commands.

The Prophet **b** prohibited prostrating to other than Allah. He said:

"No one should prostrate to any other person."

He In addition criticized Mu'ath when he prostrated before him. Since prohibiting prostrating before the creation is clearly indicated in the Prophet's Sunnah, then those who allow such acts seek to dispute the rights of Allah and His Messenger **b**. Prostrating is one of the essential acts of worship. When the polytheist allows it to the creation, he will be allowing worshipping other than Allah. The Prophet**b** was once asked, "When one sees his brother, should he bow down for him?" He said, 'No.' He was asked, 'Should he hug and kiss him?' He said, 'No.' He was asked, 'Should he shake his hand?' He said, 'Yes.'

In addition, bowing down while greeting someone

is a type of worship, just as Allah said:

﴿ وَٱدۡخُلُواْ ٱلۡبَابَ سُجَّدٗا ﴾ (٥٨) البقرة

"And enter the gate in prostration." (or bowing with humility) (2:58)

Besides, prostrating and entering through the door is not possible at the same time [the prostration mentioned in the Verse is bowing down]!

The Prophet b In addition prohibited standing up for someone just as the non-Muslims used to do. He even disallowed this act during the prayer and commanded the Muslim to imitate the leader in the prayer, that if he sits down while praying due to an illness, they all sit behind him although they are healthy. Otherwise, they will be standing while the Imam is sitting down, although their standing is for Allah. How about if standing was for other than Allah?

The ignorant misguided people have associated others with Allah in the worship, thus prostrating before other than Allah and bowing down for other than Allah. They In addition stand up before the creation just as they do when they are praying. They In addition swear, vow, shave their heads, sacrifice, perform Tawaf (circumambulation of an object or person), love, fear, and obey other than Allah, just as they do for Allah and even more. They equate Allah, the Lord of the Worlds, Whom they worship, with the creation. These are the enemies of the Messages of the Messengers of Allah ste, who equate Allah with the creation. They are the ones who will say in the Fire, while arguing with the false deities they were worshipping.

"By Allah, we were truly, in a manifest error, When We hold you (false gods) as equals (in worship) with the Lord of the Al-'Alamin (mankind, jimm and all that exists); (26:97,98)

They are In addition the people, whom Allah described, when He said:

"And of mankind are some who take (for worship) others besides Allah as rivals (to Allah). They love them as they love Allah. But those who believe, Iove Allah more (then anything else)." (2:165)

All these are among the acts of Shirk (polytheism, associating others with Allah in worship) that Allah never forgives.

The Prophet's guidance on treating those touched by the evil eye

Imam Muslim [and Ahmad, Ibn Hibban, Al-

Hakim and At-Tabarani] narrated that Ibn Ab'ass said, The Messenger of Allah **b** said:

"The evil eye is true, and (f there is anything that would precede Predestination, it would be the evil eye."

In addition, Muslim narrated that Anas "The Prophet **b** has allowed using Islamic prayer formulas *(Ruqyah, divine remedy) against fever, the evil eye and sores."

In addition, in the two sound books narrated that Abu Hurayrah said that the Messenger of Allah **b** said, "The evil eye is true." [Abu Dawood, Ibn Majah and Ahmad].

Abu Dawood reported that A'esha said:

"The person who touched others with the evil eye was commanded to perform ablution and the person whom he touched by the evil eye would wash with that water." [I\\-Bokhary, Muslim, An-Nasa'y, Ibn Majah, Abu Na'im .

Further, A'esha narrated, as the Sahihain reported:

"The Prophet **b** commanded me, or commanded, that we should use Islamic prayer formulas from the evil eye."

In addition, At-Termezey narrated that Asma' Bint

Umaya said, "I said, O Messenger of Allah b The children of Ja'far are usually touched by the evil eye. Should I perform an Islamic prayer formula for them?' He said:

"yes. If there is anything that precedes Predestination, it would be the evil eye." [An-Nasa'y and Ahmad].

In addition, Imam Malik narrated that Amir bin Rabi'ah once saw Sahl bin Hunaif take a bath and said, "By Allah! I have never seen the skin of a virgin that is softer than what I have just seen." Sahl fell to the ground. The Prophet b then came to Amir while angry and said to him:

"Why would one of you kill his own brother? Why have you not said Tabrik [Karaka Allah, (may Allah bless it)]? Take a bath for it."

Amir then washed his face, hands, elbows, knees, feet and a part of his garment in a pot for what he had done and then poured the used water on Sahl. Soon after, Sahl started moving about with the people. [An-Nasa'y, Ibn Majah, Ahmad].

Malik In addition narrated:

"The evil eye is true, so perform ablution for it."

Another Hadith narrated by Abdul Razzaq reads:

"The evil eye is true. and if there is anything that precedes Predestination, it would be the evil eye. When one is touched by the evil eye, he should take a bath for it."

At-Termezey said:

"The person who touched others with the evil eye should be commanded to submerge his hand in a pot of water and then wash his mouth, then spit the water back into the pot. He should then wash his face in the pot, then submerges his left hand it and pour some water on the right knee above the pot, and then submerges his right hand and pour water on his left knee. He should then wash his garment inside the pot and the water should not be spilled on the ground. Rather, it should be poured on top of the person whom he touched by the evil eye from behind all at once."

There are two types of the evil eye, human and Jinn related. Umm Salamah said that the Prophet once saw a young gir, who had a certain expression on her face and said:

"Seek an Islamic prayer formula for her because she is touched by the evil eye." [Al-Bokhary, Muslim, Al-'Hakim, Abu Na'im. Al-Isma'ili and At-Tabarani]

Abu Sa'id In addition narrated that:

The Prophet b used to seek refuge from the jinn and the evil eye of mankind." [At-Termezey and An-Nasa'y]

Some people who do not have sound comprehension or correct sight and hearing have rejected the fact that the evil eye causes harm, claiming that this is a superstitious, untrue belief. These people are indeed among the most ignorant people who have the least sound comprehension and the thickest minds. They are the farthest from acquiring knowledge of the soul and the heart and the effect of each on the natural world.

The best minds in every nation do not dispute the fact that the evil eye is true, although they differ on its causes and true effects. Some people say that when people who touch others by the evil eye feel evilness in their hearts, then their eyes transform the evil thoughts into harmful rays just like the type of snake that looks at its prey and causes it to perish.

Another group says that it is possible that invisible powers emit from the person who touches others with the evil eye and then enters the body of the person whom they touched and harms them.

However, other people say that Allah creates the harm on the person touched by the evil eye without any rays that emit from the eye of the person who touched him, Yet, this is the method of those who deny the existence of the various spiritual powers that exist in this world. Allah has created special powers in some of the creation that have profound effects on other creations. For instance, the soul has such a profound effect on the body that no one can deny. In addition, have you not noticed how the face of a shy person turns red if his sight falls on what is not suitable for him, and turns yellow when he looks at someone he fears? You can In addition witness the effect of the evil eye has on people and the weakness it causes in their bodies.

The evil eye is actually the effect exerted by the soul on the victim. Souls vary in their essence, powers, characteristics and qualities. Therefore, the soul of an envious person can harm a victim profoundly, and this is why Allah has commanded His Messenger to seek refuge with Him from the evil eye.

The harmful effect of an envious person on the envied person cannot be denied, except by those who are far away from reality. It is a fact that an evil envious soul touches the envied person in such an evil manner that it causes them harm. Similarly, the poisonous viper gets so enraged and evil when it meets the enemy that it has a special effect on the victim, sometimes leading to aborting the fetus or causing blindness. The Prophet gg described the short tailed viper and the striped viper as having the ability that they can affect sight and abort pregnancy. Some types of snakes have a negative effect on people by their mere sight, because of the viciousness of such creatures and the effect of this viciousness on people.

These effects that we mentioned are not restricted to physical contact, as some of those who have little knowledge in the natural world and the religion think. Rather, these effects could be caused by physical contact, sight, the soul directing its power to the victim, through imagination and evil omens, and so forth.

The envious person might be blind, yet when something is described to him or her, his envious soul affects the described object and harms it even though the blind person cannot see it. Allah said to His Prophet **b**

"And verily, those who disbelieve would almost make you slip with their eyes (through hatred) when they bear the Reminder (the Qura'an) ..."(69:51)

﴿ قُلْ أَعُوذُ بِرَبِّ ٱلْفَلَقِ ۝ مِن شَرِّ مَا خَلَقَ ۝ وَمِن شَرِّ غَاسِقٍ إِذَا وَقَبَ ۝ وَمِن شَرِّ ٱلنَّفَّـٰثَـٰتِ فِى ٱلْعُقَدِ ۝ ﴾ (١:٤) الفلق .

Say: "I seek refuge with (Allah), the Lord of the daybreak, From the evil of what He has created. And from the evil of the darkening (night) as it comes with its darkness; (or the moon as ft sets or goes away), And from the evil of those who practise witchcraft when they blow in the knots. And from the evil of the envier when he envies."

Every person who touches others by the evil eye is an envious person, but not vise versa. Since envy includes the evil eye in its general meaning, seeking refuge from it includes seeking refuge from the evil eye In addition,

The evil eye includes throwing arrows of envy that depart the envious heart and soul in the direction of the envied person, sometimes falling on its target. If the envied person is unarmed and unprepared, the evil eye will cause him harm. If the envied person is prepared and armed, the arrows might tum back on the one who threw them. This is similar to what actually occurs when one shoots real arrows. The resemblance is that this occurs through the soul while the arrows are shot in the material world, The evil eye starts when the envious person likes something then follows it with his evil thoughts and desires and then the evil eye touches the envied object.

Sometimes a person might even touch his own self with the evil eye, which is one of the worst types of envy. Sometimes one might touch others with the evil eye just by his envious nature. Some of our scholars say that such envious people should be imprisoned and should be given what they need of sustenance until they die.

The Prophetic medicine for treating sorcery (the evil eye) was of several types

Abu Dawood narrated that Sahl ibn Hunaif said:

'We come by a water spot and I went in it and took a bath, but when I finished I came down with a fever. When the Messenger of Allah b was informed, he said, 'Command Abu Thabit to

seek refuge (with Allah for Sahl) with an Islamic prayer formula.' I said, 'O my master! Does an Islamic prayer formula bring about benefit?' He said, 'There is no Islamic prayer formula except to

fend off an evil eye and against fever and a (snake or a scorpion) bite.'" [In addition, Al-Hakim narrated this Hadith].

There are several types of Islamic prayer formulas, such as reciting the first chapter in the Qura'an, the Mu'awwithatan (chapters l 13 and I 14 of the Qura'an) and Ayat Al-Kursi (2:255).

In addition, there are several types of Prophetic Islamic prayer formulas. For instance, one might recite:

"I seek refuge with Allah's Prefect Words from the

evil of what He has created."

In addition, one could recite:

"I seek refuge with Allah's Prefect Words from every devil and evil soul and from every evil eye."

In addition, one might recite,

"I seek refuge with Allah's Prefect Words, which no righteous or evil soul could ever encompass (or supercede), from the evil of what He has created, made and started; from the evil of whatever descends from the sky and whatever ascends to it; from the evil of what He has created on the earth and what comes out of it; from the evil of the trials of the night and the day; and from what comes by at night or during the day, except whoever comes with a righteous matter. O Merciful One!"

In addition, this includes the supplication:

"I seek refuge with Allah's Perfect Words from His anger and torment, from the evil of His slaves and from the whispers of the devils or that they might attend me."

In addition, one might say the following supplication:

"O Allah! I seek refuge with Your I Honorable Face

and Your Prefect Words from the evil of every creation that is only in your grasp (or control). O Allah! You expel the sins and loss. O Allah! Your soldiers will never be defeated nor will Your Promise ever be broken. All praise and glorification is due to You."

In addition, one might supplicate:

"I seek refuge with Allah's Most Exalted Face which is greater

than everything else. And with His Perfect Words that no righteous or evil being could ever overcome; and with Allah's Most Prefect Names, those which I know and those which I have no knowledge of, from the evil of what He has created, shaped and made. From the evil of every creation that I cannot overcome and from the evil of every evil creation that only You control (or grasp its forelock). Certainly, my Lord is on a Straight Path."

In addition, the Prophetic Islamic prayer formulas include:

"O Allah! You Are my Lord, there is no deity worthy of worship except You. I depend on You (for every thing). You are the Lord of the Mighty Throne. What Allah wills, occurs, and what He does not will to happen, will never exist. There is no power or strength except with Allah. I know that Allah is Able to do everything, that His Knowledge has encompassed everything and that He has kept count of everything. O Allah! I seek refuge with You from the evil within myself, from the evil and the Shirk (polytheism) of Satan, and from the evil of every creation that only You grasp its forelock. Surely, my Lord is on the Straight Path."

Or, one might recite the following supplication,

"I seek refuge with Allah, other than Whom there is no god. He is my God and the God of everything. I seek refuge with my Lord and the Lord of everything. I depend on the Ever-Living Who never dies. I seek to fend off the evil with: no power or strength except from Allah.' Allah is enough of a supporter for me, and indeed, what an Excellent Helper. Allah is enough for me from the slaves. The Creator is enough for me from the creation. The Sustainer is enough for me from the sustained. Allah is indeed enough for me.

He Who owns everything. Who grants refuge while no one can ever grant refuge against Him is indeed sufficient for me. Allah is sufficient for me. Allah's hearing who ever supplicates to Him is In addition sufficient for me. There is no goal to reach greater than

Allah. Allah, other than Whom there is no god, is sufficient for me, I depend on Him (for each and everything), and He is the Lord of the Mighty Throne."

Those who try these different types of supplication and Islamic prayer formulas will surely understand their great value and benefit, and consequently, will recognize the great need for them. These supplications will shield one from the effects of the evil eye and will fend off its harm if the evil eye touched them, but according to the degree of Faith, strength of soul, degree of reliance (on Allah) and strength of heart of whoever recites them. These supplications are types of weapons, and their effectiveness depends on the skill of whoever uses them.

If the person fears that he might touch other people by the evil eye, let him fend off its harm by saying:

The Prophet b commanded Amir bin Rabi'ah,

"Why did you not say Tabrik [Baraka Allah, (may Allah bless it)] for him?"

Further, saying "Ma sha' Allah (what Allah has willed), la quw'ata il'a bil'ah (There is no power except from Allah)" In addition helps fend off the evil eye. Hisham bin 'Urwah narrated that his father used to say, "What Allah wills will certainly come to pass, there is no power except from Allah," upon seeing something that he likes and upon entering one of his gardens.

In addition, Jibril once said an Islamic prayer

formula for the Prophet b which Muslim narrated in his sound book:

"In the Nome of Allah I say Islamic prayer formulas for your benefit, from every illness that might harm you and from the evil of every evil soul or envious person's eye. Allah will cure you, in the Name of Allah I say Islamic prayer formulas for your benefit." [At-Termezey and An-Nasa'y]

Some of our rightly guided ancestors stated that there is no harm if some Ayat (Verse) from the Qura'an were written in ink and then washed with water and that the sick person drinks that water. Mujahid issued a statement to that effect, and so did Abu Qilabah. It was In addition reported that Ibn Ab'ass once commanded that two verses from the Qura'an to be written for a woman who had hard pregnancies and that the Verses were then washed with water and she was to drink the water. In addition, Ayub said, "I saw Abu Qilabah write some Verses from the Qura'an, wash it with water and then give the water to a person who was suffering from some type of illness to drink it."

In addition, the person who touches other people with the evil eye should be commanded to wash his limbs and the end of his garments, or his sexual organ according to one opinion, from the right side. He then pours the water on the head of the person whom he touched with the evil eye from behind him without notice. This is a type of cure that the doctors cannot produce with their medicine. In addition, those who reject such type of Islamic prayer formulas would never benefit from it because they do not believe that the Islamic prayer formulas carry any benefit.

Since the doctors cannot explain many natural occurrences in the world, why would the hypocrites among them reject such powers and effects that the religion produces? Added to this is the fact that washing up with the water has a real benefit, experience testifies to its usefulness. Similarly, the anger will be washed away from the heart if one places his hand on the angry person's chest. This is similar to confronting a man who is carrying a lit torch that he wants to throw at you, but you keep pouring water on it while it is still in his hand until you extinguish it. This is why the Prophet si commanded the person who touches people by the evil eye to ask Allah to bless whatever he has envied, so that the evil thoughts that he feels go away and are replaced by the supplication, which is a type of good charity. The cure should be compatible to the disease so that it has an affect on it. It is possible that when one touches others by the evil eye that a certain power appears on the end of his garment, or his sexual organ as we stated, and that it is then transferred to the affected person or object. When it is washed by water, the evil power will be removed. Yet again, and as we have stated, this matter has a lot to do with evil spirits, which will be stopped from producing harm if washed by water. In addition, it might be that washing with water serves to cool the heart and thus cures the person who was about to touch others with the evil eye. Sometimes, when a poisonous insect bites someone and then the insect is killed, the bitten person feels a little relief afterwards. This might occur because the bitten person feels joy that the insect was killed and this feeling of elation helps to cure the poison faster. In short, when the person who touches others with the evil eye is washed, the evil that he thought of or felt will be washed away with the water.

If someone asks, "If washing with the water helps the aggressor, then what about the victim of the evil eye?"

We say that pouring the water on victims of the evil eye In addition helps cool the effect of the evil eye on the victim just as it extinguished the veiled thoughts from the aggressor's heart. Water, which is used to cool burning iron rods, is In addition often used as a medicine with which the doctors would concur. It is natural that the same water used to extinguish the evil eye is used to rid the victim of the evil eye of its effect.

Therefore, comparing the Prophetic medicine to regular medicine that doctors use is just like comparing the doctor's medicine to folk medicines. Rather, the comparison is even less appropriate, for the difference between the Prophets and the doctors is profoundly greater than the difference between the doctors and those who are not qualified to practice medicine. You should have discovered by now the brotherly relation between religion and wisdom, and that they never contradict each other. Allah guides whom He wills to the straight path and opens the doors of success to those who knock on such doors. He Alone is the Source of all bounties and irrefutable proofs. Fighting the evil eye is more likely to be successful if one conceals his blessings from the people.

For instance, AI-Baghawi narrated that once Uthman saw a handsome boy and commanded, "Blacken his cleft chin so that the evil eye does not touch him."

AI-Khattabi In addition narrated in Gharib AI-Hadith, "It was narrated that Uthman once saw a handsome boy and that he said, 'Hide his cleft chin with black color.'" Uthman wanted to hide the cleft chin of the handsome boy using black color so that he was not touched by the evil eye.

Another Islamic prayer formula that helps ward off the evil eye was related by Abu 'Abdullah AI-Tayya'hi he was once traveling for Hajj or Jihad using a good animal. There was a man in the caravan who would never look at something but would bring it to its demise. Abu 'Abdullah was then told, 'Preserve your camel from this man's eye.' He said, 'My camel cannot be touched by harm.' The person who touched with the evil eye was informed of Abu 'Abdullah's response and he waited for a chance when Abu 'Abdullah was not present and looked at the camel which soon fell on its feet! When Abu 'Abdullah came and was told that the person had touched it with the evil eye and that his camel was suffering, as was evident, he said, 'Show me the man.' When he came by him he said, 'In the Name of Allah a restraint that restrains, a hard rock and a blazing star: I ask that the evil eye returns to the person who started it and on the most dear people to him (meaning the envious person himself)"

﴿ ٱلَّذِى خَلَقَ سَبۡعَ سَمَٰوَٰتٖ طِبَاقٗاۖ مَّا تَرَىٰ فِى خَلۡقِ ٱلرَّحۡمَٰنِ مِن
تَفَٰوُتٖۖ فَٱرۡجِعِ ٱلۡبَصَرَ هَلۡ تَرَىٰ مِن فُطُورٖ ٣ ﴾ (٣) الملك

Allah said:

Then look again: "Can you see any rifts?" Then look again and yet again, your sight will return to you in a state of humiliation and worn out." (67:3,4)

Then, the person known for the evil eye lost his sight and the camel was cured.*

The Prophet's guidance on treating sickness in general with Islamic prayer formulas Muslim narrated that Abu Sa'id Al-Khudri said that Jibril came to the Prophet b and said to him:

"O Muhammad ! Are you complaining from an illness?" He said,

"Yes." jibril then said, "In the Name of Allah I say Islamic prayer formulas for your benefit, from every illness that might harm you and from the evil of every evil soul or envious evil eye. Allah will cure you, in the Name of Allah I say Islamic prayer formulas for your benefit."

If someone asks, "What do you say about the Hadith that Abu Dawood narrated:

"There is no Islamic prayer formula except for an evil eye or fever."

To answer this question we say that the Hadith does not deny that the Islamic prayer formulas can be used in other instances. Rather, the Hadith only states that the Islamic prayer formulas work best for the evil eye and fever of all kinds. What further attests to this fact is that the Hadith itself narrated that Sahl ibn Hunaif asked the Prophet s§& when he was touched by the evil eye, "Do the Islamic prayer formulas bring about benefit?" The Prophet b then answered:

"There is no Islamic prayer formula (that works

better) than in the cases of evil eye and the fever."

In addition, the various Ahadeeth in general allow Islamic prayer formulas. For instance, Muslim narrated that the Prophet a& allowed using Islamic prayer formulas in the cases of the evil eye, fever and Namlah (ant's bite or sores).

The Prophet's guidance on treating one bitten (by an animal) by reciting Al-Fatihah

In the Sahihain [In addition At-Termezey, Ibn Mdjah and Ahmad] it is narrated that Abu Sa'id Al-Khudri said, "Some of the Companions of the Prophet ^ went on a journey till they reached some of the Arab tribes (at night). They asked the latter to treat them as their guests but they refused. The chief of that tribe was then bitten by a snake (or stung by a scorpion) and they tried their best to cure him but in vain. Some of them said (to the others), 'Nothing has benefited him, will you go to the people who resided here at night, it may be that some of them might possess something (as treatment),' They went to the group of the companions (of the Prophet **b**) and said, 'Our chief has been bitten by a snake (or stung by a scorpion) and we have tried everything but he has not benefited. Have you got anything (useful)?' One of them replied, 'Yes, by Allah! I can recite an Islamic prayer formula, but as you have refused to accept us as your guests, I will not recite the Islamic prayer formula for you unless you fix for us some wages for it.' They agreed to pay them a flock of sheep. One of them then recited (The chapter Al-Fatihah): 'All the praises are for the Lord of the Worlds' and puffed over the chief who became alright as if he was released from a chain, and got up and started walking, showing no signs of sickness. They paid them what they agreed to pay. Some of them (i.e., the Companions) then suggested to divide their earnings among themselves, but the one who performed the recitation said, 'Do not divide them till we go to the Prophet sg and narrate the whole story to him, and wait for his order.' So, they went to Allah's Messenger b and narrated the story. Allah's Messenger asked:

"How did you come to know that the chapter Al-Fatihah could be recited as an Islamic prayer formula?"

Then he added:

"You have done the right thing. Divide (what you have earned) and assign a share for me as well."

It is a well-known fact that certain types of speech have a profound effect and benefit that experience testifies to. So how about the Words of the Lord of the Worlds that are as preferred to the creation's speech as Allah is preferred above His creation? Allah's Words contain the ultimate cure, the perfect immunity, correct guidance and an encompassing mercy, that if it was revealed to a mountain, it would turn to dust ın appreciation of Allah's Glory. Allah said:

"And We send down of the Qura'an that which is a healing and a meıcy to those who believe (in Islamic Monotheism)

"Allah has promised those among them who believe (i.e., all those who follow Islamic Monotheism, the religion of Prophet Muhammad **b** till the Day of Resurrection) and do righteous good deeds, forgiveness and a mighty reward (i.e.. Paradise)." s

What could one think of the opening of the Qura'an (Al-Fatihah, the first chapter) that is not comparable to any Verse or chapter revealed in the Qura'an, the Torah, the Gospel or the Zabur (that was revealed to Prophet Dawood **b**). The Al-Fatihah contains the general meaning of all the Divine Books sent down by Allah. It contains Allah's Names and Attributes, such as Allah, the Robb (Lord), Ar-Rahman (Most Merciful) and Ar-RahIm (Most Beneficent). It In addition affirms Resurrection, Allah's Oneness in Lordship. It In addition mentions the creation's dependence on Allah's help and guidance and that He Alone grants such bounties. It In addition contains the best and most beneficial supplication that the creation needs:

being guided to the Straight Path that entails

acquiring knowledge of His Names and Attributes, worshipping Him alone, obeying His Commands, refraining from His prohibitions and staying firm on this path until death. It In addition contains the kinds of creation that are divided into those who have acquired the bounty of knowing the Truth, and who prefer and implement its implications. On the other hand, there are those who have earned Allah's Anger by avoiding the truth after knowing it and there are those who are led astray from the True Path. These are the camps that the creation is divided into. In addition, the Al-Fatihah affirms Predestination and the Commandments of the religion, Allah's Names and Attributes, Resurrection and Prophethood. It In addition purifies the heart and mentions Allah's Justice and Generosity. It In addition refutes all types of innovations and evil methods. We mentioned all these virtues for the Al-Fatihah in our book that explains it, Madariju As-Salikin. Certainly, a chapter that contains all these virtues and benefits deserves to be used as a cure for disease, as well as an antidote for poisonous stings.

Indeed, Al-Fatihah is the best cure because it contains sincere servitude to Allah, praising Him, relating all bounties to Him, seeking His help and support, and invoking Him for all types of advantages, such as the correct guidance that brings about benefit and fends off torment.

It was reported that the part in Al-Fatihah that contains the Islamic prayer formula is what Allah said:

﴿ إِيَّاكَ نَعْبُدُ وَإِيَّاكَ نَسْتَعِينُ ۝ ﴾ (٥) الفاتحة

"You (Alone) we worship, and You (Alone) we ask for help (for everything)." (1:5)

Indeed, these are mighty powerful words that contain the strongest medicine contained in this chapter. These words entail sincere dependence and reliance on Allah, seeking refuge and help from Him and showing meekness and need of Him. Consequently, these words contain the best goals to seek, which is worshiping Allah Alone. In addition they contain the best method to acquire these goals, that is, invoking Allah for His support so that one achieves these goals.

While I was in Mecca, I once fell sick and had no access to a doctor or medicine. So I used to seek a cure in The Al-Fatihah by sipping a drink from the well of Zamzam that I recited the Al-Fatihah on. I found complete cure in this method and I used to rely on it whenever I felt pain. This cure always helped me.

There is a wonderful secret in using the Al-Fatihah as an Islamic prayer formula to treat poisons, and Allah has created a cure for every disease as we have stated. Venomous beasts have a special effect on their victims with their evil souls. Furthermore, the weapon that the venomous beasts use is the needle that they use to sting and inject the venom into their victims. Likewise, the person who is applying the Islamic prayer formula will have a positive effect on the person receiving the Islamic prayer formula, thus enhancing his chances of a speedy recovery by Allah's will. In this case, the victim will feel that his strength and resolve are enhanced with the Islamic prayer formula and the divine remedy, similar to the relation that exists between regular medicine and the sick person. In addition, the wetness and the air contained in the spit of the person who recites the Islamic prayer formula, that contains the supplication and the remembrance of Allah, will all enhance the chances of recovery. Since the person who recites the Islamic prayer formula recites it with both his heart and mouth, then adding some of the air and moisture that exists inside his body through the spit will maximize the effectiveness, power and strength of the remedy. Certainly, this mixture of heart and soul used in the divine remedy works just as regularmedicine works on the body.

The person who applies the Islamic prayer formula has an advantage over the evil forces (including poisonous snakes etc.,) since he adds words of the Islamic prayer formula and spit to the strength of his inner self to remove the effects of the evil forces and the venom. In addition, the more strength of heart the person has, the stronger the Islamic prayer formula he recites becomes. There is another secret behind using spit in the divine remedy, which is In addition used by the evil forces, just as Allah said,

﴿ وَمِن شَرِّ ٱلنَّفَّٰثَٰتِ فِى ٱلْعُقَدِ ﴾ (٤)الفلق

"And from the evil of those who practise witchcrafts when they blow in the knots."

The body is greatly affected by what the heart feels and so blowing the air and spitting resembles a way to intensify the effect of what the heart feels and intends. Those who work sorcery tie some knots and blow onto them words of sorcery, which work on the victim although he or she might not be present. In this way, the evil force helps transferring the words of sorcery and their effect to the victim. When the force for good retaliates by using the Islamic prayer formula and then breathing unto the victim, the more powerful of the warring parties wins. War between good and evil forces resemble real war that occurs between people. The spiritual forces essentially use and enlist physical bodies in their wars against each other. Whoever is only concerned about the material world will not feel any of this raging war since he is attached to the environment that he believes in, that is, the material world, and he is far away from the world of spiritual forces and their effect on mankind.

In short, when the good spiritual force is strong enough and feels the effects and the meanings contained in the Al-Fatihah, along with the breathing that accompanies reciting it, the Islamic prayer formula will have the intended effect against the evil forces and will thus remove their harmful effect. Allah knows best. The Prophet's guidance on treating scorpion stings.

The chapter Al-lkhlas contains the essentials of the Faith and the Creed, various aspects of Tawheed, and attesting to and affirming Allah's Oneness that entails denying all types and forms of shirk with Him. It In addition entails affirming that Allah is the Sustainer, along with asserting every type of perfection for Him. Consequently, the creation seeks Allah for each and every need. This chapter In addition denies that Allah has a parent, an offspring, or an equal, and this is why it equals one third of the Qura'an. Furthermore. Allah's Name "As-Samad (the Sustainer)" that the chapter contains includes each and every type of perfection. In addition, the chapter denies that Allah has an equal, while Allah's Name Al-Ahad (the One) In addition denies the existence of a partner with Allah. These are the three essential cornerstones of Tawheed [Allah's Oneness in Lordship and worship and in His Names and Attributes].

The Mu'awwizatan (chapters 113 and 114 of the

Qura'an) In addition includes seeking refuge with Allah from every type of evil and harm. Seeking refuge from the evil that Allah has created includes every type of evil that such creations, whether physical or spiritual, can ever produce and cause. Seeking refuge from the night when its sign, (the moon), sets, entails seeking refuge from the evil souls that thrive during the night, as opposed to the light of the day. This is because when the darkness falls and the moon sets, the evil forces come out. In addition, seeking refuge from those who tie knots and blow on them includes seeking refuge from the evil of sorcerers and their sorcery. In addition, seeking refuge from envious people means seeking refuge from the evil forces that cause harm through the envious people's bodies and sight. The second chapter (I 14) of the Moaw'azatan entails seeking refuge from the evil of humans and Jinn. Consequently, the two Moaw'azatan entail seeking refuge from every type of evil. Therefore, they have a great benefit as a shield against evil before it occurs. This is why the Messenger of Allah **b** advised 'Uqbah bin Amir to recite them after every prayer, as At-Termezey has narrated. This advice from the Prophet ^ contains a great secret and benefit that helps repulse all types of evil during the time between the prayers. The Prophet s& In addition described the Moaw'azatan when he said:

"No one who seeks refuge can ever find a refuge like them."

It was In addition reported that when the Prophet f&, was the victim of sorcery the spell contained eleven knots tied each with a special incantation blown on it, and that whenever Jibril Up recited a Verse from the Moaw'azatan, a knot was untied, until all eleven knots were untied. Then, the Prophet gig was cured, as if being released from a restraining chain.

As for using regular medicines to cure scorpion sting, salt has a great value in this regard. The author of Al-Qanoon said, "Salt should be used in a bandage with linen seeds to cure the scorpion's sting." Salt helps dissolve the poison, which has a burning pain that needs to be cooled. The cool moisture contained in the linen seed cools the pain, while the salt helps extract and remove the poison. This is one of the best and easiest types of remedies for scorpion stings, which require cooling the pain and extracting the venom. Allah knows best.

Muslim narrated that Abu Hurayrah said, "A man came to the Prophet ^ and said to him, 'O Messenger of Allah bI have suffered greatly from a scorpion that stung me last night." The Prophet b said:

"Had you said these words when you went to sleep, 'I seek refuge with Allah's Perfect Words from the evil of what He has created,' it would not have harmed you." [Ahmad]

Know that the Divine cures help after one catches a disease and In addition help prevent if from happening. If any type of harm befalls one afterwards, it will not be severe. Natural medicines, on the other hand, only help after the disease attacks. Islamic prayer formulas and the various supplications either prevent the disease from happening or make it milder after it happens, depending on the strength of soul and heart of the sick person. Therefore, the Islamic prayer formulas and supplications are used as preventive measures and In addition as a cure.

As for prevention, in the Sahihain it is narrated that A'esha said:

"Whenever the Messenger of Allah se would go to bed, he used to breathe into bis hands with

QuI huwa Allahu Ahad (AI- Ikhlas) and the Moaw'azatan." He then would wipe his face and whatever he could reach of bis body with his hands."

In addition, in the Sahihain it is narrated that the Prophet **b** said:

"Whoever reads the Iast two Verses from Chapter AI-Kaqarah (the second chapter in the Qura'an), at night, they will be enough for him."

In addition, Muslim narrated that the Prophet **b**

said:

"Whoever resided in a place and said, 'I seek refuge with Allah's Perfect Words from the evil of what He has created,' then nothing will harm him until he departs that place."

Abu Dawood In addition narrated that the Messenger of Allah ^ used to say at night when he was traveling:

O land! My Lord and your Lord is Allah. I seek refuge with Allah from your evil, from the evil of whatever is in you and from the evil of whatever walks on your surface. I seek refuge with Allah from a lion, a despot (or jinn), a snake and a scorpion and from those who reside in this land, and from the begetter (son of Adam) and that which he begot."

As for the second benefit of Ruqyah, providing a cure, we mentioned healing the ill person by reciting the Al-Fatihah and In addition reciting the Ruqyah to cure scorpion stings. The Prophet's guidance in treating the Namlah.

We mentioned the Hadith narrated by Anas & AI ^ in Sahih Muslim that the Prophet of Allah **b** allowed using the Ruqyah from every type of fever, evil eye and Namlah. .

In addition, Abu Dawood narrated that Ash-Shifaa bint Abdullah said, "The Messenger of Allah came by while I was with Hafsah and said:

"WIiy (Io you not teach her (Hafsah, his wife) the Ruqyah from Namlah as you taught her how to write." An-Namlah, literally, the ant, is called as such because it is a type of swelling that appears on the sides of the body. The Namlah is a known disease and causes a type of sting in the sides that makes one think that an ant is crawling on his side and biting him. There are three types of this disease.

Al-Khallal narrated that Ash-Shifaa bint Abdullah used to recite Ruqyah from the Namlah during the time before Islam. When she emigrated to the Prophet **b** in Medina, after she had given him her pledge of allegiance in Mecca, she said, "O Messenger of Allah! I used to recite the Ruqyah from the Namlah during the time of jahiliyyah (before Islam) and I want to read it to you." She recited it to him, "In the Name of Allah! May the harm be extracted until it goes back to where it came from without harming anyone. O Allah! Remove the harm, O Lord of the people." She used to recite it on a clean branch of wood seven times, choose a clean place, rub the branch on a clean stone with sour wine vinegar and then anoint the affected area with it. The Hadith In addition asserts the fact that it is legislated to teach women to read and write.

The Prophet's guidance in treating the snake's bite

We mentioned the Hadith in which the Prophet b said,

"There is no Ruqyah more beneficial than one recited for the evil eye and fever."

In addition, Ibn Maj'ah said that A'esha narrated, "The Messenger of Allah b allowed using the Ruqyah for the scorpions and the snakes bite." Further, Ibn Shihab Az-Zuhri narrated, "One of the companions of the Messenger of Allah was stung by a snake. The Prophet sSs said, 'Is there a person who could recite Ruqyahl' They said, 'O Messenger of Allah ! The children of Al-'Hazm used to recite a Ruqyah for snake's bite but abandoned the practice when you prohibited using Ruqyah.' He said, 'Summon 'Umarah bin 'Hazm.' When they summoned him, he recited his Ruqyah to the Prophet who said that there is no objection to it. Hence, the Prophet b allowed him to use it, and 'Umarah recited the Ruqyah on the victim.'" [Al-Bokhary, Muslim, An-Nasa'y and Ahmad].

The Prophet's guidance in treating an ulcer and various wounds

In the Two sound books is narrated that A'esha said:

"Whenever a person would complain from an ulcer (or a canker), or a wound, the Messenger of Allah b would put his finger in the soil (on the ground after inserting it in his mouth, then raise it). saying, 'In the Name of Allah: with the soil of our earth has got a moisture with the saliva of some of us, let our sick be cured, with our Lord's permission.

This is an easy, beneficial cure for the various ulcers and fresh wounds, especially when there is no available medicine. The sand, which is cold and dry and is available on all parts of the world, dries out the moisture that accumulates around the ulcer or wound. This moisture prevents quick healing by natural means, especially in warm areas. Most ulcers and wounds are In addition accompanied by a hot fever, which, when added to the irritant of warm weather, would only intensify the pain of those who are especially sensitive to heat. Since pure sand is cold and dry, more cooling than even the most effective medications for this purpose, the coolness of the sand will effectively pacify the warmth caused by the wound, especially when the sand is washed and dried. Pure sand In addition helps dry out most harmful moistures and wetness, because it is a strong drying agent against the wetness that prevents quick healing, as we stated. Further, pure sand helps cool the hotness in the ailing organ, which will strengthen its power of resistance (immunity) and thus end the pain by Allah's Leave,

The Hadith indicates that one should place some saliva on his index finger then place it on pure sand, some of which will stick on to his finger. The finger should then be placed on the affected organ or the wound, and then one recites the supplication mentioned in the Hadith. This practice joins the blessings of mentioning Allah's Name, relating all matters to Him and trusting in Him, adding both the cure and the supplication that will make the remedy even more effective.

There are two opinions regarding the Prophet's statement, "The sand of our land", if whether it entails the sand of the entire earth or just the sand of Medina. There is no doubt that some types of sand are more effective remedies for various ailments than sand from other areas. Galinus said, "In Alexandria, I saw many people who suffer from sever dropsy and an ailing spleen use the sand of Egypt as ointment on their legs, thighs, hands, backs and ribs, and they used to benefit from this remedy." He In addition said, "Hence, this ointment (muddy sand) could help cure Putrid and limp tumors." He continued, "I know of many people, whose bodies have swollen due to excessive bleeding, who benefited from remedy using mud. I In addition know of others who used it to cure terminal illnesses that attacked various organs, and the terminal ailments were eradicated." Another author said, "Sand that is imported from the area of Kannus - known as the island of Mastic - is an effective cleanser and causes the flesh to grow in and around ulcers, thus effectively eradicating them."

Since various types of sand have a healing effect, what about the sand of the best and most blessed area on the face of the earth, especially when mixed with the Prophet's saliva? Added to these blessings is the supplication that the Prophet recited and in which he mentioned the Lord's Name and related all matters to Him. We mentioned that the Ruqyah increases in effectiveness according to the strength of faith of the person who is reciting it and the response of the ill person to the Ruqyah. No sane, honorable Muslim doctor can deny this fact. However, if any of these qualities is absent, let such a person say whatever falsehood he wishes!

The Prophet's guidance on treating pain in general with Islamic prayer formulas

Muslim [Ibn Ma'jah, Ahmad and At-Tabarani} narrated in his Sahih that 'Uthman bin Abu Al-'As complained to the Prophet b from a pain in his body that he suffered from ever since he became a Muslim. The

Prophet **b** said:

Place your hand on the affected area in your body and say, 'In the Name of Allah,' thrice. Then say, 'I seek refuge with Allah's Might and Power from the evil of what I am suffering from, and because of which I have become worry. seven times."

The remedy mentioned here entails reciting Allah's Name, relating all matters to Him and seeking refuge with His Might and Power from the pain, and will surely eradicate the pain. In addition, repeating the supplication contained in the remedy frequently will make it even more effective and successful just as the case when the medication is frequently administered until the disease is fully eradicated.

In the Sahihain it is narrated that the Prophet **b** used to visit some of his family members (who were ill) and would touch them with his right hand, saying:

"O Allah, the Lord of mankind! Do away with the complaint and bring about the cure. You Alone bring the cure, and there is no cure except Your cure, a cure that does not leave illnesses."

The last Islamic prayer formula includes begging Allah by His Perfect Lordship and Mercy to bring about the cure. The Islamic prayer formula In addition affirms

return. O Allah! Reward me for the calamity that has befallen me and replace it with what is better.' Except that Allah will reward him for his calamity and will replace it with what is better than whatever he lost."

The words that are contained in the Hadith are a truly effective and are a beneficial cure for those afflicted by disasters or calamities. These words contain two major aspects that if the slaves of Allah acquire knowledge of them, they will relieve them from the shock of the disaster. First, the slave of Allah, his family and wealth are Allah's exclusive property that Allah has loaned to the slave. When Allah takes back some of what he has loaned the slave, He is the Owner who takes back what belongs to Him. Further, whatever Allah gives the save is preceded and followed by periods of non-existence, and the slave only takes temporary possession of them when they come into existence. In addition, the slaves of Allah neither create whatever they own, and they are not its true owners, nor are they capable of protecting such possessions and property. Therefore, the slaves are only hired agents who do what they are commanded, since they are not the real owners.

The slaves return is to Allah, the True Lord, and consequently, they will have to sooner or later depart this life and leave it behind. The slaves will return to Allah just as He created them the first time:

dispossessed, without a wife or a family or wealth or tribe. Only the good and bad deeds will the slaves have then. If this is the case with whatever Allah gives the slaves, its beginning and end, then why should the slaves be proud of whatever they have or get sad if they loose them? When the slaves remember their beginning and end, this thought will help them discard sadness and depression for their loss.

In addition, sadness and depression will be relieved when the slaves realize that they have neither the power to avoid whatever has befallen them, nor to bring about what was not destined for them. Allah said;

﴿ مَآ أَصَابَ مِن مُّصِيبَةٍ فِي ٱلۡأَرۡضِ وَلَا فِيٓ أَنفُسِكُمۡ إِلَّا فِي كِتَٰبٖ
مِّن قَبۡلِ أَن نَّبۡرَأَهَآۚ إِنَّ ذَٰلِكَ عَلَى ٱللَّهِ يَسِيرٞ ٢٢ لِّكَيۡلَا تَأۡسَوۡاْ عَلَىٰ
مَا فَاتَكُمۡ وَلَا تَفۡرَحُواْ بِمَآ ءَاتَىٰكُمۡۗ وَٱللَّهُ لَا يُحِبُّ كُلَّ مُخۡتَالٖ
فَخُورٍ ٢٣ ﴾ (٢٢:٢٣) الحديد

"No calamity befalls on the earth or in yourselves but it is inscribed in the Book of Decrees (Al-Lauh Al-Mahfuz) before We bring it into existence. Verily, that is easy for Allah. In order that you may not grieve at the things over that you fail to get, nor rejoice over that which has been given to you. And Allah likes not prideful boasters." (57:22,23)

In addition, the anguish caused by the calamity will be relieved when the slaves think deeply about what Allah has bestowed on them as compared to what they have lost. They will find that whatever they still have of Allah's bounty is much larger, especially since Allah has promised them what is even better than whatever they have lost, providing that they are patient with the calamity. If Allah wills, He could make the calamity even larger and more severe.

The shock of calamities could In addition be soothed by observing other people around him and realizing that wherever one looks he sees a disaster to his right and to his left. If someone searches the entire world, he will see that all of mankind is suffering some type of calamity: either losing a loved one, or from a disaster. He will In addition realize that the joys of this world are just daydreams or passing shadows, and that even if this earthly life brings a little joy, it In addition brings many tears, and if it brings a comfort for one day, it can bring about a long term disaster. Further, if this life brings some joy, it can prevent further joy from coming for a long time. In addition, no place of residence will be filled with any type of good, but could soon be filled with lessons and losses. Finally, if this life brings happiness for a day, it can be hiding the evil of the days to come.

Ibn Mas'ud said, "Every joy will be followed by sadness, and no house is filled with joy but will soon be filled with anguish."

In addition,Ibn Sirin said, "There is not a laugh but a cry to succeed it."

Further, Hind bint An-Nu'man said, "One time, we were some of the most mighty people enjoying the most respected authority. Soon after, when the sun went down, we became the fewest people. It is Allah's promise that He will not fill a house with joy but it will soon be filled with lessons (or sadness)."

Once, a man asked Hind to tell him her story and she said, "One morning, we woke up while none among the Arabs but seeks us in eagerness. When the night fell, all the Arabs felt pity for us."

Further, her sister Hurqah once cried, at a time when they were mighty. When she was asked about why she cried and if someone had bothered her, she said, "No. I saw that my family was enjoying comforts and remembered that no house is filled with joy but would one day be filled with grief."

Furthermore, Ishaq bin Tallhah said, "I came by her (Hurqah) one day and said to her, "What do you know about the lessons from the stories of the kings?' She said,

"What we enjoy today is better than what we enjoyed yesterday. We read in the books that no people of a house would enjoy a bounty, but would later on be tested with a trial. In addition, time would never show a people a joyous day but would be hiding another day that they would hate."

Curing the shock of disasters and calamities In addition comes through knowing that sadness and grief will not avert the calamity but will intensify it.

In addition, curing grief and anguish comes through knowing that missing the rewards for being patient and content, such as mercy and correct guidance that Allah has promised in return for being patient, is much larger than the calamity itself.

A part of the cure In addition comes through knowing that grief brings comfort to the heart of the enemy, grief to the friends, anger to the Lord, joy to the devil, destruction to the reward and weakness to the heart. On the other hand, when one observes patience and satisfaction, he will expel the devil and defeat his plots, will please the Lord, bring joy to the friends and sadness to the enemy. In this case, the person would say words of condolence to his friends instead of they to him. This, indeed, is the sought after perfection and firmness, unlike striking the cheeks, uttering foul words and being dissatisfied with what Allah has decided.

Curing grief after disaster strikes a so comes through knowing'that being patient and content would lead to a type of joy, tranquility and comfort that is much greater than what had been lost because of the disaster. In this case, it will be enough of a reward for the patient slave that he will acquire a house of praise that will be built for him in Paradise as a reward for praising his Lord and referring all matters to Him. Let one think about the bigger disaster the one that he had suffered or to lose thc rewards that he would have gained in the Residence of Eternity [for being patient],

At-Termezey related from the Prophet s& that he said, "On the Day of Resurrection some people would wish that their skins were sliced with scissors in the life of this world because of the reward that they witness the people who endured disasters would receive for being patient."

Some of the followers of the people of Al-Medina once said, "If it was not for the calamities of this life, we would be bankrupt of rewards on the Day of Resurrection."

In addition, curing anguish and grief entails feeling content in the heart seeking Allah's rewards, for everything can be replaced, except for Allah's Pleasure. The cure In addition entails knowing that the calamity's effect on one is all what he will gain of it. Those who are content with the calamity will gain contentment, while those who are enraged, will only gain rage. The calamity will affect one as much as he allows it. One should then choose between the best of rewards or the most evil consequences. If one feels rage and disbelief, he will be written in the record of the destroyed ones. If one feels grief and abandons an obligation or commits a prohibition, he will be written in the record of those who neglect their duty. If the calamity caused one to complain and be impatient, he will be written with those who commit injustices against themselves. If one rejects Allah's decision and questions His wisdom, he will have knocked on the door that leads to hypocrisy or will have entered through it. If one is patient and firm for Allah's sake, he will be written among the patient ones. If one feels content, he will be written among the content believers. If one praises and thanks Allah, he will be written with the thankful slaves and will be gathered under the flag of those who praise Allah. If the calamity directed one to feel eager to meet his Lord, he will be written among the sincere persons in their love for Allah.

Ahmad and At-Termezey related that the Prophet ﷺ said:

"When Allah loves a people. He tests them with trials. If they are content, then they will achieve contentment. Those who get enraged, will only reap rage."

Curing grief In addition entails knowing that no matter how much grief one feels he will sooner or later be forced to forego the matter. And then, he will not be rewarded for this forced patience.

A wise man once said, "In the first day when a calamity strikes, the wise person behaves just like the ignorant person behaves days later. Those who do not observe an honorable patience, will soon be forced to forget just as the animals do."

In addition in the Sahih it is related that the Prophet **b** said:

"Verily, patience is at the stroke of the calamity."

Further, Al-Ash'ath bin Qays said, "Observe patience with Faith and await the reward from Allah Alone. Otherwise, you will be forced to forget just as the animals do."

Among the cures of grief is that the person should know that the most useful remedies for his case are his agreeing with his Lord and God in what He has chosen for him, for the secret that love contains is that those who love agree with the loved one. Those who claim to love then disagree with what the loved one likes and seek what he dislikes will anger the loved one and will be testifying to the untruthfulness of their claimed love,

Abu Ad-Darda once said, "When Allah decides a matter, He likes that His decision is accepted." In addition, 'Imran bin Al-Husain used to say when he was ill, "The most beloved to Him is In addition the most beloved to me." Abu Al-Aliyah In addition said similar words. This remedy only works for those who have sincere love for Allah and is not suitable for just any one.

In addition, curing grief includes comparing what is more joyous, beloved and enduring: being content with the calamity or the joy of receiving Allah's reward. When one realizes and acquires the superior option, he should thank Allah for His guidance. If one chooses the lesser of the two, let him know that the affliction that his mind, heart and religion have suffered is more than the affliction he suffered through the disaster.

Curing grief In addition requires knowing that He Who has tested the slave with the affliction is the Most Wise, the Most Merciful, and that He did not test him with the affliction to destroy, punish or overwhelm him. Rather, the affliction is merely a test of his patience, contentment with Allah and faith. In addition Allah wants to hear the slave's pleas, supplications, and humility before Him, seeking refuge with Him, his heart's humbleness before Him and his explaining his grievances to Him.

Shaikh Abdul Qadir said, "My son! The affliction was not meant to destroy you. Rather, it was meant as a test of your patience and faith. My son! Fate is a lion, and lions do not eat carrion." The affliction is just like the bellows for the believer that rids him of impurities. The believer will either end up being pure gold or pure evil! When the bellows do not benefit the slave in this life, he will be faced with the mightiest bellows, hell. The slave should thus know that his being tested with the bellows of this life is better for him that being tested with the bellows of the next life! In addition, the slave has no other choice but to be tested with one of the two bellows, so let him appreciate Allah's bounty on him by testing him with the bellows of this world.

Curing grief In addition entails knowing that if it were not for the afflictions of this life, the slave would become arrogant, proud and hard-hearted, which would ultimately cause his destruction. It is the mercy of the Most Merciful that He tests the slave with afflictions sometimes so that these afflictions act as a prevention against evil manners, thus preserving the health of one's slavery to Allah. In addition they extract spoiled substances from his system. All praise is to He Who sends down mercy with afflictions, and Who tests the slaves with the bounties He grants.

If it was not for the fad that Allah treats His slaves with the remedies of afflictions and trials, they would be arrogant and would commit injustices and aggression. When Allah decides to do good for a certain slave, He tests him with pain and affliction, according to the degree of his faith. This is how Allah rids the slaves of destructive ailments (sins and lusts), until the slave is purified and correctly guided, and Allah qualifies him to the highest degree in this world: being His slave. He will In addition qualify him for the best rewards in the Life Hereafter: Gazing at Allah and residing close to Him.

Curing grief In addition entails knowing that the bitterness of this life is itself the sweetness of the Life Hereafter, as Allah will turn it to sweetness later on. In addition the sweetness of this life is itself the bitterness of the Life Hereafter. Moving away from a short-lived bitterness to acquire an eterna sweetness is surely better than vise versa.

If one does not comprehend these facts, let them remember the words of the truthful one,

"Paradise is surrounded with joys while the Fire is surrounded with lusts."

Therefore, bring yourself to what Allah has prepared for His loyal supporters - those who obey Him of eternal joy, everlasting happiness and ultimate success.

In addition consider and remember the torment, everlasting sadness and the humiliation that Allah has prepared for the evil and wasteful slaves.

"Each one does according to Shakilatihi (i.e., his way or his religion or his intentions)." (17:84)

Every person seeks what is suitable for him and what he deserves. Do not think that the cures mentioned herewith are over explained, for the utter need of them by both the doctor and the sick required explaining them in detail. Allah knows best.

The Prophet's guidance on treating sadness, grief, and depression

In the Sahihain it is narrated that the Messenger of Allah **b** said:

"There is no deity worthy of worship except Allah, the Most Great, the Most Forbearing. There is no deity worthy of worship except Allah, the Lord of the Mighty Throne. There is no deity worthy of worship except Allah, the Lord of the seven heavens, the Lord of the earth and the Lord of the Honorable Throne."

In addition, Abu Dawood narrated in his Sunan that Abu Bakrah related from the Prophet **b** that he said:

"This is the supplication of those afflicted by

distress, 'O Allah! I seek Your Mercy. Do not make me reliant on my own self for an instant, and lead all my affairs to success, there is no deity except You."

In addition, Abu Dawood narrated that Asmaa Bint 'Umays said that the Allah's Messenger s& said to her:

"Should I teach you some words that you should recite when in distress, 'Allah, is my Lord with Whom I associate nothing and no one."

Imam Ahmad narrated that Ibn Mas'ud said that the Prophet **b** said:

"Whenever a sadness or grief strikes a slave and the slave then says, 'O Allah! I am Your slave, the son of Your slave, the son of Your female slave. My forelock is in Your grasp. Your decision about me will certainly come to pass. Your judgment on me is certainly just. I ask You by every Name that is Yours and which You call Yourself by, whether You revealed it in Your Book, taught it to some of Your creation or kept in the Knowledge of the Unseen that You have. Make the Noble Qura'an the spring of my heart, the light of my chest, the eliminator of may sadness and the end of my grief. Then, Allah will remove his sadness and depression and will replace them with joy."

In addition, At-Termezey narrated that Sa'd bin Abu Waqqas related from the Messenger of Allah **b** that he said:

"The supplication of Thu An-Nun (Jonah) which he supplicated to the Lord while in the belly of the whale."

"La ilaha ilia Anta [none has the right to be worshipped but You (O Allah)], Glorified (and Exalted) be You [above all that (evil) they associate with You]! Truly, I have been of the wrongdoers."

"No Muslim man would supplicate with it concerning a matter but would be positively answered by Allah."

Imam Ahmad In addition narrated in the Musnad,

"Whenever the Prophet **b** would be concerned about a matter, he would turn to prayer."

Furthermore, Allah said:

﴿ وَٱسْتَعِينُوا۟ بِٱلصَّبْرِ وَٱلصَّلَوٰةِ ۚ وَإِنَّهَا لَكَبِيرَةٌ إِلَّا عَلَى ٱلْخَـٰشِعِينَ ﴾

(٤٥) البقرة

"And seek help in patience and As-Salat (the

dealing with His slave with injustice and for not punishing him without a reason. The fifth, the slave's affirming that it is he who has committed the injustice. The sixth, pleading to Allah by the most beloved methods to Him, by His Names, Attributes, such as Al-'Hay (The Ever Living), Al-Qayyum (Who Sustains everything and everyone). The seventh, depending and relying on Allah

Alone for everything. The eighth, the slave affirms that his hope is only in Allah. The ninth, acquiring true dependence on Allah and relating all matters to Him, while admitting that the slave's forelock is in His Hands Alone and that He does with it whatever He will. In addition, admitting that Allah's decision on the slave will certainly come to pass and that His judgment is certainly just.

The tenth, the slave's heart should enjoy the gardens of the Qura'an and should make the Qura'an just like the spring of pure water to the animals. In addition, the slave should use the light of the Qura'an to shatter the darkness of desires and lusts. The Qura'an should be one's companion when no one else is present; the comfort that relieves every type of calamity and the cure that discards every illness that attacks the slave's heart. In short, the Qura'an should be the remover of sadness and the end of depression and grief. The eleventh, turning to Istighfar, seeking forgiveness from Allah. Twelfth, repenting to

Allah. Thirteenth, performing jihad in Allah's cause. Fourteenth, performing prayer. Fifteenth, knowing all power and strength to He Who grasps them in His Hands.

How divine remedies affect diseases

Allah has created the son of Adam and his body's organs and designated a state of perfection that each organ could attain and achieve. Consequently, when the organ looses its perfection, it feels pain. Allah has In addition designated a state of perfection for the heart, the leader of the organs. When the heart looses its perfection, it will fall down with various ills and sicknesses, such as sadness, grief and anguish.

Furthermore, when the eye looses what it was created for, sight;

when the ear looses what it was created for, hearing; and when the tongue looses what it was created for, speech; then these organs will have lost their perfection.

The heart was created to acquire knowledge of its Creator and to love Him, worship Him Alone, be content with Him, to be joyous loving Him and to feel satisfied with Him. The heart was In addition created to rely on Allah, to love for His Sake, hate for His Sake, to be loyal for His Sake, to be enemies of His enemies for His Sake and to remember Him always. The heart was created to love Him more than anyone or anything else, to have Hope in Him rather than anyone or anything else and to revere Him more than anything or anyone else. There is no joy, happiness, delight or sweetness except by acquiring such qualities, which are just like food, good health and life for the heart. When the heart looses its food, health and life, then sadness, grief and affliction will attack it from all sides and will remain with it.

The worst diseases that attack the heart are Shirk (polytheism, making partners with Allah), sins, and forgetfulness, ignoring what Allah likes and is pleased with, abandoning relating all matters to Him and not depending on Him for everything. Diseases of the heart In addition include relying on other than Allah, rejecting His decisions and doubting and ignoring His warnings and promises.

When one thinks about the diseases of the heart, he will find that the reasons that we mentioned are the only ones behind these ills. Consequently, the only effective remedies for these ills are their opposites and antidotes that the Prophetic remedies contain. We stated before that the disease is removed by its opposite and that health is preserved by using what it is accustomed to which is included in the Prophetic remedies.

Tawheed opens the door to all types of good,

happiness, joy, elation and enjoyment for the slave. In addition, repenting to Allah extracts all types of harmful, sinful causes of the heart's ailment. Further, Tawheed is the diet of the heart against bad substances, for it closes the doors of evil. The doors of happiness and all types of good will be opened with Tawheed, while repentance and seeking forgiveness will close the doors of evil.

Doctors of old said, "Whoever seeks to acquire good health for the body should consume less amounts of food and drink. Whoever seeks the well being of his heart, let him abandon sin." In addition, Thabit said, "The body's well being requires consuming less food, the soul's comfort is in committing less sins and the consolation of the tongue is in uttering less speech."

Sins are just like poison to the heart - if they do not destroy it, they will weaken it. Then when the heart is weaker, it will become less efficient in fighting disease.

The biggest of the heart's ills occur by satisfying its lusts and desires, while ignoring them constitutes its biggest cure. We should In addition mention that originally, ignorance and injustice were created in the self. Because the self is ignorant, it thinks that its cure is in following its desire, although this path leads it to its destruction and demise. And because the self is unjust, it does not accept the prescription of the sincere doctor. Consequently, when the self is prescribed the ailment instead of the cure, it accepts it while refusing to take the cure when it is prescribed. And because the self prefers the illness rather than the cure, which it tries to avoid, many other illnesses and diseases will break out and by then the doctor will not be able to diagnose them and consequently, the cure will not be available. The biggest calamity of all this is that the self absolves itself of guilt and blames Fate and its Lord, inwardly in the beginning and then explicitly later on!*

When the ailing person reaches this stage, there is no hope of curing him, unless the Mercy of the Lord rushes to his aid and Allah allows him to start a new life while providing him with the required sustenance. This is why the Hadith that Ibn Ab'ass has narrated about the supplication during the time of distress contained Unity (Tawheed) of Allah in Lordship and worship, glorifying Him and mentioning His being Most Forbearing. These two Attributes (Glory and Forbearing) are necessary to add perfection to the Attributes of Ability, Mercy, Kindness and Forgiveness. In addition, the same Hadith described Allah's Lordship above the upper and lower worlds and above the Throne, which is the ceiling and the mightiest of all creation, Affirming Perfect Lordship to Allah requires worshiping Him alone in Unity (Tawheed), and loving, fearing, hoping, glorifying and obeying Him Alone. In addition, affirming Allah's Perfect Glory requires affirming and attributing every type of perfection to Him and denying every type of shortcoming and being equated with the creation. In addition, Allah's being Most-Forbearing necessitates affirming the perfection of His Mercy and Kindness towards His creation.

When the heart has access to these facts, it will seek to acquire the qualities of loving Allah and glorifying Him in Tawheed. Then, the heart will acquire and enjoy such elation and delight that will allow it to overcome the feelings of affliction, sadness and grief. It is a fact that whenever the sick person hears of what brings happiness and joy to his heart, the body will be more effective in resisting the ailment,

Furthermore, when one compares the depressing feelings while in anguish to the wonderful meanings contained in the supplication while distressed, he will find that these words are perfectly suitable to deliver the heart from its depression and substitute it with the elation that accompanies happiness and joy. Only those who have had access to such feelings and whose hearts are filled with the light of the truth that comes with these feelings will give this subject matter its due consideration.

The Prophet's statement:

be trained or at least restrained by the laws of Islam. Satan (the force of evil) appeals to our Nafs (self) and tries to encourage it to commit sins. This in turn causes negative damage to the soul, which we are responsible for.

"O the Ever-Living, the Self Subsisting! I urgently seek Your Mercy."

It has a special kind of effect in removing the grief.

Allah's Living is an attribute that includes every type of perfect quality, while the attribute "The Self Subsisting" entails Allah's perfect Actions. That is why Al-Hayy (The Ever Living), Al- Qayyum (The Self Subsisting) are included in Allah's Mightiest Name, which if He is called by it, He will answer and if He is begged by it, He will give.

Furthermore, Perfect Life is the opposite of sickness and shortcomings since the residents of Paradise do not die, they do not feel any sadness, depression or any type of ailment. When life has an end, it indicates the existence of shortcomings in actions and in ability to sustain. Being ever-living is thus suited to being ever-sustaining. The Ever-Living does not have any shortcoming in His being. The Self Subsisting Al-Qayyum, is Able to do everything He wills. This is why asking Allah by His Names Al-Hayy, The Ever-Living, Al-Qayyum, the Self Subsisting has profound effects on removing what is the opposite of life and Ability.

Related to this, the Prophet b used to ask Allah by His Lordship of Jibril, Michael and Israfil to guide him to that which the people had differed in concerning the truth, by His Will, for the heart lives by correct guidance. The three angels mentioned in the supplication are responsible for the elements and necessities of life. For instance, Jibril is responsible for delivering the revelation with which the heart lives. Michael is responsible for the sustenance, which is the life of the body. Israfil is responsible for blowing the Horn, which signals the resurrection of the souls and their being returned to their bodies. Asking Allah by His Lordship of these three angels, who are responsible for all types of life, has a special effect in acquiring what one seeks and longs for.

Therefore, invoking Allah's Name Al-Qayyum has a special effect in answering supplications and ending afflictions. The Sunan and Abu Hatim in his Sahib narrated that the Prophet $a said: "Allah's Greatest Name is in these two Verses."

﴿ وَإِلَـٰهُكُمْ إِلَـٰهٌ وَاحِدٌ لَّآ إِلَـٰهَ إِلَّا هُوَ ٱلرَّحْمَـٰنُ ٱلرَّحِيمُ ﴿١٦٣﴾ ﴾

(١٦٣) البقرة

And your Ilah (God) is One Ilah (God - Allah), La ilaha ilia Huwa (there is none who has the right to be worshipped but He), the Most Gracious, the Most

Merciful." (2:163)

And:

﴿ الٓمٓ ۝ ٱللَّهُ لَآ إِلَٰهَ إِلَّا هُوَ ٱلۡحَيُّ ٱلۡقَيُّومُ ۝ ﴾

(١:٢) آل عمران

"Alif Lam Meem. Allah! La ilaha ilia Huwa (none has the right to be worshipped but He), Al-Hayyul-Qayyum (the Ever Living, the One Who sustains and protects all that exists)." (3:1 -2)

At-Termezey commented that this is an authentic Hadith.

In the Sunan and the Sahih of Ibn Hibban it is In addition narrated that Anas said, "A man once supplicated, 'O Allah! I ask You by Your owning the praise, there is no deity worthy of worship except You, the Mannan (Munificent), Who created the heaven and the earth. O Owner of the praise and Honor. 'O Hayy, Qayyum.

The Prophet **b** said:

"He has asked Allah by His Greatest Name, which if He is called by it He answers, and if He is asked He gives."

This is why the Prophet used to say when making Du'a,

"O Hayy, O Qayyum." The Prophet's statement:

"O Allah, I seek Your Mercy. Do not make me rely on my own self for an instant, and lead all my affairs to success. There is no deity worthy of worship except You."

This supplication entails invoking Allah, Who grasps all good in His Hands. It In addition includes depending on Allah Alone, relating all matters to Him Alone and pleading to Him to lead the slave's matters to success.' It

In addition includes asking Him not to allow the slave to rely on his own self, and invoking Him by mentioning His Oneness. All these have a special effect in removing grief. Such is the case with the Prophet's statement:

"Allah is my Lord, I associate none with Him."

As for the Hadith that Ibn Mas'ud narrated:

"O Allah, I am Your slave, the son of Your slave..."

It contains what no one book can explain of divine knowledge and the secrets of the slavery to Allah. The

Hadith includes attesting to the slavery of the person and the slavery of his father and mother to Allah, that the forelock of the slave is in the Hands of Allah and that He does what He will with the slave. The slave cannot bring about benefit, harm, life, death or resurrection without Allah. When the slave's forelock is in someone else's hand, the slave does not own anything regarding himself. Rather, he is a prisoner in the grasp, power and authority of his owner.

The Prophet b In addition stated that:

"Your decision on me will certainly come to pass, and Your judgment on me is certainly just."

This portion of the Hadith contains two major aspects of Unity (Tawhid). First, the Hadith affirms Predestination and that Allah's decisions will certainly come to pass on His slaves and that the slave can neither escape them nor fend them off.

Allah's decisions are certainly just and thus do not contain any injustice in them for His slave. Rather, Allah's decisions always conform to justice and kindness. In addition, injustice is a shortcoming that constitutes a need of some sort, an ignorance or abuse. Such behavior can never occur by He Who has encompassing knowledge of everything, Who does not need anything or anyone, while everything and everyone stand in need of Him, and Who is the Most Just Disposer of affairs. No part of Allah's decisions can ever be empty of Wisdom and Perfection, just as none of it can ever escape His Power and Will. Allah's Wisdom is encompassing, just as His Power and Will are, and this is the reason why the Prophet Hud b said when his people wanted to scare him with their idols:

"I call Allah to witness and bear you witness that I am free from that which you ascribe as partners in worship. With Him (Allah). So plot against me, all of you, and give me no respite I put my trust in Allah, my Lord and your Lord! There is not a moving (living) creature but He has the grasp of its forelock. Verily, my Lord is on the Straight Path (the truth)." (11:54-56)

This Ayah indicates that although Allah owns the forelock of His slaves and does what He wills regarding their affairs, He is on the Straight Path, meaning He never decides anything regarding them that is not full of wisdom, justice, kindness and mercy. The Prophet's statement:

"Your Decision regarding me will certainly come to pass"

It is similar to what Allah said:

"There is not a moving (living) creature but He has the grasp of its forelock." (1:55)

In addition, the Prophet's statement:

"Your judgment on me is certainly just,"

It is In addition similar to what Allah said:

"Verily, my Lord is on the Straight Path (the truth)." (I 1:55)

Then, the Prophet s& begged Allah by the Names that He has called Himself with, those which the slaves know and those which they do not know, such as the Names that He has kept with Him and did not allow any angel or Messenger to have access to. This type of supplication is one of the best and dearest to Allah, along with being the most beneficial in achieving what one seeks and longs for.

The Prophet a& then asked Allah to make the Qura'an in his heart just like a spring is to the animals. He In addition asked Allah to make the Qura'an a remedy for his sadness and grief, so that it works just as medicine works when it removes an ailment, allowing the body to regain its health and youth. He In addition asked Allah to make the Qura'an the remover that clears rust and impurities from the heart. This remedy, when the ailing person uses it with a sincere heart, will certainly remove the ailment and will replace it with complete recovery, health and energy.

As for the supplication that Zhin An-Nun (Jonah) has made, it contains an affirmation of Tawhid (Unity) and praises Allah's perfection. In addition, it contains the slave's affirming his own injustice and the sins that he has committed, making the supplication an especially effective remedy for sadness, grief and anguish. It is In addition a very effective means of approach to Allah that ensures deliverance of what one seeks. Tawheed (Unity) and praising Allah include affirming all types of perfection for Allah and denying every type of shortcoming from approaching Him. One's affirming his injustices indicates the slave's faith in the religion and belief in reward and punishment. It In addition leads the slave to being humble and to repent to Allah, asking Him to forgive his faults and affirming his slavery and meekness to Allah. There are four matters that the slave would be begging Allah with in this supplication: Tawheed (Unity), praising Allah, affirming one's slavery to him and admitting one's mistakes.

As for the Hadith narrated by Abu Umamah,

"O Allah! I seek refuge with You from sadness and anguish,"

It contains seeking refuge with Allah from eight matters. There are four pairs of things that are related: grief and anguish, inability and laziness, cowardice and miserliness, and preponderance of debts and dominance of men. When a hated matter reaches the heart, it will be either a current concern, which will cause sadness, or it will be an anticipated matter of concern and anguish, which might affect the slave's important interests.

When one does not attain his vital interests, it will be because he is unable or unwilling to seek such interests. When one does not bring about benefit to others and to himself, it will be because he is either a coward or miserly and unwilling to spend from his money. When one falls under domination, it will be because of his being indebted, or because he is overwhelmed by other people unjustly. The Hadith includes seeking refuge from all types of evil.

Seeking forgiveness has a profound effect on repelling grief, anguish, sadness and depression. This is a fact agreed upon by those of wisdom of every nation. This is because sins and errors bring about grief, anguish, fear, sadness, distress, and ailments of the heart. After a while, those who are used to committing evil and sins will get bored with them. Then, they will commit these errors to drive away the depression and loneliness that they feel. Since these are the effects of sins and errors on the hearts, then the only remedy for this condition includes seeking forgiveness and repenting (to Allah).

As for the prayer, it has a profound effect on bringing relief and comfort to the heart, along with strengthening it and bringing about joy and elation to it. The prayer is the connection of the heart and soul with Allah and brings about feelings of joy by drawing closer to Him, remembering Him, feeling happy by speaking to Him, standing before Him, and using one's entire body and strength in implementing one's slavery to Him. The prayer In addition entails giving each organ and limb its due right of its slavery, while freeing the heart from remembering the creation, dealing with it or talking of it. The attention of the heart and limbs will thus be concentrated on the Lord and Creator, along with being free from the irritation caused by his enemy (Satan) while in prayer. This is why the prayer is one of the best types of medicines, remedies, and nutrition and is only suitable for healthy hearts. As for ailing hearts, they are just like ailing bodies, not fit for normal good foods.

The prayer is one of the best methods to acquire the good of this life and the life hereafter while fending off the harm of this and the next life. It In addition discourages people from falling into sin, cures diseases of the heart, fends off the ailments of the body, brings light to the heart and the face and elevates the energy of the limbs and the soul. It In addition brings about sustenance, fends off injustice, helps the oppressed, dissipates the lusts of the hearts, preserves one's bounty, fends off torment, brings about mercy, relieves calamity and helps against many ailments that attack the internal organs.

Ibn Majah narrated in his Sunan that Abu Hurayrah said, "The Messenger of Allah s& saw me while I was asleep suffering from a pain in the stomach. He said to me:

" 'O Abu Hurayrah! Does your stomach bother you (he said it in Persian)?' I said, 'Yes, O Messenger of Allah ! He said, 'Stand up and pray, because the prayer is a cure.'"

It was In addition reported that these words are not the Prophet's words but Abu Hurayrah said them to Mujahid,

When the hypocrite doctor's heart is not pleased with all these facts, we talk to him in medical terms. We say to him that the prayer is an exercise for the body and soul, as it entails various movements and positions, such as standing up, bowing down, prostrating, sitting on the ground, moving between these positions during which most of one's joints are used. In addition, most of the internal organs are exercised in the prayer, such as the stomach, the intestines and the rest of the body organs that are responsible for food and digestion. Who can deny that these acts and movements strengthen the body, especially when the soul is strengthened and relieved during the prayer? In this case, the body will be strengthened and the pain will subside.

The disease of hypocrisy and rejecting what the Messengers were sent with and preferring atheism has no cure except for Fire.

Allah said:

Fire (Hell). None shall enter it save the most wretched. Who denies and turns away." (92:14-16)

As for the effect of Jihad on repelling sadness and grief, it is well established, when the heart is forced to tolerate evil succeeding and becoming dominant and apparent, its sadness, depression, fear and distress increases. But when the soul performs Jihad for Allah's sake, Allah will turn that sadness and grief into happiness and strength. Allah said:

"Fight against them so that Allah will punish them by your hands and disgrace them and give you victory over them and heal the breasts of a believing people. And remove the anger of their believers') hearts. Allah accepts the repentance of whom He wills. Allah is All-Knowing, All-Wise." (9:14,15)

No act is more capable of removing the heart's grief, sadness and anguish more than jihad.

As for the effect of saying "there is no deity worthy of worship except Allah" in removing depression, it is a fact because these words include referring all matters, power and strength to Allah Alone. They In addition include submitting all matters to Allah, not denying Him any supremacy over any matter and referring the Ability to make any changes in this and the higher worlds to Allah Alone. Nothing can super-cede these words in this regard.

It was said that there is no angel who descends from or ascends to the heaven without uttering the words, "there is no power or strength except from Allah". Finally, these words have an especially profound effect in repelling the devil.

The Prophet's guidance on curing fear and insomnia

At-Termezey narrated in his Sunan that Khalid once complained to the Prophet $se that he does not sleep well at night. The Prophet s& said:

"When you go to bed say, 'O Allah! The Lord of the seven heavens and what is under them, the Lord of the earths and what they carry, and the Lord of the devils and whoever they misguide! Be my supporter against the evil of all of Your creation, preventing any of them to cause me any harm or injustice. Mighty indeed are those whom You support, honorable indeed is Your praise, and there is no deity worthy of worship except You.'"

In addition, At-Termezey narrated that the Messenger of Allah ﷺ used to teach his companions these words when they face any fear.

"I seek refuge with Allah's perfect Words from His anger and torment, and from the evil of His slaves and the whisperings of the devils. I seek refuge with You, my Lord from their presence."'

Ibn Umar used to teach these words to his children and would even write them for those who were not able to memorize them. There is no doubt that such words are suitable and effective in removing and repelling all types of harm.

The Prophet's guidance on treating burns

Burns are usually caused by fire which is the substance from which the devil was created, and this is why the devil finds it befitting his nature and the evil that he seeks to achieve. Therefore, the devil helps the fire cause harm. The fire usually seeks domination and devastation. These two matters, domination and devastation, are the guidance of the devil that he calls to and with which he leads mankind to destruction. The fire and the devil both seek domination and affliction, while Allah's Pride always intervenes by extinguishing these evils and the acts of the devil.

This is why praising Allah that He is the Great has a profound effect on extinguishing the fire, for Allah's Greatness overwhelms anything and everything. When the Muslim praises Allah's Greatness, this supplication will cause the fire and the efforts of the devil to fade away and thus the fire will be extinguished, Allah willing. We have used this method before and found it to be true.

The Prophet's guidance on staying healthy

Preserving one's good health requires the help of wetness that resists heat. The wetness resists heat while the heat helps mature various substances and rids the body of its wastes. Otherwise, without wetness, the excessive heat would harm the body and would not allow its organs to function normally, while excessive dryness allows the heat to burn the body and make it dry. Each one of the two conditions, wetness and heat, thus needs the other to sustain and allow the body to function. Further, since the heat feeds on wetness, it preserves the moisture from rotting and decomposing. When one of these two conditions is more dominant than the other, the constitution of the body will be altered and changed.

As we have stated, heat decomposes wetness, compelling the body to seek to replace the lost moisture with food and drink, which In addition provides the body with sustenance. When moisture is present in excessive amounts, the heat is not able to decompose the excess wetness and thus the moisture decomposes and rots, causing harm to the body. In this case, various ailments attack the body, as much as the body and the various organs are susceptible to accept these ailments. All these facts are taken from what Allah said:

"And eat and drink but waste not by extravagance..."

Allah directs the slaves to consume what helps the body of food and drink and to replace lost energy. The amount [of food and drink] that should be consumed should not exceed what the body has lost plus what the body needs to function properly. Otherwise, the excess food will be an extravagance that brings about ailments and will not preserve the health, and such is the case when one eats excessively or does not consume sufficient amounts.

Therefore, the few words that Allah stated hold the key to staying healthy. There is no doubt that the body is always going through the process of decomposing and producing waste. The more the decomposition occurs, the less the heat will be effective, since decomposition feeds on moistures (which in turn feeds the inner heat). When the heat is weak, the digestion efficiency decreases until the moisture dissipates. Thus, the heat will be extinguished and consequently, the term (life span) that the slave was allowed in this life will come to an end.

The goal behind the person seeking a cure for himself and for others is to preserve the body until everyone reaches their final destination (death), not because preserving the necessary moistures and heat will keep the youth and health forever, for this goal is not attainable in this life. The goal that the doctor seeks to achieve entails preserving the existent wetness from what might spoil it and to preserve body-heat from what might weaken its power. The doctor thus preserves the balance between the two powers or conditions in the body, just as Allah has created the heaven and earth with justice and perfect balance. In fact, the entire creation thrives on and by justice and balance.

Those who study the guidance of the Prophet s& will find it the best guidance with which the health of the body can and will be preserved. Preserving good health depends on eating and drinking sensibly and on utilizing one's clothes, place of residence, the air, sleep, being awake, mobility, idleness, sex, extracting the excess material of the body and keeping whatever is necessary and important in the best form and shape. When these aspects are satisfied in the manner that is suitable for the body, the area, age and custom, the person is more likely to have good health and well being until it is his time to die.

Good health is one of the best bounties that Allah bestows on mankind and In addition one of His best rewards. In fact, good heath is the best earthly bounty of all, and those who have been bestowed with sound comprehension should strive to preserve their health and protect it against what might oppose or alter it.

Al-Bokhary narrated in his Sahih that the Messenger of Allah gg said:

"Two bounties regarding which many people cheat themselves. health and free time."

Further, At-Termezey narrated that Abdullah bin Mihsan Al-Ansari

said, The Messenger of Allah **b** said:

" 'He who reaches the morning while health in his body. safe in his residence and having day's sustenance, will be as if the entire life of this world was granted to him."

In addition, At-Termezey related from Abu Hurayrah that the Prophet **b** said:

"The first blessing that the slave will be asked about on the Day of Resurrection will be the saying to him, 'Have We not made your body healthy and drove away your thirst with cold water?'

This is why some of the (righteous predecessors) stated that the Verse:

﴿ ثُمَّ لَتُسْـَٔلُنَّ يَوْمَئِذٍ عَنِ ٱلنَّعِيمِ ۝٨ ﴾ (٨) التكاثر

"Then on that Day you shall be asked about the delights (you indulged in. this world)." (1O2:8)

It is referring to health.

In addition, Imam Ahmad narrated that Abu Bakr As-Siddiq said, I heard the Messenger of Allah **b** saying:

"Ask Allah for certainty and good health, for indeed, no one will have a better possession after certainty of Faith than good health."

The Prophet sg joined the well being of this life and the Next Life. Further, the slave's success cannot be complete in both lives except by joining certainty of faith and well being. Certainty of faith fends off the torments of the Next Life while well being fends off the ailments of this life that might attack the body or the heart.

An-Nas'ay narrated that Abu Hurayrah ^ <iii ^ related from the

Prophet b that he said:

"Ask Allah for forgiveness, well being and health. Indeed, no one acquires a better possession after certainty of faith than good health."

The three matters mentioned in the Hadith entail removing the ills of the past with forgiveness, of the present with well being and of the future with immunity (from error and thus from the Torment). Indeed, these words entail the continuity of well being always.

Abdur-Rahman bin Abu Laila said that Abu Ad-Dardaa said, "O Messenger of Allah b it is more beloved to me to acquire good health so that I am thankful for it rather than being tested and then observe patience. The Messenger of Allah b said:

"The Messenger of Allah b likes good health just like you."

Further, Ibn Ab'ass is reported to have narrated:

"A Bedouin man came to the Messenger of Allah b and said to him, 'What should I ask for after I finish the five prayers?' The Prophet b said, 'Ask Allah for good health.' The man repeated the question, and the Prophet as said to him after the third time. 'Ask Allah for well being in this and the Next Life.'"

If this is how significant health is, we should then mention and study the Prophet's guidance on preserving health and well being, for we will come to realize that his guidance is the most perfect in this regard. With the Prophet's guidance, one attains health of his body and heart and In addition their very existence, both in this world and in the Next Life. Allah is sought for all types of help, and our dependence is on Him, and there is neither power nor strength except from Him.

The Prophet **b** did not restrict himself to eating one type of food

This would be harmful to one's nature. In addition, the body could face weakness and even death if one consumed only one type of food. In addition, when someone is used to only one type of food his body does not accept any other type. Restricting the diet to only one type of food, even if it is the best type, is harmful and dangerous.

The Prophet a? used to eat what his people used to eat in their regular diet, such as meat, fruits, bread, dates, and other types of food that we mentioned.

When one type of food needed to be made milder

the Prophet s^ would use its opposite, such as neutralizing the hotness of ripe dates with watermelon. If he did not find what neutralized the effect of a type of food, he would eat of it the necessary amount without excessiveness.

When the Prophet b would not like a food, he would simply refrain from eating it and would not force himself to have it. This is a great aspect of preserving the health. When one eats what he does not have an appetite for, the food's harm will overweigh its benefit.

Abu Hurayrah said, "The Messenger of Allah b never criticized a food. If he had an appetite for it, he ate it. Otherwise, he did not eat from it," When the Prophet b was presented with lizard meat (Dhabb) he did not eat from it. He was asked, "Is it disallowed?" He said:

"No; But, this food is not among the foods that my people used to eat, and I do not have an appetite for it."

The Prophet ^ used eat a regular diet when he was offered a type of food that he was not used to eating and which he had no appetite for, he refrained from eating it. Yet, he did not prevent those who were used to that kind of food and who had an appetite for it from eating it.

The Prophet b used to like eating meat, especially the arm and the upper parts of the sheep. This is the part that was poisoned and offered to the Prophet b.

In the Sahihain it is narrated that the Prophet m, was once brought some meat and that he was given the arm, which he liked. Furthermore, Abu 'Ubaid narrated that Dhiba'ah bint Az-Zubair said that she slaughtered a sheep in her house. The Messenger of Allah b sent to her.

"Feed us from your sheep." She said to the messenger, 'Only the neck is left, and I feel shy to send it to the Messenger of Allah b.' The Prophet's emissary went back to the Prophet b to teII him what happened. The Messenger said, 'Go back to her and tell her to send it, because the neck is the part that guides the sheep and is closer to the good things and far away from the septic things.

There is no doubt that the lightest part of the sheep's meat is the neck, arm and thigh. These parts are In addition the easiest to digest and the softest on the stomach. The method the Prophet b observed in this regard satisfies the three basic rules regarding food, which are, the food being beneficial and helpful to the nature, being light on the stomach and not heavy, and being quickly digested. This is the best type of food to consume and consequently, eating a small part of this food is better than consuming a large amount of the other types of food.

The Prophet bused to like eating sweets and

honey. Meat, honey and sweets are the best foods and the most beneficial for the body, liver and various organs. In addition, eating these types of food has a profound effect on preserving the health and strength, and that is why only those who already suffering from an ailment would be harmed by consuming them.

The Prophet s& used to eat bread with whatever condiment happened to be available. Sometimes he would eat bread with meat, sometimes with watermelon and sometimes with dates. One time, the Prophet **b** placed a dried date on a piece of bread and said that this, the date, is the condiment of that, the bread. Barley bread is cold and dry while dates are hot and wet, so eating both foods together is one of the wisest decisions, especially for those used to this type of food, such as the people of Al-Medina. Sometimes, the Prophet ^ would eat bread with vinegar, saying, 'What a good condiment vinegar is.' This praise for the vinegar came because it was the only available food in the house then, not because vinegar is better than the other types of foods, as some ignorant people think. The Hadith sates that the Prophet as once came to one of his wives and asked if she had any condiment when they offered him some bread. When she said that they only had vinegar, he said, "What a good condiment vinegar is."

Eating bread with a condiment preserves the

health unlike eating only one type of food. Condiments are called as such because when they are added to the bread, the bread tastes better and the food helps preserve the health.

In addition, the Prophet ^ used to eat from the fruits that were in season in his land, as this In addition is one of the best methods of preserving health, Allah's wisdom decided that every land has its own fruits that are suitable and beneficial to that land when in season. When the people consume these fruits they will help preserve their health and well being and it serves as several medicines. On the other hand, those who refrain from eating the fruits of their area will be among the most ailing persons and the farthest from good health and well being.

The wetness that the various fruits contain represents the favorable heat of the season and the land. The stomach would then be able to bring the fruits to maturity and would fend off their harm, if one does not eat them excessively causing his nature to bear what it cannot bear. In addition, one should not spoil the food that his stomach is digesting by eating fruits, nor drink water with it. Fruits should be eaten only after the food in the stomach is digested to prevent constipation. Those who consume fruits in the proper manner, in the proper time and in the proper conditions the fruits act as a cure and a remedy for them.

The Prophet's guidance on the proper way to sit while eating

The Prophet **b** said:

"I do not eat while leaning on my side." He In addition said, "I only sit like the slave sits and eat like the slave eats."

Leaning on the side harms the stomach because it prevents the food

from going down the proper channel and reaching the stomach quickly, as it pressures the stomach and does not allow it to be open properly for the food to pass through.

Eating while leaning on something is the practice of the arrogant people and this is why the Prophet **b** said that:

"I only eat like the slave eats."

The Prophet **b** used to sit on his feet while eating. He used to place his knees on the ground and would place the bottom of his left foot on the upper part of his right foot in humility for the Lord and in respect for the food and for those present. This is the best way to sit for eating, because the organs of the body will all be in their proper position, along with observing good manners.

As we have stated, the best way to eat is sitting up with the organs of the body in their natural position. The worst way of eating is leaning on one's side because the windpipe and the chewing organs will be pressured in this position and squeeze the stomach.

In addition, the Prophet **b** could have meant that he does not sit while leaning on pillows as the arrogant do and those who want to eat more food. Rather, the Prophet as used to eat what is barely sufficient just as the slave does.

The Prophet b used three fingers while eating

This is one of the best methods of eating. Eating with one or two fingers does not help the appetite or provide sufficient amount of food in each bite, and consequently, one would only be able to finish eating after a long time. In addition, the organs responsible for handling the food would not be comfortable with the fact that they are getting so little food with each bite, in this case the organs will pass through periods of inactivity while one is still eating! If one eats one or two grains at a time, he will neither enjoy eating or feel comfortable. Eating with five fingers sends to the stomach more food than it can handle in each bite. Death might even occur if one of the organs becomes clogged with excessive food. In addition, the organs of the body will be forced to handle large amounts of food and thus the person would neither enjoy eating it nor would their body be comfortable digesting it. Therefore, the best way of eating is by using three fingers as the Prophet b and those who imitate him do.

The Prophet's guidance on certain combinations of food

The Prophet b never mixed fish and milk, milk and sour foods or two hot dishes, or two cold dishes, two sticky dishes, two constipating dishes, two laxative dishes, two heavy dishes, two liquid foods or two types of foods that produced the same condition. In addition, he did not join between two types of food that caused opposite effects, such as constipating and diarrhea, or easily digested with heavy foods broiled with cooked foods, dry with fresh foods, eggs and milk or meat and milk. In addition, he neither ate a food when it is rather hot, nor old food that was heated for him the next day. Further, he did not eat any salty or rotten foods, such as pickles. All these types of foods are harmful and cause the health to change for the worst.

The Prophet b In addition used to neutralize the harm of some foods by their opposites, as much as he could. When the food is hot, he neutralizes its effect with a cold food, and when it is dry, he neutralizes it with wet foods, such as eating ripe dates with cucumbers and dried dates with butter. He In addition used to drink the water of soaked dates to neutralize the effect of heavy foods. Further, the Prophet bused to eat dinner even if it only consisted of a few dates.

Abu Nu'aym mention that the Prophet m, used to discourage sleeping just after eating food because it will harden the heart. The doctors In addition advise the people to walk even a few steps after dinner, because sleeping just after dinner is very harmful. Muslim doctors add that one could In addition pray after eating his dinner, so that the food resides in the bottom of the stomach where it will be easily digested.

The Prophet b did not drink [water or milk] with his food, because the drink would spoil the food, especially when the water is hot or cold.

It is not preferred that one drinks water after sports activity, when tired, after sexual intercourse, before and after eating food and after eating fruit. In addition, it is not preferred that one drinks water after taking a bath and after sleeping. All these activities will harm the health and one should not think about the benefits he might gain from drinking with the food.

The Prophet's guidance on beverages

The Prophet's guidance regarding beverages was In addition the most beneficial for preserving the health. The Prophet b used to drink honey with cold water, and this is an especially effective method to preserve the heath that only the best doctors could have knowledge of. Drinking honey on an empty stomach will dissolve phlegm, purify the stomach's protective layers and dissipate its viscidity and excrements while heating it mildly. Honey In addition helps against the clogs in the stomach, kidney, liver and prostate. Honey is much more profitable to the stomach than any other sweet.

We should state that honey might harm those suffering from bile, because it aggravates it. In this case, the harmful side effect of honey is neutralized when taking it with vinegar, as this method makes the honey very beneficial. In addition, honey is much more beneficial than any other sugar based drink, especially for those who are not used to these types of sweet drinks.

When one drinks sweet drinks that he is not used to, he will not benefit as much as he will benefit from honey, as this is the role that one's customs play. The customs remove foundations and establish foundations..

When the drink is both sweet and cold, it will be most beneficial for the body and one of the best methods to preserve its health and the well being of the soul, strength, liver, and heart. In addition, when the drink is both sweet and cold, the body will be eager for it, will benefit from it, nutrition wise, and will quickly digest and transfer it to the other organs of the body.

Cold water is wet, quenches the thirst, preserves the moistures in the body, regenerate the moistures that the body has lost, softens the food and helps transfer it through the veins quickly.

The doctors differed on if water is In addition nutritional, as some of them said that it is nutritious since the body grows and becomes milder and stronger, especially when it is in need of water. They In addition said that there are several similarities between man and animals, such as growing and

becoming fairer and stronger. The plants In addition grow and have their own special kind of senses and movements. Since plants feed on water, how can anyone deny that water is nutritious, they asked?

They In addition say that they do not deny that food provides most of the nutritional intake of the body. They only deny that water is not considered of any nutritional value at all. They In addition say that the food only provides nourishment because of the watery parts it contains.

They In addition say that water is the resource of life for animals and plants. There is no doubt, they say, that the substance that is closer to the resource of life will provide more nourishment. How about if the substance is the resource of life itself?

Allah said:

"And We have made from water every living thing." (2 :3O)

They ask, how is it that the resource of life does not provide nutrition to the body?

They In addition add that the thirsty person would regain his strength and activity when he satisfies his thirst. He will In addition be able to restrict his food intake and rely on water. However, the thirsty person would not quench his thirst if he eats a large amount of food. They add, "We do not deny that water helps transfer the food to the various parts and organs of the body. We only deny the statement that water does not have any nutritional value at all."

Another group denied that water is nutritional saying that water alone does not sustain life, or help the body grow, or restore the moisture that the body has lost through heat. However, their opponents do not deny these facts. They only say every substance provides nutrition in a different way compatible to its nature. For instance, good aroma provides a type of nutrition, and this fact makes the nutritional value of the water even more apparent.

In short, when the water is cold and mixed with a sweet substance, such as honey, raisins, dates or sugar, it will be one of the most beneficial substances that enters the body and will indeed preserve health. This is why the best drink to the Prophet b was cold and sweet. Warm water begets flatulence and is not favorable for the body or the health.

Since water that is kept overnight is more favorable than recently drawn water, the Prophet ate said when he entered a garden of Abu At-Taihan:

"Do you hove any water that was kept in its skin overnight?"

He was brought some of that water and he drank from it. [Abu Dawood, bin Majah and Ahmad]. This Hadith was collected by Al-Bokhary, who narrated that the Prophet as said:

"If you have some water still in its skin (then bring me some). Otherwise we will sip (from the well).."

Water that is not freshly drawn is similar to yeasty

dough, while freshly drawn water is similar to the dough that does not contain yeast. When water is soaked overnight, its earthly and sandy pollutants will rest on the bottom. It was mentioned the Prophet as liked kept water, as 'A'esha said:

"Fresh water was being brought to the Messenger of Allah b drown from the weII designated for drinking."

The water that is kept in skins, especially leather skins, has a better taste than water kept in clay containers. This is why the Prophet ^s asked for the water that was kept in skin containers rather than the other types of containers. When the water is kept in skin containers, it will filter through the pores in the skin [thus making its taste better]. Similarly, the water that is kept in clay containers that allnw the water to filter is better than that in the clay containers that do not allow the water to filter. The Prophet s& had the best methods, the most honorable soul and the best guidance in every matter. He has showed his nation the most beneficial methods and means concerning the benefit of their hearts and bodies in this life and the Next Life.

A'esha said that the best type of drink to the Prophet b was cold and sweet. This statement might indicate that the Prophet's drink contained fresh, sweet water drawn from wells and springs. Her statement might In addition indicate that he used to drink water that is mixed with honey or soaked dates and raisins. Or, her statement could carry both meanings, which is the correct opinion.

The Prophet's statement:

"if you have some water in its skin. Otherwise we will drink from its mouth."

It indicates that it is allowed to drink the water directly from the pool or container with the mouth. Many doctors advise against this method and say that it is harmful for the stomach. It appears that the Prophet b did so only to demonstrate that it is allowed. Further, drinking with the mouth from the pool is harmful when one lays on his stomach and face, such as drinking from a river or a spring. Drinking with the mouth from an elevated pool of water while sitting up is not different from drinking using the hands,

The Prophet b guided his nation to drink while sitting down

He specifically commanded his nation not to drink while standing up, He In addition commanded those who drink while standing to vomit. Yet, he did drink while standing as is correctly reported of him.

Some people said that the Prophet's drinking while

standing overrules his command not to drink while standing. Another group said that his drinking while standing only demonstrates that this practice is only disliked not prohibited. Another group said that there is no contradiction between the two Ahadeeth. The Prophet i& drank while standing when he needed to do so, as he came to the well of Zamzam and was given a bucket of water that he drank from while standing.

Drinking while standing begets many ailments and does not quench the thirst, nor will the water settle in the stomach so that the liver transfers it to the rest of the body. In this case, the water will descend quickly to the stomach and will aggravate it, and the water will not be digested properly. However, if one does this occasionally, it will not harm him.

Drinking water in three separate breaths

Muslim narrated that Anas said that the Messenger of Allah **b** used to sip the water in three separate breaths and would say:

"This method quenches the thirst better and is more palatable and sanitary."

This Hadith indicates that the Prophet ^s used to remove the cup away from his mouth, take a breath and then drink some more. In another Hadith, the Prophet **b**

In addition, when one takes the drink in one breath, he might choke on it because of the large amount of the liquid. However, there is no fear from choking when one takes a breath while drinking. Further, when one takes a drink, the hot gases accumulating in his body will ascend from around the liver and the heart because of the cold water or liquid that is descending on the stomach. In this case, the water will come rushing down while the gases are ascending, causing flatulence and sometimes choking the person. One will not enjoy the drink in this case.

In addition, when cold water descends suddenly on the liver it will weaken it and cause a decrease in its temperature. However, when one takes the drink in separate sips, the liver will not lose its warmth and thus will not weaken. Similarly, when one pours water on a boiling pot, it will not decrease its temperature significantly,

At-Termezey narrated that the Prophet b said:

"Do not drink in one breath just as the camel does. Rather, drink twice and thrice, and mention (Allah's) Name before drinking and thank (Him) upon finishing."

Mentioning Allah's Name before drinking and thanking Him upon finishing has a significant effect in benefiting from the drink, enjoying it while fending off its harm. Imam Ahmad said, "When the food has four qualities, it will have become perfect: when Allah's Name is mentioned before having it, when Allah is thanked after finishing with it, when there are many hands to eat from it, and when it is from legal, pure sources."

Covering pots and closing water skins

Muslim narrated in his Sahih that Jabir bin Abdullah said, I heard the Messenger of Allah b say;

"Cover the pot and tie the knot of the water skin, for there is a day during the year in which a disease descends and falls in whatever pot that is not covered, or water skin, which is not tied, that it passes by."

This Hadith contains a type of divine knowledge that the doctors could never reach on their own. Laith bin Sa'd, one of the narrators of this Hadith, said, "Non-Muslims know which day it is, in January, and they try to avoid its harm."

The Prophet b commanded that the pots be covered, even with a branch, so that one makes covering it a habit. In addition, when one covers the pot with a branch, crawling insects will not fall in the food but will pass over it on the branch.

Furthermore, the Prophet ga commanded that we mention Allah's Name when covering the pot to repel Satan and insects and animals.

Drinking from the mouth of the water skin is not allowed

Al-Bokhary narrated that Ibn Ab'ass said:

"The Messenger of Allah b disallowed drinking from the mouth of the water skin."

There are many benefits in this Hadith. For instance, when one drinks from the tip or the mouth of the water skin, he will breathe in it and will give it an offensive odor. In addition, water may descend strongly and harm the stomach. In addition, there might be an insect in the water that one is unaware of, and that might harm him if he swallows it. In addition, water might be polluted with harmful substances that will enter the person's stomach while he is unaware. In addition, drinking from the mouth of the skin fills the stomach with air and thus the water will not have sufficient space.

Drinking from a chipped cup is not allowed

Abu Dawood narrated in his Sunan that Abu Sa'id Al-Khudri said:

"The Messenger of Allah b disallowed drinking from the chipped side of the cup and from breathing in the drink."

This Hadith In addition teaches the Muslim many types of good behavior. For instance, drinking from the chipped side of the cup might cause one to swallow the substances that have accumulated near the chipped side. In addition, one might not be able to enjoy his drink when he is drinking from the cup's chipped side. In addition, dirt and fat concentrate near the chipped side and are usually not fully cleaned when rinsed. In addition, the chipped side of the cup is the worst and is not beneficial. One of ours saw a man once buying inferior goods and said to him, "Do not buy it, do you not know that Allah has not blessed inferior things?" In addition, the chipped side of the cup might cause injury to the mouth.

As for breathing in the cup, it will transfer the foul odor from the person to the drink. This is why the Prophet s@ has disallowed breathing or blowing in it. In the Hadith that At-Termezey narrated, Ibn Ab'ass said:

"The Messenger of Allah ate prohibited breathing in the pot (or cup) or blowing on it."

If some asks, "What about the Hadith ın the Sahihain in which Anas narrated:

"The Messenger of Allah **b** used to take three breaths while drinking"

We say that we believe in this Hadith and that it does not contradict the Ahadeeth that we mentioned, because it only means that the Prophet **b** did not sip the drink in one breath.

The Prophet b drank milk undiluted or mixed with water

Drinking sweet milk in hot areas is very beneficial in preserving the health and providing moisture for the body and the liver. This is especially the case when the animals that produce the milk have grazed on wormwood, lavender, lavender cotton, and so forth, because their milk is both a food and a medicine.

At-Termezey narrated that the Prophet b said:

"When any of you eats food, let him say, 'O Allah! Bless it for us and give us what is better than it.' When someone is given milk, let him say. 'O Allah! Bless it for us and give us more of it.' Certainly, milk is the only food or drink that is sufficient."

Further, Muslim narrated:

"The Messenger of Allah b used to be made Nabith (some dates soaked in water) in the beginning of the night and would drink it in the morning of the next day, the next night and the next day, and another night, and the next day until 'Asr. If any of it remained, he would then give it to a servant or would order that it be poured out."

The Nabith mentioned in this Hadith is some dates

that are soaked in water to sweeten the water and it is used both in drinks and foods. The Nabith has a great benefit in strengthening the body and preserving the health. The Prophet ﷺ did not drink the Nabith that is more than three days old fearing that it might have started to decompose and become intoxicating.

The Prophet's guidance regarding clothes

The Prophet's guidance regarding clothes was the best guidance, the most beneficial for the body and the easiest to wear and take off.

The Prophet **b** used to wear an outer garment and Izar (which covered the body), as these types of clothes are the softest on the body. The Prophet ate In addition liked to wear shirts, which was preferred by him.

What the Prophet s& used to wear was the most beneficial for the body, as his clothes did not have excessively long or wide sleeves. Rather, the sleeves were to the wrists and would not be longer than the hand, as this would make them harder to wear and to move about easily. Further, the sleeves were not shorter than what we have described, so as not to expose the hands to the cold and heat,

In addition, the Prophet's shirts and garments did not reach the ankles and would usually reach the middle of his legs. Otherwise, if the clothes were longer, they will restrict the movement and make one feel restrained. They were not shorter than what we have described, so as not to expose the thighs to the heat and cold.

The Prophet's turban was not excessively big so that it did not harm the head. It was not very small either, otherwise it would not be sufficient to protect the head from the heat and cold. It was medium in size, and he used to pass a part of it under his chin to protect the neck from the heat and cold and to keep the turban firmly on the head when riding his horse or camel and when in battle.

Many people use some type of braces instead of passing the turban under the chin, although the two methods cannot be compared in terms of benefit or even beauty.

When one thinks about the types of clothes that the Prophet ag used, he will find that they are indeed among the best for the body and health and the farthest from extravagance and difficulty to wear.

Most of the time, the Prophet b used to wear Khuff (socks) while traveling, because the feet would need such types of foot covering to fend off the effects of the heat and cold. Sometimes, he would use the Khuff when he was not traveling.

The best colors that the Prophet sag used to wear were white and striped garments. He did not wear all red, black or dyed garments.

As for the red garment the Prophet **b** was reported to have worn, it was a Yemeni garment that had black, red, and white stripes. We have mentioned this before and stated that some people erred when they thought that the Prophet wore red garments.

The Prophet's guidance concerning one's place of residence

The Prophet s& had knowledge that this life-term was just a transit station in which one resides for the remainder of his earthly life and then moves on to the Next Life. It was not a part of his guidance or the guidance of his companions, and all those who followed and imitated him, to establish and be concerned with building houses, raising them, beautifying them and extending them. Rather, their places of residence were among the best transit stations that could benefit the traveler, fending off the cold, heat, people's eyes, the beasts and even the fear that it might fall down on them because of its considerable weight! In addition, their residence were neither shared by wild animals, due to their size, nor did the air and wind buffet them due to their excessive height. They were neither built underground, because this would harm the inhabitants, nor were they very high above the ground. They were on the level of the ground. These are the best types of houses, most beneficial and least cold or hot. They were not so small that the inhabitants would be irritated by their smallness, nor very spacious, for the residents would not be able to benefit from the excess space. Their homes did not contain bathrooms so that they did not bother the people with a stinking odor. The scent in their homes was fresh, as the Prophet used to like good smells and always had a good scent in his house. In fact, the Prophet's sweat was one of the best scents ever smelled, and such was the scent of his body. There is no doubt that this is the description of the best type of home, most suitable for the body and for staying healthy.

The Prophet's guidance concerning sleep

Those who read about the Prophet's guidance concerning being awake and concerning sleep will find that his sleep was the best and most beneficial for the body, the organs and one's strength. He used to sleep in the early part of the night and would wake up in the beginning of the latter part, use siwak (natural toothbrush), perform ablution and pray as much as Allah permitted him. Consequently, the body, the organs and one's strength will acquire their fair share of sleep, rest and physical activity, along with acquiring the complete rewards (from Allah). This method ensures righteousness of the heart and body in this life and the Next Life.

The Prophet ^ did not oversleep or deprive his body of necessary sleep, making his method in this regard the most perfect. He used to sleep when sleep is warranted and would lay on his right side and remember Allah in supplication until sleep overwhelmed his eyes. In addition, his body would not be burdened with overeating or overdrinking. He neither slept on the bare floor, or on high beds. Rather, he had mats made of leaves, used to lean on a pillow and would sometimes place his hand under his cheek.

We will now elaborate on the beneficial and harmful methods of sleep.

Sleep is a condition during which the body's instinctive heat becomes idle, so that the body gets some rest. There are two types of sleep, normal and abnormal. Normal sleep entails resting the inner powers and the senses. When these powers are idle, the body refrains from its usual activity and thus the vapors and wetness that were moving and decomposing while awake would ascend to the brain which is the residence of these powers. The brain then becomes idle, and this is the normal type of sleep.

Abnormal (i.e. heavy) sleep occurs because of an accident or a disease. In this case, the excess wetness will take over the brain in a manner that prevents the person from waking up easily. Or, excessive amounts of vapor and moisture ascend to the brain, just as what happens in the aftermath of overeating and overdrinking, and cause the brain to relax and thus the person goes to sleep.

There are two benefits in sleep: the senses get to rest from the fatigue that overtakes them, n this case, the senses will rest from the tiresome activity that occurs when one is awake. The second benefit is digesting food and leading the various mixtures, conditions or temperaments to maturity (processing bodily wastes). While one is asleep, his instinctive energy or heat concentrates on the digestion process and this is why the body gets cold and needs a cover while one is asleep.

The best type of sleep is for one to sleep on his right side so that the food sits in the stomach comfortably, for the stomach leans to left side as we have stated. One could In addition lay on his left side a little so that the digestion is made faster because the stomach leans on the liver. One should then turn again on his right side to help the stomach push the food down the stomach and this way one starts and ends his sleep while laying on his right side, Sleeping on the left side regularly harms the heart because the organs of the body will pressure the heart with their weight.

in the early hours of the day and in the afternoon. Ibn Ab'ass once saw his son sleeping in the early morning and said to him, "Wake up! Do you sleep at the hour during which sustenance is being divided,"

It was said that sleeping during the day is of three types: good habit, which entails sleeping around noon; careless habit, which occurs in the early morning and keeps one busy from matters of this and the Next Life; and madness, which occurs after 'Asr (afternoon). This is why some of ours said, "Those who sleep after 'Asr and lose their minds should only blame their own selves."

Sleeping during the early morning prevents sustenance from coming, in that the early morning is the time when the creation goes out to seek their sustenance. Being asleep during this time in which sustenance is being divided causes one to miss out on this chance of gaining sustenance, except when one sleeps for a necessity or a need. This type of sleep is In addition very harmful for the body because it causes numbness in the senses and spoils the stomach's contents that should be being decomposed through physical activity. Further, sleeping in the early morning hours causes numbness and a general weakness in the body, especially if one goes to sleep before relieving himself (using the toilet), moving about, performing physical activity and before having the stomach busy (by eating some food). This itself is a difficult ailment that even leads to more ailments.

Sleeping under the sun excites otherwise dormant ailments, and such is the case with sleeping while a part of the body is under the sun and a part of the body is under the shade. Abu Dawood narrated that Abu Hurayrah said that the Messenger of Allah b said:

"If one of you was in the shade and then the shade recedes and exposes a part of the body to the sun while the other part is still under the shade, let him move from that place." [Al-Hakim].

Ibn Majah and Abu Dawood a so narrated:

"The Messenger of Allah b disallowed sitting between the shade and the sun."

This Hadith indicates that it is not allowed for one to sleep while partially in the shade and partially in the sun.

Further, in the Sahihain it is narrated that Al-Bara bin 'Azib said that the Messenger of Allah b said:

"Whenever you go to bed perform ablution like that for the prayer, lie on your right side and say, 'O Allah! I surrender myself

to You. turn my face towards You, entrust all my

affairs to You and depend upon You for Your Blessings both with hope (in You) and fear of You. There is no fleeing from You, and there is no place of protection and safety except with You O Allah! I believe in Your Book (the Qura'an) which You have revealed and in Your

Prophet (Muhammad) whom You have sent.' Make these words the last of your speech, because if you die on that very night, you will die on the Fitrah (i.e. or the religion of Islam)."

In addition, Al-Bokhary narrated that 'A'esha said:

"When the Messenger of Allah **b** would pray the two (voluntary) Rak'ah of Dawn, he would lay on his right side."

It was said that the wisdom behind sleeping on the right side of the body is that the person does not oversleep. Since the heart leans towards the left side, then sleeping on the right side prevents the heart from residing in its normal place thus causing the sleeping person to wake up when he feels restless. Sleeping on the left side makes the heart comfortable and thus the person oversleeps and misses out on the affairs of his life and religion.

Since seeping is similar to death, it is not possible or suitable for the Ever-Living Who does not die. Further, sleeping is not suitable for the residents of Paradise. In addition, while asleep, people need to be protected from every type of harm or affliction, and since only Allah is Able to fulfill this need, the Prophet ﷺ has taught us to supplicate to Allah with words of reliance, fear and eagerness before going to sleep. With these words, one invokes Allah's prefect protection for himself and for his body, The Prophet ﷺ In addition directed us to remember our faith in Allah and making such words the last of our speech at night. Since one might die in his sleep, he then will enter Paradise if these words of faith were the last words he uttered in this world.

The Prophet's guidance in this regard has included the benefits of the heart, body and soul while awake and asleep and for this life and the Next Life. Allah's peace and blessings be on he whose nation has acquired all types of good through him.

The Prophet's statement:

"I submit myself to You."

This means I surrender myself to You just as the owned slave surrenders his freedom to his master.

Further; turning the face towards Allah means directing one's full attention to the Lord with sincerity with the intention and while affirming being a slave, humble and obedient to Him. Allah said:

﴿ فَإِنْ حَآجُّوكَ فَقُلْ أَسْلَمْتُ وَجْهِىَ لِلَّهِ وَمَنِ ٱتَّبَعَنِ ﴾

(٢٠) آل عمران

"So if they dispute with you (Muhammad b say; "I hove submitted myself to Allah (in Islam), and (so have) those who follow me."(3:2O)

The face is the most honorable part of the body and the residence of the senses and awareness.

Referring matters to Allah means submission and contentment in the heart, while being pleased with what Allah decides and chooses of what He wills and with what He is pleased with. Referring all affairs to Allah is one of the honorable parts of slavery to Allah.

Leaning one's back to Allah indicates the strength of one's depending on and trust in Him. He who leans his back to a firm foundation will not have fear of falling down,

The heart has two types of strength, seeking, which is In addition eagerness, and running away, which is In addition fear. The slave seeks his interest and runs away from whatever might harm him. Therefore, the Prophet s& has joined both powers in this Hadith by saying, "With eagerness and fear."

The Prophet ^ then praised the Lord by stating that the slave has no refuge or resort from Allah except Allah. Allah is the One Whom the slave seeks refuge with so that He saves him from Himself, n another Hadith, the Prophet **b** said:

"I seek refuge with Your Pleasure from Your Anger, and with Your Pardon from Your Torment, and I seek refuge from You with You."

Therefore, Allah Alone grants refuge to His slave and saves him from His torment, which a so occurs by His will. Torment and Favor are both from Allah Alone. Further, the slave asks Allah for support against what He has (of Torment and trials) and seeks Him Alone for his safety. He

Alone ıs the Lord of everything and nothing occurs except by His will.

﴿ وَإِن يَمْسَسْكَ ٱللَّهُ بِضُرٍّ فَلَا كَاشِفَ لَهُۥٓ إِلَّا هُوَ ۖ وَإِن يُرِدْكَ بِخَيْرٍ فَلَا رَآدَّ لِفَضْلِهِۦ ﴾ (١٠٧) يونس

"And if Allah touches you with hurt, there is none who can remove it but He..." (1O:1O7)

And:

﴿ قُلْ مَن ذَا ٱلَّذِى يَعْصِمُكُم مِّنَ ٱللَّهِ إِنْ أَرَادَ بِكُمْ سُوٓءًا أَوْ أَرَادَ بِكُمْ رَحْمَةً ﴾ (١٧) الأحزاب

"Say: 'Who is he who can protect you from Allah if He intends to harm you. or intends mercy on you?' " (33:17)

The Prophet b then ended the supplication by affirming faith in Allah's Book and Messenger, which holds the key to the ultimate safety and success in this life and the Next Life. This is the Prophet's guidance concerning sleep.

The Prophet's guidance on waking

The Prophet b used to wake up when the rooster crowed and would then praise Allah, affirm His Greatness and Oneness, supplicate to Him, and he would use siwak (natural toothbrush). He would then perform ablution and stand before his Lord reciting His Speech (the Qura'an), praising Him and hoping in Him with eagerness and fear, What actions can be more preserving for the health of the heart, body. soul and genera strength and that acquires the favors of this life and the Next Life than these actions?

The Prophet's guidance on physical activity

As for the Prophet's guidance while busy and while free, we will mention a part of the Prophet's guidance that will satisfy us that his guidance in this regard was the most perfect.

It is a fact that the body relies on food and drink for its survival. It is In addition a fact that not all of the food and nourishment is digested when consumed. Rather, a part of it remains, and as time goes by, these substances accumulate in various qualities and quantities in the body. These accumulations harm the body because they cause clogs in different vessels and make the body feel heavy. If one gets rid of these substances by extracting them with medication, the body is harmed because most of these medications are toxic to varying degrees; In fact, the medication extracts the beneficial substances along with the harmful ones. As for the quality of these substances, the body is harmed when they heat up, spoil, become cold or weaken the natural heat and energy from fully maturating the excess substances.

The clogs caused by the residual substances are harmful whether they remain in the body or get extracted. Moving about is one of the best methods to deny these substances the chance to accumulate. Moving heats the organs and dissipates the leftover substances disallowing them from accumulating by the passage of time. The body will In addition get used to being energetic and light through physical activity and would optimize the intake of food, firm up the joints and strengthen the muscles and the ligaments. Moderate physical activity immunizes the body against most ailments and mood changes, providing the activity is done at the right time and under the proper circumstances.

Physical activity should be practiced after one has digested their food. In addition, moderate physical activity is that which gives the cheeks color and which nourishes the body. As for the activity that causes sweat it is too excessive.

Any organ that is used regularly in a type of physical activity will get stronger, especially during enjoyable sports in which the organ is used. Those who practice sports regularly will strengthen their bodies and those who nourish their memory their memory will get it stronger. Every organ has its own suitable sport or physical activity. For instance, the chest needs recitation, where one should start speaking with a low tone and then increases the volume of his tone. Hearing needs to hear various sounds and voices, gradually from the softer to the louder voices. The tongue needs to speak, and the eye needs to see while the legs need to walk while increasing the pace of walking gradually.

Horse riding, archery, wrestling and running are sports for the whole body. These types of sports dissipate chronic ailments, such as leprosy, dropsy and constipation.

Furthermore, the heart needs a type of sport that entails learning, behaving, and feeling happiness, joy, patience, firmness, courage, forbearing, performing righteous good deeds, and so forth. Patience, love, courage and kindness are among the best types of sports or physical activity for the inner-self. When the heart learns these types of physical activities little by little, these attributes will firmly reside in the heart and will be characteristic of that person.

In short, when you learn the Prophet's guidance in this regard you will realize that it is the most perfect and beneficial and that it preserves good heath and the power of the body. It is In addition beneficial for the worldly affairs and the Next Life.

In addition, there is no doubt that prayer preserves the health of the body and helps dissolve its excess and residual substances. It In addition preserves faith and brings happiness for this and the Next Life. Standing up in prayer at night In addition preserves health. Prayer In addition helps against acute ailments and energizes the body, heart and soul profoundly. In the Sahihain it is narrated that the Prophet **b** said:

"Satan ties three knots at the back of the head of any of you if he is asleep. On every knot he reads and exhales the following words, 'The night is long. so stay asleep.' When one wakes up and remembers Allah, one knot is undone. When one performs ablution, the second knot is undone. When one prays, the third knot is undone and one gets up energetic with a good heart in the morning. Otherwise one gets up lazy and with a mischievous heart."

The Islamic commandment of Fasting In addition preserves the health and is a type of physical activity for body and soul, No one whose character is not spoiled could ever deny these facts.

As for Jihad and what it entails of various movements and activities, it is one of the best preservers of strength, good health, firmness of the heart and body and extracting unwanted residual substances that accumulate in the body. jihad In addition helps remove sadness, grief, anguish and depression. Only those who have tasted this cure know these facts. Hajj and performing the rest of its obligations, horseracing, helping other people achieve their needs and rights, visiting the sick, following funerals, walking to the mosque to perform jumu'ah and congregational prayers, performing ablution and taking a bath all have similar effects and benefits.

All the acts that we mentioned will help preserve the health and aid the body towards the healthy passing of liquid and solid wastes. There is an added benefit in these acts as they help acquire the good of this life and the Next Life and fend off harm.

Now, we should realize that the Prophet's guidance in all of this is the best guidance. His guidance is superior regarding the treatment of the heart and the body, preserving their well being and fending off harm from them. There is no more proof for those who have been given the correct guidance than what we have already mentioned. Indeed, all success comes from Allah Alone.

The Prophet's guidance concerning sexual activity

His is the most effective guidance, as it preserves the health, completes satisfaction, and acquires the goals that this activity was meant to achieve.

Sexual intercourse is meant to achieve three essential goals:

Reproduction and the preservation of mankind until the number of souls that Allah has ordered to come to this world is fulfilled and completed. Second, expelling the water (semen), which would cause harm if it remains inside the body. Third, satisfying sexual desire and enjoying sex and the bounty that it represents. The last essential goal is the only one that will be satisfied in Paradise, because there will be no reproduction in Paradise nor accumulation of sperm that needs to be discarded.

The best doctors state that sex is one of the best methods to preserve good health. Galinus said, "The essence of the sperm consists of heat and air, and it is hot and wet because it is produced from the pure blood that feeds the essential organs,"

If this is how significant sperm is, one should realize that it should not be used or spent except to achieve reproduction or to legally rid the body of it when it gets old. When the sperm is congested in the body, it will cause certain ailments, such as obsession, madness, and epilepsy. Discarding it, on the other hand, helps cure many of these ailments. When the sperm is kept in the body for a long time, it becomes spoiled and turns into a toxic material that can cause certain ailments. This is why sometimes sperm is expelled from the body naturally.

Some of ours said, "Man should take care of three things: he should not ignore walking, so that when he needs it one day he is able to do it; he should not refrain from eating, because the intestines will shrink; he should not refrain from sexual activity, because if the well's water is not drawn out, it will drain."

In addition, Muhammad bin Zakariyya said, "Whoever ignores sex for a long time, his nerves will weaken, and their flowing will be blocked, and his penis will shrink. I have seen some people who did not have sex claiming to observe some kind of abstinence and their bodies became colder, their movements restricted and unexplainable depression touched them. Further, their appetite and digestive powers In addition decreased."

Sexual activity helps lower the gaze, repulse lust, allows one the ability to refrain from illegal sexual activity and In addition achieves these goals for the wife. When one uses his sperm in a legal manner, he will benefit himself and his wife in this life and the Next Life.

This is why the Prophet **b** used to fulfill his legal sexual desire, as he used to say:

"I was made to like women and perfume from your world."

Further, the Prophet **b** encouraged his nation to marry:

"Get married, because I will compete by your numbers with the other nations."

In addition, Ibn Ab'ass said: "The best of this

nation are those who have the largest number of wives (up to four)." * In addition, the Prophet **b** said:

"I marry women, eat meat, sleep, stand in Qiyam, fast and break my fast. Whoever ignores my Sunnab is not from my people."

Furthermore, he **b** said:

"O young men! Get married whoever can afford it, because it helps lower the gaze (from looking at what is prohibited) and protects the sexual organ (from illegal sexual activity). Those who cannot afford it should fast because fasting will cure them."

In addition, when Jabir married a matron woman, the Prophet **b** said:

"Why not have a virgin who fondles you and you fondle her."

In addition, Ibn Majah narrated in his Sunan that Ibn Ab'ass related from the Prophet **b** that he said:

"We do not see a better resort for those who love each other than marriage."*

Muslim In addition narrated in his Sahih that Abdullah bin Umar related from the Prophet **b** that he said:

"The Life of this world is enjoyment, and the best enjoyment in the life of this world is a righteous wife."

The Prophet ^ used to encourage his nation to marry beautiful virgin women who are In addition religious. An-Nasa'y narrated that Abu Hurayrah said, The Messenger of Allah **b** was asked, 'Who among women is the best?' He said:

"The one who would please him (her husband) if be looks at her, obeys him if he commands her and avoids disobeying him in what he hates concerning herself and his money."

In the Sahihain it is In addition narrated that the Prophet **b** said:

"The woman is married for four reasons: her wealth, position, beauty and religion. So marry the religious woman, may your hand be filled with sand (a good expression)."

The Prophet **b** In addition used to encourage marrying women who bare children and did not like marrying women who cannot bare children.

Abu Dawood narrated that Ma'qil bin Yasar said, "A man came to the Prophet **b** and said, 'I know of a beautiful, rich woman whom I want to marry, but she does not bare children. Should I marry her?' He said, 'No.' The man came a second time, and the Prophet s& did not allow him. On the third time, the Prophet said:

"Marry the kind woman who bares children, for I will compete concerning your large numbers with to the other nations."

At-Termezey related from the Prophet b that he said:

"Four are among the tradition of the Prophets: marriage, using siwak (natural toothbrush), wearing perfume and dyeing with Henna."

The husband should first fondle his wife before having sex with her, by kissing her and sucking her tongue sometimes. The Messenger of Allah b used to do the same with his wives. Abu Dawood narrated in his Sunan:

"The Prophet bused to kiss 'A'esha and suck her tongue."

In addition, jabir bin 'Abdullah narrated:

"The Messenger of Allah b did not allow sexual intercourse before fondling (the wife)."

Sometimes, the Prophet sag would sleep with all

of his wives in one night and would only take one bath afterwards. Sometimes, the Prophet b would take a bath after sleeping with each of his wives. Muslim narrated in his Sahih that Anas said, "The Prophet b would sometimes sleep with all of his wives and take one bath afterwards." In addition, Abu Dawood narrated in his Sunan that Abu Rafi' the Prophet's servant, said, "The Messenger of Allah y&, once slept with all of his wives and took a bath after each time. I said, 'O Messenger of Allah b why not take only one bath afterwards?' He said,

"This is more pure, cleaner, and better."

It is allowed for those having sexual intercourse to have sex for a second time after they perform ablution. Muslim narrated in his Sahih that Abu Sa'id Al-Khudri said that the Messenger of Allah b said:

"When one of you sleeps with his wife and then wants to repeat, let him perform ablution."

Taking a bath or ablution after sex refreshes the energy and the strength and cleans whatever has remained during sex (semen, for example). It is In addition an act of purity and cleanness. The inner heat will In addition get back to its normal level of activity after it had been excited during sex. In addition, taking a bath satisfies what Allah prefers of cleanliness and discards its opposite (impurity), which Allah hates. Thus, taking a bath after sex is one of the best acts that preserves ones health and strength.

Sex is best after your food has been digested

At that time the bodies' inner coldness, hotness, dryness and wetness are moderate. Sex is harmful when the stomach is full more than it is empty. Such is the case when the body feels excessive wetness, as compared to dryness, and heat as compared to coldness. In addition, one should have sex when the desire is ignited and thus the body is naturally ready to have sex, not because one just thought about it.

One should not ignite his sexual appetite when it is not naturally excited and should not force himself to have sex. In addition, when one feels that his sexual appetite is ignited, he should have sex to satisfy it. One should avoid having sex with an old woman, the very young who are not ready yet for sex or do not desire it, an ailing woman, a woman who isn't comely or a hated woman. Having sex in such cases will weaken the strength and the sexual drive.

Some doctors made an error when they stated that having sex with a matron women is better for the health than with a virgin. This statement defies what the best minds have stated and goes against the nature of mankind in general. When one marries a virgin, his heart will be fully dedicated to her and will be filled with her love, In addition, he will not divide the type of love he reserves for her with any other women (who he marries later on). This is why the Prophet **b** said to Jabir 'is **a virgin?"**

The women of Paradise, the Horn's, have not been touched by any person before their future, believing husbands in Paradise, a bounty from Allah that makes them more appealing. In addition, A'esha once said to the Prophet **b** ;

"If you pass by a tree that has been grazed on and a tree that is still untouched, which one would you allow your camel to graze on?" He said, "The tree that is still untouched by grazing."

She meant that he did not marry a virgin woman except her.

Having sex with a woman that one loves will not weaken the body and will expel the semen more effectively. Having sex with a woman that one does not like will weaken his strength and will not expel sufficient amounts of the semen congested in the body.

Having sex with a woman who is having her period is not allowed in the religion and by the nature of things, as it is very harmful and all doctors warn against it.

Furthermore, we should state that the best sexual position is for the man to get on top of his wife after having fondled and kissed her. This is why the woman is sometimes called "Firash (mat, or bed)". The Prophet once said,

"The son belongs to the Firash."

This (a sexual position that we mentioned above) is a part of man's being responsible for the woman, as Allah said:

﴿ ٱلرِّجَالُ قَوَّٰمُونَ عَلَى ٱلنِّسَآءِ ﴾ (٣٤) النساء

"Men are the protectors and maintainers of women." (4:34)

In addition, Allah said:

﴿ هُنَّ لِبَاسٌ لَّكُمْ وَأَنتُمْ لِبَاسٌ لَّهُنَّ ﴾ (١٨٧) البقرة

"They (women) are labooson [i.e. body cover, or screen, or Sakan, (i.e., you enjoy the pleasure of living with her) for you, and you (men) are Libas for them." (2:187)

The favored sexual position that we mentioned is taken from the beautiful description the Ayah gave for the wife and her husband of being the garment or the cover for each other.

The worst sexual position is for the woman to get on top of the man during sex, because it is against the natural way that Allah has created men and women and males and females. In this case, the man will not be able to ejaculate all of the semen and whatever remains will get soiled and harm his body. In addition, this position might allow some harmful moisture to descend from the woman's sexual organ to the penis. In addition, the womb would not be able to hold on to the semen in this position and thus conception will be more difficult. Further, the woman is and should be the receiving party and when this position is turned around and she becomes the giver, the act will go against the natural way.

It was reported that the People of the Scripture used to have sex with their wives while leaning on their sides, saying that this position is the most comfortable for the women.

As for Quraish and the Ansar, they used to have sexual intercourse with their woman from behind (in the vagina), and the Jews criticized them for this practice. Afterwards, Allah revealed:

﴿ نِسَآؤُكُمْ حَرْثٌ لَّكُمْ فَأْتُوا۟ حَرْثَكُمْ أَنَّىٰ شِئْتُمْ ﴾ (٢٢٣) البقرة

"Your wives are a tilth for you, so go to your tilth, when or how you will..." (2:223)

In the Sahihain it is In addition narrated that Jabir ^ Ai ^ said, "The Jews used to say that if a man had sex with his wife from behind in the womb the offspring would be cross-eyed. Then Allah revealed:

"your wives are a tilth for you, so go to your tilth, when or how you will..." (2:223)

In another narration of this Hadith by Muslim, the Prophet as commented (on the Ayah),

"If you wish from behind and if you wish from the front, but only in one valve (i.e. the vagina)."

Anal sex with the wife was never allowed by any Prophet, and it is a grave error that some people relate that some of the Salaf allowed men to have anal sex with their wives.

Abu Dawood narrated in his Sunon that Abu Hurayrah related from the Prophet at that he said:

"Cursed be the person who has sex with a woman in her anal canal."

In addition, Ahmad and Ibn Majah narrated that the Prophet b said:

"Allah does not look at the person who has sex with his wife in her anal canal."

At-Termezey and Ahmad mentioned another narration of this Hadith in which the Prophet b said:

"Whoever has sex with a woman during her period or in her anal canal, and whoever goes to a soothsayer and believes in him will have committed disbelief in what Allah has sent down to Muhammad."

In another narration of Al-Bayhaqi, the Prophet b said:

"Whoever has sex with a man or a woman in the anal canal will have committed Kufr (disbelief)."

Furthermore, it was narrated that the Messenger of Allah b said:

"Allah is not shy to say the truth; Do not have sex with women in their anal canals."

In addition, At-Termezey narrated that Talq bin Ali said that the Messenger of Allah b said:

"Do not have sex wIth women in their anal canals. Allah does not shy away from saying the truth."

Further, Ibn 'Adi narrated in his book, Al-Kamil,

that Abdullah bin Mas'ud related from the Prophet ^ that he said:

"Do not have sexual intercourse with women in the anal canals."

Abu Than' In addition related from the Prophet b that he said:

"Whoever has sexual intercourse with men or women in their anal canals, will have committed disbelief."

In addition, Isma'il bin Aiyash narrated that Jabir said that the Prophet bsaid:

"Be shy with Allah, but Allah is not shy to say the truth: Do not have sex with women in their anal canals."

In addition, Ad-Darqutni narrated this Hadith using another chain of narrators and it reads:

"Allah is not shy to say the truth: anal sex with women is not allowed."

Al-Baghawi In addition narrated that once Qatadah was asked about the person who has sex with his wife in her anal canal, and Qatadah related from the Prophet s& that he said:

That is the smalI sodomy (or homosexuality.

Imam Ahmad In addition narrated that Ibn Ab'ass said:

"Your wives are a tilth for you ..." (2:223)

"The Ayah, was revealed regarding some people from the Ansar. They came to the Prophet ^ and asked him and he said, 'Have sex with your wife however you like, but avoid anal sex.'"

In addition in the Musnad Imam Ahmad it is narrated that Ibn Ab'ass said that Umar bin AI-Khattab came to the Prophet **b** and said: "O Messenger of Allah **b** I am destroyed." The Prophet m, said, "What has destroyed you?" 'Umar said, "I turned over my Firash (mount, woman) last night (had sexual intercourse from the back in the vagina)." The Prophet **b** did not answer him. Soon after, Allah revealed:

"Your wives are a tilth for you, so go to your tilth, when or how you wish (2:223)

The Prophet **b** said:

"Do it from the front and from behind if you wish, but avoid menstruation and the anal canal."

Furthermore, At-Termezey narrated that Ibn

Ab'ass related from the Prophet b that he said:

"Allah does not Look at a man who had anal sex with another man or with a woman."

'Uqbah bin 'Amir In addition narrated that the Messenger of Allah b said:

"Cursed be whoever has sex with women in their anal canals."

Furthermore, Musnad Al-Harith bin Abi Usamah narrated that Abu Hurayrah and Ibn Ab'ass said, "The Messenger of Allah b gave us a speech just before he died and it was the last speech the Prophet b gave in Al-Medina until he went to Allah. He said:

"Whoever had sex with a woman in her anal canal, or with a man, or with a male child, will be gathered on the Day of Resurrection with an odor emitting from him that is more foul than rotted carrion. The people will be bothered by his smell until he enters Hellfire. In addition Allah will destroy his rewards and will not accept from him a prayer or a fast. He will In addition be entered into a coffin of fire and the coffin will be shut closed on him using nails of fire."

Abu Hurayrah commented, "This is for whomever did not repent (from sodomy)."

"A man came to the Messenger of Allah **b** and asked him about having sex with women from the rear. The Prophet **b** said, 'It is allowed.' When the man left, the Prophet $a summoned him and asked him. What was your question? In which of the two holes it from is the rear in the vagina, then it is allowed. As for having sex in the anal canal from the rear. no. Allah is not shy to say the truth. Do not have sex with women in the anal canal." Furthermore, Allah said:

"Then go in unto them as Allah has ordred for you."

Mujahid said, "I asked Ibn Ab'ass about the meaning of what Allah said:

"Then go in unto them as Allah has ordained for you."

He said, 'Have sex with her in the same place where you were not allowed when she is menstruating."

All bin Abi Talhah commented, "Meaning in the vagina."

The Ayah has indicated that it is not allowed to have sexual intercourse in the anal canal in two different ways.

First, Allah has only allowed having sex in the

place where the offspring is created not the anus, which is a harmful place. The place of offspring is mentioned in what Allah said:

﴿ فَأْتُوهُنَّ مِنْ حَيْثُ أَمَرَكُمُ ٱللَّهُ ﴾ (٢٢٢) البقرة

"As Allah has ordained for you (go in unto them in any manner as long as it is in their vagina)." (2:222)

Having sex with the wife from the rear in the vagina is In addition entailed in the Ayah, because Allah said:

﴿ فَأْتُوا حَرْثَكُمْ أَنَّىٰ شِئْتُمْ ﴾ (٢٢٣) البقرة

"So go to your tilth, when or how you wi7I." (2:223)

It means that from wherever you wish, from the front or the rear. In addition, Ibn Ab'ass said: meaning the vagina.

Allah has disallowed vaginal sex with the woman when there is a temporary harmful condition (menstruation). So what about anal sex in the place of harm which will In addition harm the cause of reproduction. In addition, anal sex with the woman will surely encourage the man to have anal sex with young boys.

In addition, the wife has a right on her husband to have natural sexual activity and anal sex does not satisfy this right nor fulfill her desire.

Further, the anal canal was not created for this act nor is it suitable for it, unlike the vagina. Those who refrain from sex in the vagina and perform anal sex will have deviated from Allah's Wisdom and Commandments.

In addition, anal sex is very harmful for the man and this is why the wisest doctors advise against it. The vagina has a special quality in extracting the semen and relieving the man from it. The anal canal, on the other hand, does not help extract all of the semen because it is not in its nature.

Anal sex is In addition harmful to the man because it requires tiresome movements and because it goes against his nature.

The anus is In addition the place of dirt and filth. Yet, the man faces it with his face and embraces it [during anal sex]!

Anal sex is In addition very harmful for the woman because it is unnatural, abnormal and not suitable for what she was created for.

Anal sex In addition causes depression and distress, along with the people feeling hateful and estranged with both parties to the anal sex.

Anal sex In addition blackens the face, causes distress in the chest, extinguishes the light of the heart and gives the face a darkness that will become a trademark for those who do anal sex.

Anal sex In addition causes hatred (between the participants to the act) and will soon lead both participants to part from each other.

Anal sex In addition causes the nature of both participants to be terminally spoiled, unless they repent to Allah with a sincere heart.

Anal sex In addition erases all the good qualities and replaces them with their opposites. It In addition dissipates the affection and good relations between the two parties, who will soon curse and hate each other.

Anal sex is In addition one of the major reasons behind the destruction of the bounties and the coming of torment and disaster. It In addition leads to being cursed and hated by Allah, as He will ignore those who indulge in this act and would not look at them. What good can such people ever gain later on and what evil could they wish to avert? What kind of life can they live after Allah's curse falls on them, along with His hatred towards them, His ignoring them and His shunning them?

Anal sex a so dissipates shyness, and shyness is the life of the heart. When the heart looses shyness, it will like the disliked and dislike the liked. Thus, the heart will have fallen into utter ruin and destruction.

Anal sex In addition alters human nature from the path that Allah has created it for, to a type of lower animal behavior. Rather, it is even lower. When the nature is altered and changed, the heart, the deeds and the guidance will In addition be altered. One will then like the evil things and deeds, leading him to fall into total disarray regarding his condition, deeds, and speech.

More than any other act, anal sex In addition causes one to have rude behavior and makes him dare to commit evil.

Anal sex In addition brings one humiliation, degradation and disgrace more than any other act.

Finally, anal sex causes the slave hatred and dislike, and the people will feel despise and disgust with him, as is evident ail around us.

May Allah's peace and blessings be on he whose guidance gives those who follow it the happiness of this and the Next Life. On the other hand, destruction and demise of this and the Next Life are the result of deviating from his guidance and what he was sent with.

There are two types of harmful sexual activity

One type that the religion declares harmful and another type that defies nature.

The harmful sexual intercourse that the religion prohibits is in grades, some are worse than others. Temporarily prohibited sexual activity is less dangerous than those totally prohibited. For instance, sex is disallowed during the Fast, Ihram, I'tikaf, menstruation, and so froth. There is no punishment prescribed when one violates this type of limited prohibition. The second type, which is totally prohibited, falls under two categories, prohibited for eternity, such as marrying whom one is not allowed to marry, which is one of the worst types of illegal sexual activity. This category requires capital punishment according to a segment of the scholars, such as Ahmad bin Hanbal. There is an authentic Hadith that upholds this ruling too. The second category is totally prohibited but not for eternity, such as committing adultery or fornication with whom one is theoretically eligible for marriage. In the case of adultery, it will be violating two rights: Allah's right and the husband's right. If the woman was forced to this act, it will be a violation of three rights (Allah's, her husband's and her own). If she had a family and relatives, they will be ashamed by the rape, and thus a fourth right would be violated. If the

woman was not allowed for the man even theoretically, a fifth right will be violated. The harm of this type of act varies according to the grade of prohibition it violates.

There is a type of sexual activity that is harmful for one's nature, whether due to the form or the manner it takes. For instance, having excessive sexual intercourse will weaken the strength and harm the nerves. It will In addition cause convulsive shaking, facial paralysis and spasms. It In addition weakens the eyesight and the rest of the powers of the body, along with weakening the instinctive heat and energy, widening the body vessels and exposing them to accumulating harmful substances.

The best time to have sex is after the food has been digested in the stomach, but not when the stomach is empty for it weakens the instinctive heat. In addition, one should not have sex when he is full, because in this case sexual intercourse causes clogs, nor when one is tired, after taking a bath, after vomiting or when one is nervous, sad, depressed distressed or very happy.

The best time to have sex is after the night falls, especially when the food had been digested. One then takes a bath or ablution and sleeps afterwards he regains his strength. One should not indulge in activity after sex because it is very harmful in this ...

The Prophet's guidance on treating passion

This is a disease that attacks the heart. Yet, it ... different type of disease concerning its symptoms, causes, and cure. When this ailment becomes acute, the doctors will not be able to cure it nor will the one afflicted be able to bear its effects.

Allah has mentioned the subject of passion concerning two types of people: women and lovers of beardless boys. For instance, Allah mentioned the story of the wife of Al-'Aziz (Ruler of Egypt) and the Prophet Yusef **b**. He In addition mentioned the second type about the people of the Prophet Lut **b** He said about them when the angels came to visit the Prophet Lut **b**

"And the inhabitants of the city came rejoicing (at the news of the young men's arrival). [Lut (Lot)] said: 'Verily, these are my guests, so shame me not. And fear Allah and disgrace me not.' They (people of the city) said: 'Did we not forbid you from entertaining (or protecting) any of the 'Alamin (people, foreigners and strangers from us)?' [Lut (Lot)] said: 'These (the girls of the nation) are my daughters (to marry lawfully), if you must act (so).' Verily, by your life (O Muhammad **b**), in their wild intoxication, they were wandering blindly." (15:67-72).

There is a false claim that was started by those who do not give the Prophet a& his due respect and appreciation, stating that the Prophet b once saw Zainab bint jahsh* and said, "All praise be to He Who changes the hearts as He wills!" They In addition claim that the Prophet m was inflicted with this disease, passion, and that his heart liked her. Yet, they claimed, he commanded Zaid to keep her and not divorce her, until Allah revealed:33

"And (remember) when you said to him (Zaid bin Harithah AI ^ ii — the freed-slave of the Prophet) on whom Allah has bestowed grace (by guiding him to Islam) and you (O Muhammad b, too) have done favour (by manumitting him): 'Keep your wife to yourself, and fear Allah.' But you did hide in yourself (i.e., what Allah has already made known to you that He will give her to you in marriage) that which Allah will make manifest, you did fear the people (i.e., their saying that Muhammad (married the divorced wife of his manumitted slave) whereas Allah had a better right that you should fear Him." (33:37)

Those who uttered this false claim In addition claimed that the Ayah is talking about passion. Consequently, some of them collected a book about passion in which they mentioned several Prophets who were afflicted with this disease, including the Prophet b This is an utter ignorance of such people of the Qura'an and the Messengers and a misunderstanding that alters the true meaning of Allah's Words. Further, this false claim accuses the Prophet ^ with what he is truly innocent of.

Zaid bin Harithah whom the Prophet had adopted before Islam until he was called Zaid bin Muhammad, married Zainab bint Jahsh. Zainab was not humble with her husband and he asked the Prophet's advice if he should divorce her. The Messenger of Allah b said, to him:

"Keep your wife to yourself, and fear Allah."

The Prophet ^ thought that if Zaid would otherwise divorce her, he would marry her after him. But, the Prophet **b v** hid this thought in his heart because he feared what the people might say if he married the ex-wife of his adopted son. This is why Allah mentioned in this Ayah His favors on the Prophet **b** and commanded him not to fear what the people might say in doing what Allah has allowed for him. Allah In addition reminded him that it is He whom the Prophet as should fear, so he should not be hesitant in doing what Allah has allowed for him because of fear of what the people might say.

Further, Allah informed the Prophet ^ that He has given Zainab to him in marriage after Zaid had divorced her so that his nation imitates him when they know that the man is allowed to marry the ex-wife of his adopted son. This is why Allah said:

"But there is no sin on you if you have not gone in them (to marry their daughters), and the wives of your sons who (spring) from your own loins (are forbidden for you to marry)...." (4:23)

And in this chapter (4:4O), Allah said:

"Muhammad (**b**) is not the father of any of your men." (33:4O) While in the beginning of the chapter Allah said:

"...nor has He made your adopted sons your real sons. That is but your saying with your mouths." (33:4)

Therefore, think deeply about Allah's defense of the Prophet as that refuted the false accusation directed at him. All success comes from Allah. Yes, the Prophet of Allah **b** used to love his wives, especially A'esha the most beloved to him among them. Yet, his love for them did not reach the evil of perfect love, which he reserved for his Lord. The Prophet **b** once said:

"If I was going to take an intimate friend from the people of the earth, I would have taken Abu Bakr."

And in another narration, he said:

"Your friend (himself, Muhammad) is the intimate friend of the Most Beneficent."

Having passion towards images only afflicts empty hearts

This affects hearts that are deprived of the love of Allah, ignoring Him and preferring someone else. When the heart is full of the love of Allah and eagerness to meet Him, this love will fend off the disease of love and passion for images. This is why Allah said about Prophet Yusef **b**

﴿ وَلَقَدْ هَمَّتْ بِهِۦ ۖ وَهَمَّ بِهَا لَوْلَآ أَن رَّءَا بُرْهَـٰنَ رَبِّهِۦ ۚ كَذَٰلِكَ لِنَصْرِفَ عَنْهُ ٱلسُّوٓءَ وَٱلْفَحْشَآءَ ﴾ (٢٤) يوسف

"Thus it was, that We might turn away from him evil and illegal sexual intercourse. Surely, he was one of Our chosen, (guided) slaves." (12:24)

This indicated that sincerity is a cause and a remedy that drives away passion which might lead to sin and fornication, which is the culmination of passion. When the cause behind the disease is repelled, the effects of the disease will In addition be repelled.

Some of ours once described passion that it is the

act of a heart that is empty of everything except what it has a passion for. Allah said:

"And the heart of the mother of Musa (Moses) became empty [from every thought, except the thought of Musa (Moses)]. She was very near to disclosing his case." (28:1O)

This Ayah indicated that the heart of Moses's mother was empty of every concern except for Moses, because of her great love for him and her heart's affection for him. Passion has two parts, loving an object and an eagerness to possess the loved object. When one of these two parts does not exist, then passion does not exist either.

The ailment of passion has caused bafflement to many wise people and some of them issued some statements in this regard that should not be taken seriously.

We say that Allah's Wisdom has decided regarding His creation that there are similarities that occur between things and people, and that things and people are driven to their likes and to avoid what is not similar to them. The secret to the harmony that occurs in the world is due to the similarities between various creations. Various things [and people] thus lean towards similar objects, while dissimilar objects ignore each other. Allah said:

﴿ ۞ هُوَ ٱلَّذِى خَلَقَكُم مِّن نَّفْسٍ وَٰحِدَةٍ وَجَعَلَ مِنْهَا زَوْجَهَا لِيَسْكُنَ إِلَيْهَا ۖ فَلَمَّا تَغَشَّىٰهَا حَمَلَتْ حَمْلًا خَفِيفًا فَمَرَّتْ بِهِۦ ۖ فَلَمَّآ أَثْقَلَت دَّعَوَا ٱللَّهَ رَبَّهُمَا لَئِنْ ءَاتَيْتَنَا صَٰلِحًا لَّنَكُونَنَّ مِنَ ٱلشَّٰكِرِينَ ﴾ (١٨٩) الأعراف

"It is He Who has created you from a single person (Adam), and (then) He has created from him his wife [Hawwa' (Eve)], in order that be might enjoy the pleasure of living with her." (7:189)

Allah has made this the reason why man feels attracted and consequently passionate, for woman. She is similar to him in essence. The reason for the attraction [between men and women] is not only the beauty of the image, but the similarity in the habits, guidance and mannerism, all of which help ignite passion.

In the Sahih it is narrated that the Prophet said:

"The souls are similar to recruited soldiers. Those who recognize

each other will be intimate and those who do not recognize each other will be apart."

In addition, Imam Ahmad narrated in his Mosn'ad the reason behind this Hadith, "A woman in Mecca used to be able to make people laugh and when she came to Al-Medina she resided with a woman who In addition used to be able to make people in Al-Medina laugh. The Prophet **b** said:

"The souls are just like recruited soldiers."

The religion of Allah gives the same rulings to similar matters and thus does not differentiate between similar matters nor join between dissimilar matters. Those who think to the contrary are mistaken due to their lack of knowledge of the religion, or lack of effort on their part to acquire knowledge on the subject of similarities and dissimilarities. Or, their error comes from relating to the religion what is not a part of it without the authority that can justify it. With Allah's Wisdom and justice, His creation and command have been established by equating similar things and differentiating between dissimilar things. This fact is true both in this life and on the Day of Resurrection. Allah said:

﴿ ۞ ٱحْشُرُوا۟ ٱلَّذِينَ ظَلَمُوا۟ وَأَزْوَٰجَهُمْ وَمَا كَانُوا۟ يَعْبُدُونَ ﴿٢٢﴾ مِن
دُونِ ٱللَّهِ فَٱهْدُوهُمْ إِلَىٰ صِرَٰطِ ٱلْجَحِيمِ ﴿٢٣﴾ ﴾ (٢٢:٢٣) الصافات

(It will be said to the angels): "Assemble those

who did wrong, together with their companions (from the devils) and what they used to worship. Instead of Allah, and lead them on to the way of flaming Fire (Hell): ..." (37:22,23)

In addition, Allah said:

﴿ وَإِذَا ٱلنُّفُوسُ زُوِّجَتْ ﴿٧﴾ ﴾ (٧) التكوير

"And when the souls shall be joined with their partners (the good with the good and the bad with the bad)." (81:7)

This indicates that each person will be tied to his likes. Those who have love for each other for Allah's sake will be together in Paradise, while those who love each other for the devil's sake will be together in Hell. One is with those whom he likes, whether he likes it or not. Al-Hakim narrated that the Prophet ^ said:

"If a man loves a people, he will be gathered with them (on the Day of Resurrection)."

There are several types of love. The best and most honorable of them is love for the sake of Allah, which requires loving what He loves and In addition loving Him and His Messenger.

Another type of love is that which occurs when

... it have a similar religion or way, or sect, or relation, or craft, or a goal that they ... Another type of love is what occurs when one ...quire a matter that the loved object has, position, money, knowledge, or any other ... he seeks. This is material love that dissipates ...al is reached. Indeed, he who likes you for a ...er... purpose goes away when his goal is ...omplished.

The love that results because of the similarities ...een the two parties does not fade away unless there is ...ason that makes it fade away. This type of love ...tes passion because it is a love that the soul and the ...eart share. No other ailment can cause more profound ...fects on those afflicted, of obsession, weakness, concern and even destruction, like passion.

If one says that since the reason behind affection is what you have stated, the souls being connected and compatible, why is it not always exchanged between the two parties? Sometimes, love is one sided, although you stated that the reason for it is the similarity and the compatibility between the souls.

The answer is that there are reasons that arise and prevent the love from being exchanged by both sides. One-sided love is the result of one of three reasons: a deficiency in the love because it is accidental and not real.

In this case, the loved person might even feel dislike for the other party. Second, sometimes the loved person might be the cause for the love to be one-sided, such as a deficiency in his mannerism, shape, path, actions, appearance, and so forth. Third, due to a specific reason that prevents the loved person from sharing the same feelings with the other party.

When these reasons are not present, and the love is thus real, love will be shared by both parties.

Arrogance, envy, loving various positions and enmity by the disbelievers were the main reasons the Messengers were not more beloved by them than their own selves, families and offspring. When these barriers were removed from the hearts of the Messengers' followers, their love for the Messengers was indeed more than the love they had for their own selves, wives, children and wealth.

Attainment of one's love object is its cure and other cures for love

The subject is that since love is one of the ailments in general, it does have a cure or several cures. If the lover has a legal path to take to attain his loved object, it will be his cure. In the Sahihain it is narrated that Ibn Mas'ud said that the Prophet **b** said:

"O young people! Whoever amongst you can afford marriage, let him marry. Those who cannot afford it should resort to fasting, for it will be a cure for them."

The Prophet b has directed the people to the best methods to obtain what they love, a major and a minor method. He ordered the men to resort to the first choice, marriage, which is the perfect cure for this disease. Thus, people should not prefer other solutions to the solution that the Prophet b recommended.

Ibn Majah narrated that the Prophet b said:

"We never saw anything like marriage for lovers."

This is the meaning that Allah indicated when He allowed in marriage both free and slave women when needed: Allah said:

"Allah wishes to lighten (the burden) for you; and man was created weak (cannot be patient to leave sexual intercourse with woman)." (4:28)

Therefore, Allah mentioned man's weakness in this Ayah and stated that He has made matters easy for him by allowing him to marry as many as he wishes, two, three or four. He In addition allowed him slave women in marriage if he wishes, so as to treat this ailment, passion, to cure the weakness in mankind and as an act of mercy [from Him] to His slaves.

When no legal method exists for the lover to attain his love object

If there is no legal method that the lover can attain his loved object or because of his inability to do so, or both, then passion will become a difficult disease in this case and the afflicted person needs to feel that he cannot satisfy it. It is a fact that when the heart feels hopelessness in something, it will no longer seek to acquire it,

If the disease, passion, still exists even under these hopeless conditions, then the nature of the person would have deviated and the person needs to try another solution, that is, attending to his state of mind. The person afflicted by passion should convince himself that his heart's affection with what it cannot attain constitutes madness, and that this case is similar to whoever loves the sun, the only way to acquire it is to ascend to it! Everyone understands this is madness.

If one cannot attain his loved object because of a legal barrier that the religion erected, he should convince himself that acquiring his passion is not feasible because Allah did not allow it to happen. He should know that for his safety he should abandon such a matter and be certain that it is virtually impossible that he will ever attain it.

If one's whose heart orders him to do evil does not comply with these cures, let the slave abandon the matter for fear of losing whoever is more beloved to him, more beneficial and who offers a longer period of contentment and joy. In this case, the afflicted person will come to realize the difference between the two objects. Therefore, one should not prefer the joy of an hour that would soon turn to pain compared to eternal joy that is incomparable. The reality of the short-lived joy is that it is a daydream or a mirage that will soon end and fade away, but the responsibility would remain.

In addition, one should realize that this might lead to a hateful loss that is worse for him than losing the coveted object, and thus his loss would multiply, losing the coveted object and acquiring a hateful outcome. When one realizes these facts, then losing the coveted object becomes less serious in his heart and being patient becomes more worthwhile. The mind, religion, honor and human nature then require the afflicted person to be patient in the face of losing a lesser loved object, for in this case, patience would soon earn him joy, contentment and happiness. On the other hand, one's ignorance, transience, injustice and immaturity orders him to prefer the lesser coveted object whatever the cost. Those whom Allah gives immunity will be saved from this end.

When one's heart does not accept this solution and

dislikes using the remedy that we mentioned, let him think about what evil repercussions satisfying his lusts would bring about and what gains it would cause him to lose. He should realize that satisfying his lust is the major cause of an evil outcome in this life, as it prevents the slave from using his mind that is the controller of his actions and which should be used to lead him to benefit instead.

If one's heart still does not accept the remedy we mentioned, let him remember the shortcomings and unlikable characteristics of the coveted object, so that he might dislike the object, as well. When one thinks about this subject, he will realize that such shortcomings supercede the good qualities that made him like that object. Let him In addition ask the neighbors of his loved one about what he does not know of their attributes and behavior. It is a fact that as much as the good qualities drive loved ones closer, the shortcomings drive them apart. Then, one should weigh the two sides and choose the best and most beloved path to take. He should not be among those who are deceived by the color of an otherwise leprous skin. Let one think beyond the beautiful exterior to the true reality of things. Let one look beyond the beautiful shape to the inner evil of the heart.

If all of these remedies do not work, there will be no resort except seeking Allah Who answers the calls of those in distress when they invoke Him. Let him throw himself before His Door seeking His help with humbleness, humility and meekness.

Those who are led to this type of success should act honorably and keep their affair a secret, so as not to expose the loved one to the people and cause them harm, or else he will be committing a transgression and an injustice.

The Prophet's guidance on preserving the health with perfume

Good scents and perfumes are nutrition for the soul, and the soul is the dynamo of the rest of the body's powers. Perfume helps the brain, the heart and the internal organs and brings comfort to the heart and the soul. Perfumes are In addition the most suitable and favorable remedy and substance for the soul. In addition, there is a close connection between the good soul and scented perfumes. This is why perfumes were among the dearest substances in this world to the heart of the most pure of all people, the Prophet i&.

Al-Bokhary narrated that the Prophet ^ used to always accept perfume when presented to him. In addition, Muslim narrated that the Messenger of Allah b said:

"He who is offered Raihan (basil) should not refuse it, because it is easy to wear and has a good scent."

Further, Abu Dawood and An-Nasa'y narrated that the Prophet **b** said:

"Whoever is offered some perfume should not refuse it because it is light to wear and has a good scent."

Ibn Abi Shaibah In addition narrated that the Messenger of Allah **b**had a container that had some perfume and he used to perfume himself with it. The Prophet **b** In addition said:

"Allah has a right on every Muslim that he takes a bath (at least once) in every seven days and if be has perfume to wear some of it."

Furthermore, the angels like perfume while the devils dislike it, because the dearest scent to the devils are foul odors, while good souls like good scents. Every soul leans towards and deserves what it likes. Evil men are suitable for evil women and vise versa, while good men are suitable for good women and vise versa. Although this statement applies to men and women in general, it In addition applies to every type of deed, speech, food, drink, clothing and scent.

The Prophet's guidance on preserving the health of

the eyes

Ibn Ab'ass narrated:

"Whenever the Messenger of Man used to wear kohl, he would use it thrice in the right eye - beginning with it and finishing with it - and twice in the left eye."

In addition, Abu Dawood narrated that the Prophet **b** said:

"Those who use Kohl should use it an odd number of times."

One should use an odd number of times when applying Kohl in both eyes, thrice in the right eye and then twice in the left eye. Or, one should use the Kohl thrice in each eye, as Imam Ahmad has stated.

Kohl preserves the health of the eye, strengthens and clears the sight and removes harmful substances, along with adding a touch of beauty to the eye. When one uses kohl before he goes to sleep, it is beneficial for the eye, especially since the eyes will not be moving and thus the kohl will have its most favorable affect. The ithmid type of kohl is especially effective in this regard.

Ibn Majah narrated in his Sunon that Abdullah bin Umar related from the Prophet **b** that he said:

"Use Ithmid (antimony), because it clears the eye and grows the eyelashes." [AI-Hakim}.

In addition, Ibn Majah narrated in his Sunan that Ibn Ab'ass related from the Prophet **b** that he said:

"The best of your kohl is the Ithmid (antimony), because it dears the sight and causes the eyelashes to grow."

[At-Termezey, Ibn Majah, Ibn Hibban, AI-Hakim, At-Tabamni and Abu Nairn}.

ALPHABETICAL LISTING*

THE LETTER HAMZAH

I. Ithmid (Antimony)

The Ithmid is the black Kohl stone. The best type of Ithmid is found in Asfahan (Iran), but it is In addition found in western areas. The best type of Ithmid is that which fragmentizes quickly and which has shiny morsels. In addition, the interior of the Ithmid is polished and does not contain any impurities.

The Kohl tends to be cold and dry and it is beneficial to the eye in that it strengthens it and In addition strengthens the eye nerve. Ithmid dissolves excess flesh around ulcers and closes the wound while cleansing the area around them. Ithmid In addition relieves headaches when it is blended with pure watery (not thick) honey. When Ithmid is ground and mixed with tender fat and then used as a bandage over fire burns, it prevents blisters from appearing and In addition helps cure the skin damage that occurs in cases of bums by fire. Ithmid is the best type of Kohl used for the eye, especially for old people whose eyesight has weakened. In this case, it is better that Kohl is mixed with some Musk.

2. Utruy (Citron)

In the Sahih it is narrated that the Prophet b said:

"The example of the believer who reads the Qura'an is the example of the Utrujj: its taste is delicious and its scent is pleasant."

The Utrujj has many benefits. There are four elements in the Utrujj, the peel, heart (or pulp), the pith and the seed. Each of these four elements has its own tendency: the peels, for instance, are hot and dry, while the pulp is hot and wet. The Utrujj pith is cold and dry, while its seed is hot and dry.

The peel of the Utrujj has many benefits. For instance, when its is placed within the clothes it prevents molding. The peel's scent refreshes decaying and polluted air. The peels of the Utrujj In addition improve the flavor of the foods and dissipate foul scents. In addition, when the peels are mixed with the food they help the digestive process. The author of the Qanoon said, 'The pith of the {Utrujj) peels benefit in cases of snake bite, while the peels are used in bandages for snakebite. The ashes of the peels are used as an effective ointment against leprosy.'

The pulp of the citron (Utrujj) soothes the heat of the stomach, helps those who suffer from bile and subdues hot vapors. Further, Al-Ghafiqi said, "Eating the (citron) pulp relieves hemorrhoids."

The extract of the pith contained in the citron constipates, relieves bile, soothes hot pulsation, controls bilious vomiting, and when taken as a drink or a Kohl, relieves jaundice. The extract of the pith is In addition a good appetite stimulant, constipates and helps in cases of bilious diarrhea. The citron pith extract In addition soothes the lust of the woman and relieves and combats skin spots when used as a lubricant. It In addition cures herpes. The proof of the pith's effectiveness against ink is that when it touches the ink on the clothes, it effectively removes the stain. The pith contained in the Utrujj In addition soothes and has a chilling effect, cools the hotness of the liver, strengthens the stomach, eliminates bile and the accompanying depression and In addition quenches the thirst.

The seeds of the Utrujj have a decomposing and drying effect. Ibn Masawaih said that Utrujj, "When the skin of the seed is removed and cooked and taken as a drink with warm water, helps against deadly poisons when one drinks as much as two measures, each around twenty-five grams. When the seeds are ground and placed on a sting, they In addition help. The seeds In addition constipate and add good scent to the taste. Most of these benefits are In addition present in its pulp."

It was In addition said that, "The seeds help

against scorpion stings when two measures of it are taken with warm water, and In addition when it is ground and placed on the affected area." It was In addition said, "Its seeds help against all types of poisons and all types of venomous stings."

It was In addition reported that one of the Persian rulers was angry with his doctors and that he ordered them be jailed. He gave them the choice to have only one type of food and they chose the Utrujj. They were asked, "Why did you choose it in particular?" They said, "Because it turns into a type of perfume shortly, its sight is pleasant, its peel smells good, its pulp is a fruit, its pith is a food, its seeds an antidote and it contains fat."

Truly, such a beneficial substance deserves to be compared with the best of creation, meaning the believer who recites the Qura'an. We should mention that some of people used to like looking at the Utrujj because its sight is pleasant and comforting.

3. Aruzz (Rice)

There are two fake Ahadeeth regarding rice. The first, "If it was a man it would be forbearing." The second Hadith, "Everything that the earth produces has a disease and a cure, except the rice, for it is a cure and has no disease (or side effects)." We mentioned these incorrect Hadiths so that the people do not relate them from the

Prophet by mistake.

Rice is hot and dry and it is the most nutritious cereal after wheat. Rice is a beneficial substance as it tightens the intestinal cavity and coats and strengthens the stomach. The doctors of India claim that it is the most beneficial food when it is cooked with cows' milk. Rice is nutritious, enriches the body, increases semen production and purifies the color.

4. Arz (Pine)

Arz is In addition called Sanawbar. The Messenger of Allah **b** mentioned the pine, when he said:

"The example of the believer is the example of the green plant that the wind twists, sometimes leaving it straight and sometimes bending it. The example of the hypocrite is the example of the Arz, it will be standing on its roots then all of a sudden it is completely dry!"

The seed of the Arz is hot and wet. It is a relaxing and maturating substance, and has a sting that can be prevented if the Arz seeds are soaked in water. Further, the Arz seeds are difficult to digest but are nutritious, help relieve coughing and dries the moisture or vapor that accumulates in the lungs. They In addition energize semen production but constipate, unless one In addition eats bitter pomegranate seeds with them.

5. The izkh'er (Lemon Grass)

In the Sahih it is narrated that the Prophet a| said in Mecca about its plants:

"Do not cut its plants."

Al-Ab'ass said, "Except for izkh'er, O Messenger of Allah b for their (the people of Mecca) servants use it and it is In addition used for their houses." The Prophet $a said: "Except izkh'er."

Lemon grass is hot in the second degree and dry in the first degree. It is a light substance that opens clogs and the veins' orifices. It In addition increases urine and menstruation-flow, dissolves the stones and the hard tumors in the stomach, liver and kidneys, either as a drink or as a bandage. The stems of the lemon grass will strengthen the column of the teeth and the stomach, calm nausea and constipate the stomach.

The Letter B'aa

I. Bittikh (Watermelon)

Abu Dawood and At-Termezey narrated that the Prophet b used to eat watermelon with ripe dates, saying:

"The hotness of this substance (dates) neutralizes

the coolness of that (watermelon)."

There are several Ahadeeth regarding watermelon none of them are authentic, except the Hadith that we mentioned above.

Green watermelon is cold and wet and is sweet. It In addition works as a cleanser (for the stomach and the intestines). Watermelon departs the stomach more quickly than cucumber and quickly blends with whatever substances are present in the stomach. It is beneficial to eat watermelon when it is warm, but when it is cold it is better to have it with some ginger to offset its harm.

Watermelon should be eaten before the meals. Otherwise, it will cause nausea. Some doctors said that when watermelon is, "Eaten before the meal, it cleanses the stomach and removes ailments."

2. B'alalh (Dates)

An-Nas'ay and Ibn Majah narrated in their Sunan that A'esha said that the Messenger of Allah **b** said:

"Eat fresh dotes with dried dates, for when Satan sees the son of Adam eating fresh and dried dates he comments, 'The son of Adam remained until he started eating the new and the old together."

In another narration, the Prophet **b** said:

eat them with dried dates, or honey and butter.

3. Busr (Green Dates)

In the Sahih it is narrated that when the Prophet **b** Abu Bakr and Umar were guests of Abu Al-Haitham bin At-Taihan he brought them a cluster of dates, which is similar to a cluster of grapes. The Prophet **b** said:

"Why do you not choose some ripe dates for us?"

Abu Al-Haitham replied, "I wanted you to choose whatever you like of its green and ripe dates."

Busr is hot and dry, and its dryness is more than its hotness. In addition, the Busr dries out excess moisture, coats the stomach, relaxes the bowels and helps the gums and the mouth. The most beneficial type of Busr is the tender and sweet Busr. Yet, eating excessive amounts of Busr (green dates) regularly causes obstructions or clogs in the intestines.

4. Boydh (Eggs)

Fresh eggs are better than old eggs, and the best kind of eggs is chicken eggs. The eggs are mild but incline slightly towards being cold.

The author of the Qonoon said, "The yolk is hot and wet and makes the blood sanitary, but is not nutritious. It is In addition digested quickly when it is still soft." Another person said, "Egg yolk relives the pain, polishes the throat and the trachea, helps the throat and relieves coughing and the ulcers of the lungs, liver and prostate, It In addition eliminates coarseness, especially when blended with the grease of sweet almonds. It In addition maturates and softens whatever is in the chest and softens the roughness of the throat."

When the albumen is used as an eye drop, it cools the hot tumors in the eye and relieves the pain. When it is used as an ointment and placed on the face, it prevents sunburn. In addition, when the albumen is used as an ointment and placed on the forehead, it helps in cases of dysentery.

The author of the Qonoon mentioned eggs in the medicines and remedies of the heart. He In addition said, "Its yolk has a strong effect in strengthening the heart. Egg yolk has three beneficial uses: it turns into blood quickly, it does not produce extensive wastes, and the blood that it produces is light and similar to the blood that feeds the heart. Further, the egg yolk is the most adequate substance against the diseases that affect the essence of the soul."

5. Basal (Onions)

Abu Dawood narrated in his Sunon that 'A'esha

was asked about Basal and she said, "The last mea that the Prophet b had included onions in it."

In the Sahihain it is In addition narrated that the Prophet sg disallowed those who eat onions from entering the mosque.

The Basal is hot in the third degree and has an excess wetness, helps against pollution and prevents hot wind (meaning in the stomach). It In addition excites the sexual drive, strengthens the stomach, helps semen production, makes the color lighter, dissolves the phlegm and cleanses the stomach.

Onion grains help against vitiate (lack of pigment in certain areas of the skin) and are used as an ointment around the area affected by alopecia (A skin disease characterized by loss of hair, partial or total). Further, warts will dissipate effectively when onions are blended with salt (and used as an ointment on the warts). When someone feels nauseous after taking a laxative, smelling onions will help against vomiting. In addition, the onion will dissipate the smell of laxatives, and when onion water (extract) is administered through the nose, it will clear the head. Used as ear drops, onion extract In addition helps against weak hearing, Tinnitus, pus and water that accumulates in the ear. In addition, onion grains are used as an eyeliner, to dry out the water that attacks the eye, i.e. cataracts, when the grains are blended with honey and used on the white part of the eye.

Cooked onions are nutritious and help against icterus, jaundice, coughing and roughness in the chest. It is In addition diuretic and relaxes the bowels. It In addition heals dog bites when its water (extract) is blended with salt and rue and squeezed on the affected area. Finally, it will open the orifices of the hemorrhoids when used as suppository.

Onions cause migraines, headaches, flatulence and bring darkness to the sight.

Eating onions in excessive amounts or regularly causes forgetfulness, affects the mind and changes the odor of the mouth and the taste of food. It In addition bothers those in your presence and the angels. Cooking onions dissipates these side effects of the onion. The Sunan narrated:

"The Prophet ordered those who eat onion and garlic to kill them (make them milder) by cooking."

In addition, chewing rue leaves dissipates the odor of the onions.

6. Bazinj'an (Eggplant)

There is a fake Hadith that states that eggplant

materializes the goals anticipated from eating it. This statement is not suitable to be related from a sane person let alone the Prophet SB.

There are two types of eggplants: white and black. There is a difference of opinion on if it is hot or cold, although we think it is hot. Eggplants cause black bile, piles, clogs, cancer and leprosy. Eggplants In addition spoil ones color, make it black and cause bad breath. White eggplants do not have these side effects.

The Letter T'aa

I. Tamr (Dried Dates)

In the Sahih it is narrated that the Prophet **b** said:

"Whoever ote seven dates in the morning from the area of 'Aaliyah will not be harmed by poison or magic the rest of that day."

He In addition said:

"The people of a house where there are no dates are hungry."

In addition, the Prophet icterus ate dried dates with butter, with bread and alone. Tamr is hot in the second degree and either wet or dry in the second degree.

Dried dates strengthen the liver, relax the bowels, increase semen production, especially when taken with pine, and relieve soar throat. As for those who are not used to eating dried dates, such as the residents of cold areas, dried dates cause them clogs, harm the teeth and cause headaches, unless they are eaten with almonds and poppy.

Dried dates are among the most nutritious fruits, their essence is hot and wet. In addition, when one eats dates in the beginning of the day, they help kill worms. Although dried dates are hot, yet they have the strength of an antidote against worms, killing or at least decreasing their numbers, especially when dried dates are taken frequently on an empty stomach. Dried dates are a fruit, a type of food, a cure, a drink and a sweet.

2. Tin (Figs)

The Sunnah does not mention figs because they did not grow in that area of the Hijaz or Al-Medina. Figs require an environment that is different from that in the areas where dates grow. Allah has sworn by the Tin in His Book because of its tremendous benefits and uses,

Tin is hot and either dry or wet. The best type of figs are the white kind when they are ripe, as they cleanse the sand that accumulates in the liver and prostate and serve as a preventive substance against poisons. Figs are more nutritious than all other type of fruit, and help relieve the roughness in the chest, throat and trachea. It In addition cleanses the liver and the spleen, purifies the phlegm that accumulates in the stomach and provides good nourishment for the body. Yet, it makes one more susceptible to lice if eaten excessively.

3. Tharid (Meat and Bread Dish)

In the Sahihain it states that the Messenger of Allah b said:

"The virtue of 'A'esha as compared to other women, is like the virtue of Tharid as compared to the rest of the foods."

Tharid is composed of some bread, which is the best food, and meat, which is the best flavoring. When these two are combined together, no other food can surpass them.

There are conflicting opinions regarding which is better, the bread or the meat. The correct opinion is that bread is used more while meat is better and superior to bread. In addition, the meat resembles the true essence of the human body more than any other food. It is In addition the food of the people of Paradise. Allah said about those who sought to eat herbs, cucumbers, Fum (wheat or garlic), lentils and onions,

﴿ أَتَسْتَبْدِلُونَ ٱلَّذِى هُوَ أَدْنَىٰ بِٱلَّذِى هُوَ خَيْرٌ ﴾ (٦١) البقرة

"Would you exchange that which is better for that which is lower? (2:61)

Many among the scholars said that Fum is wheat. Hence this Ayah states that meat (quails) is better than wheat. Allah has the best knowledge.

The Letter Ieem

I. jummar (Palm Pith)

In the Sahihain it is narrated that 'Abdullah bin Umar said." "While we were sitting with the Messenger of Allah **b** he was brought a jummar of a date tree. The Prophet **b** said:

'There is a tree that resembles the Muslim as its leaves never fall."

jummar is cold and dry in the first degree, and it seals the ulcers and relieves hemorrhage, diarrhea, yellow bile and blood pressure. In addition, the jummar is not harmful, but is not nutritious and is difficult to digest. The jummar is all benefit and this is why the Prophet said it resembled the Muslim, because of his tremendous usefulness and goodness.

2. Gubn (Cheese)

In the Sunan of Abu Dawood it is narrated that Abdullah bin 'Umar said that the Prophet ai. was brought some cheese while in the area of Tabuk and that he asked for a knife, mentioned Allah's Name and then cut it. In addition, the Companions used to eat cheese in Iraq and Sham (Greater Syria) areas. Unsalted cheese is good for the stomach, easy on the body organs, produces flesh and relaxes the stomach. Salted cheese, on other hand, is less nutritious and is bad for the stomach and the intestines. Old and grilled cheese heats the stomach and is beneficial in cases of ulcers and diarrhea.

Cheese is cold and wet and is better when it is grilled because the fire makes it milder, softer and better tasting and scented. The old salted cheese is hot and dry, and boiling In addition makes it softer and less sour because the fire extracts the hot residue from the cheese. Salted cheese makes the body weak and causes stones in the liver and prostate. It is In addition bad for the stomach, and mixing it with what people think will make it milder is even worse because these substances allow the cheese an easy access to the stomach.

The Letter H'aa

1.Henna

We mentioned the benefits of henna' before and mentioned the Ahadeeth on this subject.

2. Habbah Sawdaa (The Black Seed)

In the Sahihain it is narrated that Abu Hurayrah related from the Prophet ^ that he said:

"Use the Black Seed, because it contains a cure for every type of ailment, except for death." [At-Termezey, Ahmad and Ibn Hibban].

The Black Seed (or Habbat Al-Barakah) is called Shuneiz in Persian, black cumin and Indian cumin. Al-Harbi narrated that Al-Hasan said, "It is the mustard seed" while Al-Harawi said that it is the green seed which is the seed of the terebinth. These are not correct opinions, because the Prophet b stated that it is the Black Seed, which is the Shuneiz as we stated.

The Black Seed has many benefits, as indicated by the Prophet's statement:

"It is a cure for every type of disease." This statement is just like what Allah said:

﴿ تُدَمِّرُ كُلَّ شَيْءٍ بِأَمْرِ رَبِّهَا ﴾ (٢٥) الأحقاف

"Destroying everything by the Command of its Lord!" (46:25) Its means destroys everything that is prone to destruction.

The Black Seed helps against all types of cold ailments. In addition, the Black Seed helps introduce the effective ingredients of cold medications to the areas affected by hot and dry ailments, as it helps the body absorb the medicine quickly when taken in small dosages.

The author of the 'Qanoon' and other people stated that saffron blended with camphor has similar effects, because saffron helps the camphor reach the affected area quickly. There are several types of plants that have similar effects as saffron. It is possible that the hot substance benefits in cases of hot diseases. For instance, the Anzarut, which is a type of eyeliner, is mixed with other remedies for Ophthalmia, conjunctivitis, and so forth. Ophthalmia is a hot tumor as the doctors agree. In addition, sulfur is a remedy for hot mange.

Shuneiz is hot and dry in the third degree, eliminates flatulence, extracts the helminthes (worms), relieves leprosy, and phlegmy fevers, opens clogs, decomposes accumulating gas and excess moisture in the stomach. When the Shuneiz is ground, blended with honey and drunk with some warm water, it will dissolve the stones that appear in the kidney and the prostate, and it is In addition diuretic. It increases the flow during menstruation and the production of milk if it is drunk for several days. When it is heated with vinegar and placed on the stomach, it will eliminate helminthes (worms). When it is blended with wet or cooked colorynth water, it is more effective in removing helminthes (worms). It In addition clears up, decomposes and relieves cold symptoms when it is ground in a rag and inhaled through the nose on a regular basis until the ailment is cured.

Black seed oil helps against snakebites, hemorrhoids and spots. When around twenty-five grams of it is drunk with water it will help against gasping and hard breathing.

When the black seeds are cooked in vinegar and then one rinses his mouth with it, it will relieve toothache resulting from sensitivity to cold. When one inhales powdered black seed, it will help against water that accumulates in the eye. When it is used in a bandage while blended with vinegar, it heals spots and exposed skin ulcers and decomposes the acute mucus tumors and In addition hard tumors.

The oil of the Black Seed In addition helps against facial paralysis when administered by the nose. When one drinks around twenty-five grams of its oil, it helps against spider bite. When it is ground finely and blended with the oil of the green Seed and used as ear drops, only up to three drops, it helps against cold symptoms, flatulence and various clogs.

When the Black Seed is fried and finely ground, soaked in oil and then drops are administered in the nose, it will help against cold conditions accompanied by intensive sneezing,

When the Black Seed is burned and mixed with melted wax along with henna or iris oil, it helps remove the ulcers that appear on the skin of the legs, after washing the skin with vinegar.

When the Black Seeds are crushed in vinegar and laid on leprous skin, the skin affected by black pigmentation and on the head that is affected by dandruff, it helps relieve these ailments.

When the Black Seeds are ground finely and one swallows around twenty-five grams of it each day with cold water, it instantly helps against the bite of rabid dogs, and might prevent death as a result of hydrophobia. When one administers the oil of the Black seed in the nose, it will help against facial paralysis and tetanus by eliminating their causes. Finally, when the Black seeds are burned, they help repulse the venomous beasts.

When Persian kohl is dissolved in water and then placed on the interior of the throat and then the Black seeds are sprinkled on it, it acts like an effective remover of hemorrhoids. There are many other benefits for the Shuneiz. We should state that the dose should be around twenty-five grams, as some people claim that using excessive dosages of it might cause death.

3. Harir (Silk)

We mentioned that the Prophet : **b** allowed Az-Zubayr and Abdur-Rahman bin 'Awf to wear silk because of a rash that they suffered from. We mentioned the benefits of the silk in that chapter.

Every day [that the fever lasts], one should swallow the paper with some water.

An Amulet for sciatica

One should write, "In the Name of Allah. O Allah, Lord of everything, Owner of everything and Creator of everything! You have created me and the sciatic nerve. Do not give it power over me, nor allow me to cut it. Heal me completely and eradicate the illness. There is none who can heal except You."

An Amulet for bleeding veins

At-Termezey narrated that Ibn Ab'ass said that the Messenger of Allah **b** used to teach them to recite [the following Ruqyah], against fever and various pains, 'In the Name of Allah, the Most Great. I seek refuge with Allah, the All-Mighty, from the evil of bleeding veins and from the evil of the fire's heat."

An Amulet for Toothache.

One should write on the cheek that is closer to the pain, "In the Name of Allah, Most Gracious, Most Merciful.

"It is He Who has created for you (the sense of) hearing (ears), eyes (sight), and hearts (understanding). Little thanks you give."

Or,

﴿ ۞ وَلَهُۥ مَا سَكَنَ فِي ٱلَّيۡلِ وَٱلنَّهَارِۚ وَهُوَ ٱلسَّمِيعُ ٱلۡعَلِيمُ ١٣ ﴾

(١٣) الأنعام

"And to Him belongs whatsoever exists in the night and the day, and He is the All-Hearing, the All-Knowing." (6:13)

An Amulet for abscess

One should write [this amulet and place it] on the abscess,

﴿ وَيَسْـَٔلُونَكَ عَنِ ٱلْجِبَالِ فَقُلْ يَنسِفُهَا رَبِّى نَسْفًا ﴿١٠٥﴾ ﴾

طه (١٠٥)

"And they ask you concerning the mountains: say, "My Lord will blast them and scatter them as particles of dust. Then He shall leave them as a level smooth plain." (2O:1O5, O6)

4. *Hurf* (Cress)

Abu Hanifah Ad-Daynoory said, "Cress seeds are used in remedies and are In addition called Ath-Thuffaa, which the Prophet *s&,* mentioned. Its plant is called Al-Hurf while Rashad seeds is its popular name." In addition, Abu Ubayd said that Ath-Thuffaa is the Hurf.

The *Hadith* that Abu Hanifah referred to is what Abu Ubay and other scholars have related from Ibn Abbas that the Prophet **b** was reported to have said:

"What a cure do the two bitter *remedies carry: the Thuffaa and aloe."*

Cress is hot and dry in the third degree, and it heats and relaxes the stomach, removes different types of worms, decomposes the spleen tumors, excites the sexual drive and heals the ulcers of mange and herpes.

When the cress is used as a bandage along with honey, it will decompose spleen tumors. When it is cooked with henna, it will extract harmful accumulations in the chest, while taking it as a drink helps against venomous bites and stings.

When it is burned, its smoke repulses venomous beasts and prevents the hair form falling. In addition, when it is mixed with barley flour and vinegar and used as a bandage it helps against decomposes hot tumors.

Further, when it is used as a bandage with water, it brings the pustules to maturity and helps against flabbiness in various organs, strengthens the sexual drive and works as an appetite stimulant. It In addition helps against asthma, hard breathing, relieves the thickness in the spleen, purifies the chest and increases the menstrual flow. It In addition helps against sciatic nerve and the cavity of the hip, due to the extraction power of the cress when one drinks it or is injected with it. It In addition purifies the chest and the lungs from phlegm.

When cress is crushed and taken in a drink with warm water, it will work as a laxative, decomposes flatulence and helps against the pain caused by constipation. Further, cress In addition helps against leprosy when it is crushed and used in a drink.

In addition, when the cress is blended with vinegar and used as an ointment on leprous skin and on white pigmentation disorder, it helps relieve these conditions. It a so relieves headaches that are caused by colds and by phlegm accumulation. When it is fried and drunk (with water), it constipates, especially when it is not crushed, as its consistency will be softened when it is fried.

Galinus said that the strength of the cress, "Is similar to the effectiveness of mustard grains. Hence it could be used to heat the pain in the hip, which is known as Noso and headaches, as each of these symptoms requires heat, similar to mustard seed. Sometimes, cress is mixed with other remedies and used to treat asthma, as it is known that it dissolves thick mixtures, again just as mustard seed does. It is similar to mustard seed in every respect."

5. *'Hulbab* (Fenugreek)

The Prophet *s* was reported to have visited Sa'd bin Abi Waqqas **b** .mi once when he was ~~ill~~ while in Makkah and he asked that a doctor be brought to examine him. They brought Al-Harith bin Kaladah who examined him and said, "There is no harm with him, just cook some fenugreek with dates and let him eat them." Sa'd was reported to have done that and was then healed.

Hulbah is hot in the second degree and dry in the first degree.

When the fenugreek is cooked in water, it will soften the throat, chest and the stomach. It In addition relieves coughing, dryness, asthma, hard breathing and increases the sexual drive. It In addition relieves flatulence, phlegm, piles and the various accumulations in the intestines. It In addition dissolves the phlegm from the chest and helps against gastric ulcer and lung diseases. *'Hulbah* is used to heal the intestines, mixed with some ghee and fanith.

When five measures of fenugreek is taken in a drink, it will increase the flow of menstruation, and when it is cooked and the hair is washed with it, it will make it curly and will combat dandruff.

When the flour of the fenugreek is blended with some vinegar and natron and used as a bandage on the tumor of the spleen, it will dissolve it. In addition, the woman who suffers from pain in the vagina due to a tumor will benefit if she sits in the water in which the fenugreek was cooked.

When it is used as a bandage and placed on hard, cold tumors, it will help dissolve these tumors. In addition, when its water is drunk, it will help against the pain in the stomach that results from accumulating gaseous materials and will cleanse the intestines.

When one eats the *Hulbah* cooked in honey, dates or figs on an empty stomach, it will dissolve the phlegm that accumulates in the chest and stomach, and will In addition help against coughing that accompanies such ailments.

Hulbah In addition relieves urine retention and works as a laxative. When it is placed on the erratic nail, it will heal it, while its oil helps against cracked skin due to extreme cold, when it is mixed with wax. There are many other benefits for the *Hulbah* (fenugreek).

Some doctors stated, "If the people had knowledge of its benefits, they would buy it with its weight worth of gold."

The Letter k'aff

I. Khubz (Bread)

In the *Sahih* it is narrated that the Prophet ^s said:

"On the Day of Resurrection, the earth will look like one piece of bread which the Most Mighty would prepare with His Hand as a residence for the people of Paradise."

A fake Hadith disallows cutting bread with a

knife. In addition another fake Hadith disa ws cutting meat with a knife. Muhanna said that he asked Imam Ahmad about the *Hadith* related from A'esha that narrates that the Prophet as disallowed using a knife to cut meat, because it is an act of non-Arabs. Imam Ahmad said that it is not correct and that it contradicts the *Hadith* narrated by 'Amr bin Umayyah and Al-Mughirah. The *Hadith* that he referred to is what 'Amr bin Umayyah related that the Prophet sag used to cut some pieces of ewe meat with a blade. In addition, Al-Mughirah narrated that when he asked the Prophet ^ to be his guest, he ordered that a piece of meat be broiled and he then started cutting the meat with a blade.

The best type of bread is yeasty and kneaded

The next best is furnace bread, then oven baked bread, then bread cooked under hot ashes, using fresh flour.

The most nutritious kind of bread is semolina bread, because it digests slowly and because it does not have excessive amounts of bran, then chalky bread and lastly black bread.

The best time to eat the bread is in the last part of the day when it is baked. In addition, unlike dry bread, soft bread is lighter, more nutritious, humidifying and digests faster.

Wheat bread is hot in the second degree and is mild concerning wetness and dryness, unless dried by fire.

Wheat bread In addition fattens the body rapidly. The Qatayif (similar to pancakes) cause a thick condition, while breadcrumbs provoke swelling in the stomach and digests with difficulty. Further, bread made with milk causes clogs and is difficult to digest, although it is nutritious.

Barley bread is cold and dry in the first degree and it not as nutritious as wheat bread.

2. *Kh'al* (Vinegar)

Muslim narrated in his *Sahih* that Jabir bin 'Abdullah said, "The Messenger of Allah **b** asked his wife for food and she said that I have vinegar. He asked for some of it and started eating from it while saying:

" *"What an excellent food is vinegar." (He ate it with bread.)*

Khall is a substance that is both hot and cold, although coldness is usually more apparent. It is In addition dry in the third degree and a strong drying agent. Vinegar In addition soothes the body and softens the nature,

Wine vinegar helps against gastric inflammation and bile and prevents the harm of toxic medications. It In addition decomposes milk and the blood when coagulated, and helps the spleen, coats the stomach, constipates, quenches the thirst and prevents tumors from occurring. It In addition helps the digestion process, works against phlegm, softens thick foods and softens the consistency of the blood.

When vinegar is drunk with salt, it will help against poisonous mushrooms. When vinegar is sipped, it will dissolve the clogs that occur in the blood in the lower jaw. When one rinses his mouth with warm vinegar, it relieves toothache and strengthens the gingival.

Vinegar In addition helps against a septic finger when it is anointed with it, and relieves pustules, hot tumors and fire burns. Vinegar is an appetite stimulant, softens the stomach, and favorable for young people and for those who live in warm areas.

3. *Khilal* (Toothpick)

Toothpicks are helpful for the gingival and teeth and preserve their health, and help keep the breath fresh. One of the best types of toothpicks are those made from olive wood. It is not advised to use reed, myrtle, or basil to pick the teeth.

The Letter D'al

I. Duhn (Fat or Grease)

Fat closes the pores of the body and prevents the skin from decomposing. When it is used after one takes a bath with hot water, it will humidify the body and polish it. When the hair is anointed with grease, it will beautify it and make it longer. It In addition helps against measles and most other ailments that could affect the hair.

At-Tirmidhi narrated that Abu Hurairah related from the Prophet afe that he said:

"Use grease *in your food and as an ointment."*

In the warm areas, such as Hijaz, grease works as one of the best preservers of health and as a remedy, making it necessary for the residents of such areas. As for those who live in cold areas, it is not as necessary for them. We should mention that using grease on the head on a regular basis causes harm to the sight.

The most beneficial simple kinds of grease are regular oil, then fat and then sesame oil.

As for the compound greases, some kinds are wet and cold, such as the essence of violet, which helps against hot headaches and brings sleep to the eye. It In addition moisturizes the brain, helps against cracks (or fractures) and excessive dryness of the skin. It is a so a beneficial ointment against mange and dry rashes, along with helping the joints be flexible. It is In addition suitable for those who tend to be hot during the summer.

Some types of compound greases are hot and wet, such as ben-tree grease, which is the extract of white seeds that look like dusty pistachio and which is greasy and fatty. This type of grease relaxes the nerves and helps against spots and lack of pigment in certain areas of the skin. It In addition draws thick phlegm, softens dry ligaments and heats the nerves. It In addition cleans the teeth, makes them shiny and helps them against corrosion. In addition whoever anoints his head and face with ben-tree grease will not come down with measles or cracks. Anointing the sexual organs and groins with it In addition helps against the coldness of the kidneys and dripping urine.

The Letter Thal

1. *Tharirah* (Hemarthria/Arum)

In the *Sahihain* it is narrated that A'esha said that during the Farewell *Hajj,* she perfumed the Messenger of Allah **b** with *Tharirah* for his *Ihram* and otherwise.

We mentioned the *Tharirah* and its benefits

before.

2. *Zubab* (Flies)

We mentioned the *Hadith* by Abu Hurairah *is* in the *Sahihain* about the Prophet's command to dip the housefly in the food or drink when it falls in it to get the antidote that its wing carries. This antidote works as the antidote of the poison that the fly carries on the other wing. We In addition mentioned the benefits of the flies before.

3. *Zahab* (Gold)

Abu Dawud and At-Tirmidhi narrated that the Prophet s& allowed Arfajah bin As'ad, who lost his nose during the battle of Kulab and had to use a nose made of silver that later rotted, to wear a nose made of gold. Arfajah is only mentioned in this one *Hadith.*

Gold is the joy of the life of this world and the precious material possession of this existence that brings joy to the hearts and strength to the back. It is In addition Allah's secret on His earth. Gold's condition is suitable in all types of environments and has a soft hotness that is used in various light and soothing remedies. It is In addition the most mild of all minerals.

When gold is buried in the ground, sand does not

affect it adversely. When gold is used in certain remedies, it helps cure weak hearts and the fibrillation that accompanies black bile. It In addition helps against obsession, sadness, depression, fear and love. It brings fatness to the body, dissipates pallor and lightens the color. It In addition helps against leprosy and the various other ailments including black bile. Drunk or used as an ointment, gold is an effective ingredient in the remedies for treating alopecia (a skin disease characterized by loss of hair, partial or total), and viper stings. It In addition clears the eye and strengthens it, and helps against several ailments while brining strength to the various organs of the body.

Foul breath would dissipate if one holds some gold in his mouth. In addition, those who have a disease that requires cauterization and use gold for this purpose it will heal quickly and the wound would not be covered with blisters. In addition, when gold is used as kohl, it purifies and strengthens the eyes. Further, when a golden ring is heated and applied on pigeon wings, the pigeons will be accustomed to their homes and will not abandon them.

Gold is especially effective in strengthening the hearts and this is why it was allowed in times of war and in times of peace, except when there is proof to the contrary. At-Tirmidhi narrated that Buraydah Al-'Asri said, "The Messenger of Allah si entered (Mecca) the Day of *Al-Fath* (conquering of Mecca) with gold and silver on his sword."

Gold is such a beloved object to the hearts that when they acquire it, it will be sufficient for the people to forget the other beloved objects of this earthly life.

Allah said:

﴿ زُيِّنَ لِلنَّاسِ حُبُّ ٱلشَّهَوَٰتِ مِنَ ٱلنِّسَآءِ وَٱلْبَنِينَ وَٱلْقَنَٰطِيرِ ٱلْمُقَنطَرَةِ مِنَ ٱلذَّهَبِ وَٱلْفِضَّةِ وَٱلْخَيْلِ ٱلْمُسَوَّمَةِ وَٱلْأَنْعَٰمِ وَٱلْحَرْثِ ﴾ (١٤) آل عمران .

***"Beautified for men is the love of things they covet; women, children, much of gold and silver (wealth), branded beautiful horses, cattle and well-tilled land."* (3:14)**

In addition, in the *to sound books* is narrated that the Prophet **b** said:

"If the son of Adam had a valley of gold, he would seek a second. If he bad two, he would seek a third. Nothing fills the stomach of the son of Adam except dirt, and Allah forgives those who repent."

Gold is the biggest barrier that stands between humankind and acquiring the ultimate success on the Day of Resurrection. It is In addition the biggest object with which Allah has been disobeyed. Because of gold, relations of the womb were severed, blood was shed, prohibitions were violated, rights were unjustly taken and slaves committed injustice against each other. Gold is the reason behind liking the life of this world and its shortness, and the cause behind disliking the Next Life and what Allah has prepared in it for His loyal supporters. With gold, so many truths were and are buried, so much falsehood was and is brought to life, so many unjust people were and are given support and so many innocent people were and are being dealt with unjustly.

The Letter R'aa

I. Rutab (Ripe Dates)

Allah said to Mary:

﴿ وَإِنَّ رَبَّكَ هُوَ يَحْشُرُهُمْ ۚ إِنَّهُۥ حَكِيمٌ عَلِيمٌ ﴿٢٥﴾ وَلَقَدْ خَلَقْنَا
ٱلْإِنسَٰنَ مِن صَلْصَٰلٍ مِّنْ حَمَإٍ مَّسْنُونٍ ﴿٢٦﴾ ﴾ (٢٥:٢٦) الحجر .

"And shake the trunk of date palm towards you. it will let fall fresh ripe dates upon you. So eat, drink, and be glad. Moreover, if you see any human

being, say: 'Verily, I have vowed a fast unto

The Most Gracious (Allah) so I shall not speak to any human being this day." (19: 25, 26)

In addition, in the *Sahihain* it is narrated that Abdullah bin Ja'far said:

I saw the Messenger of Allah b eating cucumbers with ripe dates."

Abu Dawud In addition narrated in his *Sunan* that Anas said:

"The Messenger of Allah b used to break his fast on some ripe dates, and if he did not have any, on dry dates. Otherwise, if be did not have dry dates, he would have several sips of water."

Ripe dates are just like water, hot and wet, and they are favorable for and strengthen the cold stomach, increase the production of semen and fertility, are suitable for cold temperaments and are very nutritious.

Ripe dates are the best types of fruit for the people of Al-Medina specifically and for all others in general where ripe dates grow. It is In addition a very beneficial fruit for the body, although ripe dates spoil quickly in the stomach of those who are not used to eating them and thus produce putrid blood. In addition, eating excessive amounts of ripe dates cause headaches and black bile and harms the teeth. Oxymel (Sakanjabin) helps neutralize the irritants that accompany eating ripe dates.

When the Prophet **b** used to break his fast, he used to eat first ripe or dry dates, or would drink some water. This is a wise decision, because fasting empties the stomach of food. Thus the liver would not find any sufficient energy that it could transfer to the various organs. Sweets are the fastest food to reach the liver and are favored by the liver, especially when one eats ripe dates, in which case the liver accepts it even more favorably, benefits from it and then transfers the benefit to the rest of the organs of the body. If there are no ripe dates available, one should eat dried dates because they are sweet and nutritious. Otherwise, some sips of water would extinguish the heat of the stomach and the Fast The stomach's appetite would then increase and become ready to accept (and digest) food.

2. Roihon (Myrtle / Basil)

Allah said:

﴿ فَأَمَّآ إِن كَانَ مِنَ ٱلْمُقَرَّبِينَ ۝٨٨ فَرَوْحٌ وَرَيْحَانٌ وَجَنَّتُ نَعِيمٍ ﴾

(٨٩:٨٨) الواقعة

"Then, if he (the dying person) be of the Muqarrabun (those brought near to Allah), (There is for him) rest and provision, and a Garden of Delights (Paradise)." (56:88,89)

And He said:

﴿ وَٱلْحَبُّ ذُو ٱلْعَصْفِ وَٱلرَّيْحَانُ ﴿١٢﴾ ﴾ (١٢) الرحمن .

"And In addition corn, with (its) leaves and stalk for fodder, and sweet-scented plants." (55:12) Muslim narrated that the Prophet **b** said:

"Whoever was presented with Rayhan should not refuse it, because it is easy to wear and has a good scent."

Ibn Majah narrated in his Sunon that Usamah related from the Prophet **b** that he said:

"Is there anyone who is ready to enter Paradise, for Paradise is all good (and pure). It is, by the Lord of the Ka'bah, a shining light, a twinkling Raihan, a luxurious palace, a running river, a ripe date, and a beautiful, pretty wife. It has many suits, eternal residence in a good plac of dwelling, fruits, vegetables, comfort and bounty in an exalted, comfortable dwelling."

They said, " 'Yes, O Messenger of Allah **b** We are

ready for it!' He said, 'Say, by Allah's Leave.' They said, By Allah's Leave.' "

Every plant that has good scent is called *'Raihan* . Therefore, every area gives a certain plant that name. For instance, the people to the west, as well as, the Arabs call the aromatic plants *Raihan*. The people in Iraq and Sham call the Hibk (a type of mint) a *Raihan*.

Raihan or myrtle is cold in the first degree and dry in the second degree. Yet, it is a compound of several qualities, most of which consist of earthly cold essence. Myrtle In addition consists of a soft hot substance. Myrtle dries the head nicely and is effective as a constipating agent.

Myrtle prevents bile diarrhea and dissipates hot and wet vapor when one smells its scent. Its scent In addition brings relief to the heart and prevents various ailments, especially when the plant is spread around the house.

In addition, myrtle heals the tumors that occur in the two ureters when it is coated on them. When fresh myrtle leaves are ground, blended with vinegar, and then placed on the head, they will stop nose bleeding. When dried myrtle leaves are crushed and the powder is sprinkled on wet ulcers it will heal them and will help weak organs when used as a bandage, relieve septic finger and heal spots and the ulcers on the hands and feet,

When myrtle is used to rub the body, it eliminates sweat, dries the excess wetness and dissipates underarm odor. When one sits in the water that myrtle was cooked in, it will help against infections on the buttocks and vagina and will heal weak joints and broken bones, when it is poured on the wound.

In addition, myrtle helps eliminate dandruff, the wet ulcers, and the spots that appear on the head. It In addition helps the hair against falling and gives it a black color. When myrtle leaves are ground with a little water and then blended with some oil or rose grease and then used as a bandage, it will be suitable against fresh (or humid) ulcers, canker sores, erysipelas (skin infection), acute tumors, urticaria (hives) and hemorrhoids.

Myrtle seeds In addition help against hemoptysis (spiting up blood) of the chest and lungs. It In addition coats the stomach, does not harm the chest or the stomach, and cleanses them. It In addition helps against diarrhea and coughing, and this is a special quality for myrtle that is rarely found in other medications. Myrtle seeds In addition help urine production and heal vesica (bladder) infections, spider bites and scorpion stings. Using myrtle roots to clean between the teeth is harmful, though.

Persian *Raihan,* which is In addition called *Hibq,* is hot, and when its scent is smelled, it helps against hot headaches when water is sprinkled on the *Hibq* and then is allowed to cool down. It is In addition said that this kind of myrtle is cold, but it looks like it has some of the four types of temperament. It In addition helps bring sleep to the eye.

The seeds of Persian myrtle relieve diarrhea of the bile, stomach, strengthen the heart and help against black bile ailments.

3. *Rumman* (Pomegranate)

Allah said:

﴿ فِيهِمَا فَٰكِهَةٌ وَنَخْلٌ وَرُمَّانٌ ﴿٦٨﴾ ﴾ (٦٨) الرحمن

"In them (both) will be fruits, and date palms and pomegranates." (55:68)

In addition, "Ali was reported to have said: "Eat *Rumman* with its pulp, because it coats the stomach."

Sweet pomegranate is hot and wet, good for the stomach, and strengthens it because of its being a mild constipating agent. It is In addition good for the throat, chest and lungs, along with relieving coughing. The water (or juice) in the pomegranate softens the stomach and is a nutrient for the body. It In addition digests quickly because it is light and produces heat along with some air in the stomach. It helps increase the semen production and is not favorable for those who have fever. Pomegranate has a special quality, that is, when one eats bread with it, it prevents it from being spoiled.

Bitter pomegranate is cold and dry and constipates mildly. It is In addition good for overheated stomach and helps produce more urine than the other types of pomegranate. It In addition softens bile symptoms, relieves diarrhea, prevents vomiting and is slightly tarry. It In addition stops the heat in the liver, strengthens the organs, helps against bilious shaking, heartaches and the ache of the tip of the stomach. It. In addition helps the stomach, rids it of excrements, extinguishes the bile, and benefits the blood.

When pomegranate's juice is extracted and is cooked with some honey until it becomes like an ointment and used as eye drops, it will clear the yellow color from the eye and will dissipate the thick wetness. When it is placed on the gingival (gums), it will help against the rashes that appear on the gingival. In addition, pomegranate juice extracted with the rind will work as a laxative and will rid the body from septic bilious moistures, along with helping against short-term fever.

As for sour pomegranate, its qualities are in the middle between the two other kinds we mentioned, although this kind leans more towards being sour. Pomegranate seeds that are mixed with honey will alleviate septic finger and malignant ulcers. Pomegranate flowers In addition help heal wounds. It is said that if one swallows three pomegranate flowers each year, he will be ımmune from ophthalmia (conjunctivitis) for an entire year.

The Letter Zal

1- Zait (Olive Oil)

Allah the Glorified said:

﴿ يُوقَدُ مِن شَجَرَةٍ مُّبَٰرَكَةٍ زَيْتُونَةٍ لَّا شَرْقِيَّةٍ وَلَا غَرْبِيَّةٍ يَكَادُ زَيْتُهَا يُضِيٓءُ وَلَوْ لَمْ تَمْسَسْهُ نَارٌ ﴾ (٣٥) النور .

"Lit from a blessed tree, an olive, neither of the east (i.e. neither it gets sun-rays only in the morning) n r of the west (i.e. nor it gets sun-rays only in the afternoon, but it is exposed to the sun all day long), whose oil would almost glow forth (of itself), though no fire touched it." (24:35)

At-Tirmidhi and Ibn Majah narrated that Abu Hurairah related from the Prophet b that he said:

"Eat the Zait and use it as an ointment, because it is produced by a blessed tree."

Al-Bayhaqi and Ibn Majah In addition narrated that 'Abdullah bin 'Umar said that the Messenger of Allah **b** said:

"Eat oil and use it as an ointment because it is from *a blessed tree (olive tree)"*

Zait is hot and wet in the first degree. In addition, the quality of the oil depends on the tree that produces it. For instance, the best type of olive oil is that squeezed from ripe olives, while oil from unripe olives is cold and dry. Red olives produce oil that is between these while black olives produce hot and wet oil. Olive oil helps against poisons, works as a laxative and rids the body of worms. Old olive oil leans more towards being hot and decomposing. When the oil is blended with water, it becomes less hot, milder, and thus more beneficial. All kinds of olive oil soften the skin and slow the aging process. The salty water blended with oil helps burned skin against blistering. It In addition strengthens the gingival.

2. *Zubd* (Butter)

Abu Dawood narrated in his *Sunan* that the two children of Busr said, "The Messenger of Allah **b** came by us and we offered him some butter and dried dates, as he used to like eating butter and dried dates."

Butter is hot and wet and has many benefits, such as maturing the mixtures (bodily wastes) and decomposing them, along with relieving the tumors that appear next to the ears and ureters (tubes leading from the kidney to the bladder). When butter is used, alone it In addition heals mouth cankers and the various other types of tumors that attack children and women. When one licks butter, it will help against lung hemoptysis (spitting up blood) and will mature the tumors of the lungs.

Butter softens the nature, the nerves and the hard tumors that result from black bile and phlegm and relieves the dryness in the body. When butter is laid on the place where children's' teeth emerge, it will help the teeth grow. Butter In addition soothes the coughing that accompanies colds and dryness. It In addition heals herpes and the roughness in the body and works as a laxative. Yet, butter reduces the appetite and the sweetness of honey and dates.

The wisdom behind the Prophet sag eating dried dates with butter is that they would neutralize the effect of each other.

3. *Zabib* (Raisins)

The best type of *Zabib* is the largest in size, the

fattest and that has thin skin and small seeds, especially when the seeds are removed before eating them. Raisins are hot and wet in the first degree, while their seeds are cold and dry.

Raisins are similar to the type of grape they are made of, as sweet raisins are hot, sour raisins are cold and constipating and white raisins are more effective constipating agents. Raisin pulp is suitable for the windpipe and relieves coughing, liver, and prostate pain. It In addition strengthens the stomach and soothes the intestinal cavity.

Sweet raisin pulps are more nutritious than grapes, but less nutritious than dried figs. In addition, raisin pulps possess maturing qualities and mildly constipate. In general, raisins strengthen the stomach, the spleen and the liver and benefit tile throat, chest, liver and prostate.

The best way to have raisins is to eat them without the seeds. Raisins provide good nutrition arid do not cause clogs like dates do. Eating raisins with their seeds I increase the nutritious intake and will benefit the stomach, liver and spleen. When one is suffering from loose nails and places raisin pulps on them, they will! Remove the nails quickly. Sweet, seedless raisins benefit for who suffer from excessive wetness and phlegm and help the liver.

Raisins In addition help memo-y power, as Az-Zuhri said, "Those who seek to memorize the *Hadith*: should eat raisirs." In addition, it was reported that Abdullah Ibn 'Abbas described the raisins that, "Their seeds are an ailment while their pulp is cure.

4- *Zanjabil* (Ginger)

Allah said:

﴿ وَيُسْقَوْنَ فِيهَا كَأْسًا كَانَ مِزَاجُهَا زَنجَبِيلًا ﴿١٧﴾ ﴾ (١٧) الإنسان

"And they will be give) to *drink there of a cup (of wine) mixed with anjabtl (ginger)."* (76: 17)

Abu Nu'aym In addition narrated in his book on the Prophetic medicine that Abu Sa'id Al-Khudri said:

Ginger is hot in the second degree and wet in the first degree. It heats the body, helps the ingestion process. softens the stomach mildly, helps open the clogs of the liver that are caused by coldness and wetness and helps against the wetness that causes sight impairment, when it is eaten or used as kohl. Ginger In addition strengthens the sexual power and decomposes the thick gases accumulating in the intestines and the stomach.

In general, ginger is good for the cold temperament of the liver and the stomach. When one takes some ginger along with two measures of sugar and some hot water, it will work as a laxative and will rid the body of harmful excrements. Ginger is an effective ingredient in the ointments that dissolve the phlegm.

Sour ginger is hot and dry and it excites the sexual drive, increases semen production, heats the stomach and the liver, helps the digestion process, dries the phlegm that prevails in the body and increases the memory power. It is In addition suitable for the coldness in the liver and stomach and washes the harmful effect of eating fruit. It In addition makes the scent better and fends off the harm of thick, cold foods.

The Letter Seen

1. Senna

We mentioned Senna before and stated that it is In addition called Sanut. There are seven opinions regarding what the word Senna means.

Senna is said to mean honey, the thick juice that appears on the surface of the butter and which looks like black stripes, cumin like seeds, Persian cumin. dill, dried dates or fennel.

2. *Safarjal* (Quince)

Quince is cold and dry, constipates and benefits the stomach. Sweet quince is cold and dry and is somewhat mild. Sour quince constipates more than sweet quince and is colder and drier. All types of *Safarjal* quench the thirst, stop vomiting, help produce urine and constipate. *Safarjal* In addition helps against stomach ulcers, hemoptysis (spitting up blood), diarrhea and nausea. *Safarjal* In addition prevents the ascending of gaseous material when one eats it after the meal. In addition, the ashes of washed *Safarjal* leaves and stems are similar to zinc in benefit.

Consuming Safarjal before the meal constipates, while consuming it after the meals softens the stool and helps the digestion process. Eating excessive amounts of *Safarjal* harms the nerves and causes painful constipation. *Safarjal* helps extinguish the yellow bile of the stomach.

When the quince is broiled, it will become softer and milder. When one removes the pips of. the quince, stuffs them with honey, dips them in a paste and then broil them under hot ashes, they will become very beneficial.

The best way to eat the quince is broiled or cooked in honey. The seeds of *Safarjal* In addition help against dryness in the throat, the windpipe and several other ailments. Its oil stops sweating and strengthens the stomach. *Safarjal* jam In addition strengthens the stomach and the liver and relieves the heart and the soul.

3. *Siwak*

In the *Sahihain* it is narrated that the Prophet **b** said:

"If it was not for the fact that my nation would not be able to bear it, I would have ordered them to use Siwak before every prayer."

In addition, in the *Sahihain* it is narrated that:

"Whenever the Prophet as would wake up at night, he would clean his mouth with Siwak."

Al-Kukhari In addition narrated that the Prophet b said:

"*Siwak* cleans the mouth and pleases the Lord." Further, Muslim narrated that:

"Whenever the Prophet b would enter his house, he would first use the Siwak."

There are many other *Ahadith* on this subject.

An authentic *Hadith* In addition stated that just

before he died, the Prophet b used the *Siwak*. The Prophet b said:

I have troubled you by frequently stressing using the *Siwak.*" The best type of *Siwak* is made from Arak trees. Further, one should not use an unknown tree for *Siwak* for it might be poisonous. In addition, *Siwak* should be used moderately, because it might cause the coating of the teeth to wear away and thus the teeth will be susceptible to the hot vapors or gasses that ascend from the stomach and to all kinds of dirt. When the *Siwak* is used moderately, it will polish the teeth, strengthen the roots of the teeth, help the tongue, prevent plaque, perfume the breath, clear the mind and strengthen the appetite.

The best way to use the *Swak* is by soaking it in rose water. In addition, the best type of *Siwak* is made from walnut stems. The author of At-Taysir said, "It was said that when one uses the *Siwak* once every five days, it will clear the head, sharpen the senses and alert the mind."

Siwak is beneficial for many reasons, such as perfuming the breath, strengthening the gingiva, clearing the phlegm and the sight and preventing cavities. It In addition preserves the health of the stomach, clears the voice, helps the digestion process, helps make the speech clear and encourages one to recite the Qura'an, remember

Allah and pray. *Siwak* In addition fights sleepiness, pleases the Lord, delights the angels and increases the number of the good deeds.

Siwak is preferred at any time, especially before the prayer, ablution, when waking up and when the mouth emits foul odor. It is In addition preferred for those who are fasting and all other people at all times. There are *Ahadith* that allow this practice for those who are fasting, because it is beneficial for them and pleases the Lord. Pleasing the Lord when one is fasting is even more desired than at other times. In addition the *Siwak* cleans the mouth, and cleanliness for the fasting person is one of his best deeds.

In the *Sunan* it is narrated that 'Amir bin RabT'ah said: "I saw the Messenger of Allah **b** on numerous occasion using the *Siwak* when he was fasting."

AI-Bukhari In addition said that Ibn 'Umar said that the Prophet sg used the *Siwak* at the two ends of the day.

There is a consensus that the fasting person rinses his mouth while performing ablution, and rinsing the mouth is an obligation or a more preferred act than using the Siwak. In addition, Allah does not have a use for the people to worship him while their mouths are emitting foul odor, nor is it an act of worship. When the Prophet mentioned that the odor that the mouth of the fasting person emits is better in His Sight than the scent of *Musk*, he meant to encourage the practice of fasting, not the practice of allowing the mouth to emit foul odor. Hence, the fasting person needs the *Siwak* more than anyone else. In addition, Allah's Pleasure is much better than His preferring the odor that the mouth of the fasting person emits.

Further, Allah prefers using the Siwak more than for the odor that comes out of the mouth of the fasting person to remain.

In addition, using *Siwak* does not prevent the good scent that Allah creates in the fasting person's mouth on the Day of Resurrection. Rather, the mouth of the fasting person will smell better than Musk on the Day of Resurrection as a sign of his observing the Fast, even if the Siwak removed the odor that used to come from his mouth. Similarly, whoever suffers a wound [for the sake of Allah] in this life is commanded to remove the blood from his body in this life, but his wound would still have the color of blood on the Day of Resurrection.

Furthermore, the *Siwak* does not completely remove the odor of the mouth for the fasting person because its reason still remains, that is, the stomach being empty of food. Only the effect of this fact will be lessened from the teeth and gums.

The Prophet b taught his nation the preferred and the disliked acts of the Fast. He did not mention the *Siwak* among the disliked acts although he knew they were using it. Rather, he encouraged them in general to use the *Siwak* and they saw him using it himself at innumerable times, knowing that they would imitate him. Never did he discourage them from using the *Siwak* in the afternoon (when they are fasting). It is a fact that the Prophet ^g is required to offer the religious ruling when it is needed.

4. Somn (Shortening)

There is a weak *Hadith* that narrates that the Prophet as encouraged the Muslim to drink cow milk, because it is a remedy and because the butter of that milk is a cure, while stating that cow meat is an ailment, The chain of narrators for this *Hadith* is not authentic.

Somn is hot and wet in the first degree, it is mild, and helps eliminate the various tumors that attack the soft parts of the body. Somn is stronger than butter as a maturing agent, Galinus said that he used shortening to cure the tumors that occur in the ear and the tip of the nose. In addition, when the base of the teeth is anointed with shortening, the teeth will emerge faster.

When shortening is blended with honey and bitter almonds, it will clear the chest and the lungs and will dissipate various ailments; Shortening is harmful for the stomach, especially if the person has a mucus condition.

When the shortening made of cow and goat milk is mixed with honey, it helps against toxic materials and snake and scorpion stings. Ibn As-Sunni mentioned that 'Ali said that the people never use a better remedy than shortening.

5. Samok (Fish)

Imam Ahmad and Ibn Majah narrated that 'Abdullah Ibn 'Umar said that the Prophet **b** said:

"We were *allowed two dead animals and two bloods: fish and locust, and liver and spleen."*

There are many kinds offish, the best of which is the most delicious, the best scented, moderate in size, which has fine scales, the softest meat, which live in fresh water that flows on pebbles and which eat plants and not organic waste. The best areas for the fish to live are those with the freshest water that runs through rocks, then the areas that have sandy ground void of filth or wastes and which are mildly calm and exposed to the sun and wind,

Sea fish are In addition soft and delicious. The meat of sea fish that has soft skin is cold and wet, difficult to digest and produces excessive amounts of phlegm, but In addition produce acceptable temperament, increase semen production and fertility and suit hot conditions.

The best kind of salted fish is the most recently salted. Salted fish is hot and dry, and the older they get the hotter and drier they become. Silurid (similar to catfish) is very viscous, and the Jews do not eat this type of fish. Yet, soft Silurid meat softens the stomach, and when it is salted, kept and then eaten, it will clear the windpipe and make the voice finer. When it is ground and used as an external ointment, it will extract the wastes that accumulate inside the body, as it has the quality of extracting such substances,

Sitting in the salty water of Silurid relives the effects of newly formed ulcers and extracts the harmful substances to the surface. Salty water of Silurid In addition relieves sciatic nerve ailment when one is injected with it.

The best part of fish meat is closer to the tail, and the soft and fatty fish meat produces fatness and flesh.

In the *Sahihain* it is In addition narrated that Jabir bin Abdullah said, "The Prophet **b** sent us with three hundred riders under the leadership of Abu 'Ubaidah bin Al-Jarrah. We went by the seashore and were soon very hungry until we ate tree leaves. The sea then threw out a whale that is called 'Anbar. We ate from it for a half a month and In addition used its fat in our food. Abu

Ubaidah then took a rib of the fish and asked a man to ride on his camel and .then pass under the rib, which he easily did."

6. Silqh (Chard)

At-Tirmidhi and Abu Dawud narrated that Umm AI-Munthir said, "The Messenger of Allah **b** came by along with Ali when he was still recovering from an illness. Then, we had some hanging clusters of dates. The Messenger of Allah **b** started eating from it, and he (Ali) joined him. The Messenger of Allah **b** then said to him:

"You are still recuperating, until 'Ali stopped eating.' I then made some barley with chard and brought it to them. The Prophet b said, to 'Ali 'Eat from this: this more beneficial for you.'"

Silqh is hot and dry in the first degree and has a soothing coofness in it. Chard In addition decomposes and opens the clogs. The *black chard* constipates and helps against alopecia (A skin disease characterized by loss of hair, partial or total), spots, *dandruff and warts if* its water is used as ointment. It In addition kills lice and is used as ointment when blended with honey to cure herpes. *Silqh* In addition opens the clogs in the liver and spleen.

The black chard constipates as we have stated, especially when taken with lentils, both of which are not suitable for the stomach. However, white chard with lentils softens the stomach and is used as a laxative and is used to treat hemiplegia (Paralysis affecting only one side of the body), when blended with food aliments and condiments. Yet, it is not nutritious, produces harmful mixtures and burns the blood. Eating it with vinegar and mustard helps neutralize these side effects. Finally, eating it excessively causes constipation and flatulence.

The Letter Shin

1. *Shuneiz* (The Black Seed)

We talked about the Black Seed before under the letter 'Hoo.

2. *Shubrum* (Euphorb)

At-Tirmidhi and Ibn Majah narrated that the Messenger of Allah b asked Asma' bint 'Umais

"How do you treat *constipation? She said. 'with Shubrum'. The Prophet* its said, 'Hot and too strong of a *laxative."*

Shubrum is a small tree that sometimes grows to be as tall as a man. The *Shubrum* has red branches with some whiteness, while the tips of its branches end with a cluster of leaves, *Shubrum* flowers are small and yellowish with some whiteness. When its flowers they fall small stems that have small grains and which look like terebinth replace them. The color of these stems is reddish and has red peels that cover its ribs. The parts of the *Shubrum* that are used are its peels, ribs and stem extract,

Shubrum is hot and dry in the fourth degree and drives away the black bile, yellow water and phlegm. It In addition causes nausea and distress. Using it in excessive amounts might even case death. When intending to use the *Shubrum,* it should first be soaked in milk for a day and a night, and the milk should be changed twice or thrice during the day. Then, the *Shubrum* should be dried in the shadow, blended with roses, tragacanth (In addition known as goats' horn), and then consumed with honey water or grape juice.

Two to four small measures of the *Shubrum* constitute one dose. We should state that Hunain said, "As for *Shubrum* milk, I do not see any goodness in it and thus do not recommend it. Common doctors have killed many people with it."

3. Sho'fr (Barley)

Ibn Majah narrated that "Aishah said: "When a member of the family of the Messenger of Allah **b** would fall sick, he would order that barley soup is made and then the ill person would be commanded to have some of it. He used to say, 'It strengthens the heart of the sad person and relieves the heart of the ill person, just as one of you would wash the dirt off of her face with water.' "

We mentioned that the remedy mentioned in this *Hadith* entails boiled barley water which is more nutritious than its flour. Barley water helps against coughing and throat roughness, relieves the irritant excess excrement, produces more urine, cleanses the stomach, quenches the thirst and extinguishes heat. It In addition provides comfort and has a decomposing quality.

This remedy entails preparing a portion of a good type of barley and five times as much water, placing them in a clean pot and cooking them under moderate temperature until only two fifths of the mixture remains in the pot. The resulting soup is then purified and used as much as needed.

4. Shown (Roasted Meat)

Allah said that when Prophet Ibrahim had the honorable guests:

"And he hastened to entertain them with a roasted calf." (I 1:69) Ibrahim had roasted the calf on heated stones.

At-Tirmidhi narrated that Umm Salamah said that

she once brought the Prophet s& a roasted piece of meat and that he ate from it and then stood up to pray without repeating the ablution. At-Tirmidhi then commented that this *Hadith* is authentic. At-Tirmidhi In addition narrated that Abdullah bin Al-Harith said, "We ate some roasted meat with the Messenger of Allah as inside the mosque." Further, At-Tirmidhi narrated that Al-Mughirah bin Shu'bah said, "I was a guest of the Messenger of Allah b one night and he ordered that a piece of meat be roasted and then took the blade and started to cut pieces of it for me. Then, Bilal came to make the call to prayer and the Prophet s& dropped the blade and said, 'What is the matter with him?'"

The best type of roast is the meat of a one-year old sheep, then a fat sheep. This type of food is hot and wet, produces black bile, but is one of the most nutritious foods for healthy, ill and recovering persons alike. Cooked meat is better, lighter on the stomach and has more wetness. Fried meat is less beneficial while meat dried in the sun is the worst kind. In addition, roasting meat on burning stones is better than flame broiled meats.

5. *Sha'hm* (Fat or Grease)

In Al-Musnad it is narrated that Anas said that a Jewish man asked the Prophet ste to be his guest and that he offered him some barley bread and melted grease.

In the *Sahih* it is In addition narrated that Abdullah bin Mughaffal said, "On the Day of Khaibar, a bag full of grease was lowered and I took possession of it and said, 'By Allah! I will not give anyone any of it!' When I turned around I found that the Messenger of Allah ^ was laughing and did not comment.' "

The best type of grease is that taken from a grown animal. Grease is hot and wet but less wet than clarified butter. This is why when both grease and clarified butter are melted, grease hardens faster.

Grease helps against throat roughness, it represses and causes rotting. To neutralize the harmful effects of grease, one should use lemon, salt and ginger. In addition, goat grease constipates more than any other type of grease, while Billy goat grease is more decomposing and helps against stomach ulcers. Goat grease helps against stomach ulcers and is used as an injection to relieve excoriation (the rubbing away of skin from injury or disease), and (spasms of the bladder or anus).

The Letter Sod

I. The So/at (The Formal Prayer)

Allah said:

﴿ وَٱسْتَعِينُوا۟ بِٱلصَّبْرِ وَٱلصَّلَوٰةِ ۚ وَإِنَّهَا لَكَبِيرَةٌ إِلَّا عَلَى ٱلْخَـٰشِعِينَ ﴾

(٤٥) البقرة .

"And seek help in patience and As-Salat (the prayer) and truly, it is extremely heavy and hard except for Al-Khashi'un [i.e. the true believers in Allah - those who obey Allah with full submission, fear much from His punishment, and believe in His Promise (Paradise) and in His Warnings (Hell)]." (2:45)

And:

﴿ يَـٰٓأَيُّهَا ٱلَّذِينَ ءَامَنُوا۟ ٱسْتَعِينُوا۟ بِٱلصَّبْرِ وَٱلصَّلَوٰةِ ۚ إِنَّ ٱللَّهَ مَعَ ٱلصَّـٰبِرِينَ ﴿١٥٣﴾ ﴾ (١٥٣) البقرة

***"O you who believe! Seek help in patience and As-Salat (the prayer). Truly, Allah is with As-Sabirun (the patient)."* (2:153)**

In addition, Allah said,

﴿ وَأْمُرْ أَهْلَكَ بِالصَّلَوٰةِ وَاصْطَبِرْ عَلَيْهَا ۖ لَا نَسْـَٔلُكَ رِزْقًا ۖ نَّحْنُ نَرْزُقُكَ ۗ وَالْعَـٰقِبَةُ لِلتَّقْوَىٰ ﴿١٣٢﴾ ﴾ (١٣٢) طه

"And enjoin As-Salat (the prayer) on your family, and be patient in offering them [i.e. the Salat (prayers)]. We ask not of you a provision (i.e. to give Us something: money): We provide for you. And the good end (i.e. Paradise) is for the Muttaqun (the pious)." (20:132)

Furthermore, in the Sunon it is narrated;

"Whenever the Messenger of Allah would be concerned about a matter, he would turn to prayer."

We In addition mentioned using the prayer as a cure for various types of illnesses before these illnesses progress.

The prayer brings about sustenance, preserves the health, discards harm, eradicates illness, strengthens the heart, radiates the face with light, brings joy to the soul and dissipates laziness. In addition, the prayer energizes the limbs, sustains power, opens the chest, nourishes the soul, brings light to the heart, protects the bounty, shields from the anger (of Allah), brings about blessings, takes one away from Satan and draws him closer to the Most Beneficent.

In general, the prayer has a profound effect in preserving the health of the body and the heart. The prayer In addition discards harmful substances. No two persons would catch a type of disease or suffer an affliction, but whoever prays among them would suffer the minimal effects of the illness or the affliction.

The prayer has a profoundly wonderful effect in repelling the evils of this life, especially when the prayer is given its due right inwardly and outwardly. Certainly, the evils of this life and the Next Life would be most effectively repelled while their good would be most effectively brought forth through prayer. The secret in this is that the prayer is the connection with Allah. The closer the connection is between the slave and his Lord, the more open the doors of all types of good will be for him, while closing the ways to evil. In this case, the tools of success will descend on the slave from his Lord, along with good health, many bounties and riches, comfort, delight, joy, happiness and the good things of life,

2. Sabr (Patience)

Sabr, patience, is one half of Faith, which is half patience and half praise and thankfulness. Some of the

So/of said, "Iman has two halves, one half patience and one half praise (and appreciation)." Allah said:

﴿ فَقَالُوا رَبَّنَا بَٰعِدْ بَيْنَ أَسْفَارِنَا وَظَلَمُوا أَنفُسَهُمْ فَجَعَلْنَٰهُمْ أَحَادِيثَ وَمَزَّقْنَٰهُمْ كُلَّ مُمَزَّقٍ ۚ إِنَّ فِي ذَٰلِكَ لَآيَٰتٍ لِّكُلِّ صَبَّارٍ شَكُورٍ ﴿١٩﴾ ﴾ (١٩) سبأ

"Verily, in this are indeed signs for every steadfast, grateful (person)." (34:19)

To Faith, *Sabr* is just like the head to the body. There are three types of Sabr. First, there is the Sabr while performing Allah's Commands, so that one does not ignore [or get bored with] them. There is a Sabr with shunning the prohibitions, so that one does not violate them. There is In addition a Sabr with the appointed destiny and decisions of Allah, so that one is not enraged because of them. When one acquires all three types of Sabr, his Sabr will be complete and the delight of this and the Next Life will be whole, along with gaining and winning in both lives. No person shall achieve these great prizes except by passing on the bridge of Sabr, just as no person will reach Paradise except by passing over the Sirot (the bridge over hell). Umar said, "We achieve the best living by Sabr."

When one thinks about the grades of perfection achieved in this life, he will realize that all of them are connected to *Sabr*. On the other hand, when one thinks about the blame worthy types of failure that one can and should avoid, he will realize that they are all connected to impatience. For instance, courage, honor, generosity and preferring others with good things are patience for a short time only (meaning this life is short).

Much of the illnesses and the sicknesses that attack the body and the heart are a result of impatience. In addition, *Sabr* is the best preserver for the health of the heart, the body and the soul, as it is the great distinction and the biggest cure. If *Sabr* only carries the reward of Allah being with the patient slaves and His love for them, it would be sufficient. Allah loves *Sabr* and supports its people:

"Certainly, victory comes with patience"

In addition, patience is good for its people.

﴿ وَإِنْ عَاقَبْتُمْ فَعَاقِبُوا۟ بِمِثْلِ مَا عُوقِبْتُم بِهِۦ ۖ وَلَئِن صَبَرْتُمْ لَهُوَ خَيْرٌ لِّلصَّٰبِرِينَ ۝١٢٦ ﴾ (١٢٦) النحل

"But if you endure patiently, verily, it is better for As-Sabirun (the patient)." (16:126)

Further, patience is the tool to achieve success.

﴿ يَـٰٓأَيُّهَا ٱلَّذِينَ ءَامَنُوا۟ ٱصْبِرُوا۟ وَصَابِرُوا۟ وَرَابِطُوا۟ وَٱتَّقُوا۟ ٱللَّهَ
لَعَلَّكُمْ تُفْلِحُونَ ﴿٢٠٠﴾ ﴾ (٢٠٠) آل عمران

"O you who believe! Endure and be more patient (than your enemy), and guard your territory by stationing army units permanently at the places from where the enemy can attack you, and fear Allah, so that you may be successful." (3:2OO)

3. Sobir (Aloe)

Sabir has many benefits, especially the Indian *Sabir,* as it rids the body of bilious excrements in the brain and the optic nerves. When the *Sabir* is used as an ointment on the forehead and the cheeks, after blending it with rose oil, it helps relieve headaches. It In addition helps relieve the sores and cankers that appear in the mouth and nose and helps against black bile and depression.

The Persian *Sabir* sharpens the mind and brings firmness to the heart, and In addition releases from the body bilious mixtures and the phlegm that accumulates in the stomach, when one takes two spoons of *Sabir* mixed with water.

Caution: drinking *Sabir* in cold weather might cause diarrhea with blood.

4. *Sawm* (Fasting)

Fasting is a shield from many illnesses of the soul, the heart and the body and has tremendous benefits. Fasting In addition preserves the health and rids the body of harmful substances while preventing it from consuming what might harm it, especially when one fasts in the best times that the religion states or when the body needs it. Fasting relieves the muscles and the rest of the body and ensures regenerating its strength. Fasting In addition has a characteristic that should make one eagerly prefer it, that is, bringing joy and relief to the heart sooner or later (i.e. on the Last Day). Fasting is the best resort for those suffering from excess bodily moistures and substances and In addition protects and preserves their health.

Fasting is a type of spiritual and physical remedy. When the fasting person observes various rulings and guidelines regarding the Fast, his heart and body will benefit from the Fast the most. In addition, the body will get rid of the harmful foreign substances that his body is susceptible to receive, along with getting rid of the harmful substances that have already penetrated the body. The Fast In addition helps the fasting person to stay away from what he is supposed to avoid and to implement and seek the goals behind the Fast and what it is supposed to achieve for him. Fasting does not only entail abstaining from food and drink. There is another goal that fasting seeks to achieve which made it an act that Allah will specify its reward [only on the Day of Judgment]. The Fast is In addition a shield between the slave and what might harm his body and soul sooner or later, and this is why Allah said,

﴿ يَٰٓأَيُّهَا ٱلَّذِينَ ءَامَنُواْ كُتِبَ عَلَيۡكُمُ ٱلصِّيَامُ كَمَا كُتِبَ عَلَى

ٱلَّذِينَ مِن قَبۡلِكُمۡ لَعَلَّكُمۡ تَتَّقُونَ ﴿١٨٣﴾ ﴾ (١٨٣) البقرة .

"O you who believe! Observing As-Saum (the fasting) is prescribed for you as it was prescribed for those before you, that you may become Al-Muttaqun (the pious)." (2:183)

Fasting is a shield and a protection making it a type of tremendously beneficial diet. Another goal that the Fast seeks to achieve is the heart being busy with Allah, thus enlisting and recruiting the various powers of the body to implement what Allah loves and the requirements of worshiping Him. We mentioned some of the secrets of the Fast when we mentioned the Prophet's guidance on this subject.

The Letter Dhad

1. *Dhabb* (Lizards)

In the *Sahihain* it is narrated that Ibn 'Abbas said that the Messenger of Allah ^ was asked if eating the Dhabb was disallowed, because he did not eat from it when it was presented to him. The Prophet $s replied:

"No. But this food is not found in my *people's land and I do not have the appetite to eat it."*

The *Dhabb* was then eaten in the presence of the Prophet b In addition, the *Sahihain* it is narrated that Ibn 'Umar related from the Prophet sg that he said:

"I neither allow it nor disallow it."

The meat of the *Dhabb* is hot and dry and strengthens the sexual drive. When it is ground and placed on a thorn that pierced someone's skin, it will extract the thorn.

2. *Dhifdi'* (Frog)

Imam Ahmad said, "(Killing) frogs is not allowed for medicinal purposes, because the Messenger of Allah s® has disallowed killing them." Ahmad was referring to the *Hadith* that he narrated in his *Musnad* in which

Uthman bin Abdur-Rahman said that a doctor mentioned using frogs for medicinal purposes, and the Messenger disallowed killing them.

The author of 'Al-Qanoon said, "Eating the meat or the blood of the frog might cause swellings in the body, pale color and [uncontrollable] ejaculation until death. This is why the doctors hesitate to use it formedicinal purpose because of its harm." There are two types of frogs, land and water frogs. Some of the land frogs are POISONED.

The Letter To'

1 *TaJb* **(Perfume)**

The Messenger of Allah b said:

"From your world, women and Tatb (perfume) were made beloved to me and the comfort of my eye is the prayer."

The Messenger of Allah ^ used to frequently use *Tatb* and did not like foul odors.

Taib (perfume) is the fuel of the soul, which is the engine of the powers of the body. Therefore, various strengths and powers in the body are nurtured in the presence of *Taib*. Similarly, the powers of the body are nurtured by consuming food and drink, feeling comfort and elation, being close to loved ones, receiving good news and by the absence of hateful, disliked persons whose presence is heavy on the heart. Indeed. associating with disliked persons weakens the strength and causes sadness and depression, just as the effects that fever and foul odor have on the body. This is why the companions of the Messengers were disallowed from acquiring the characteristics that would bother the Prophet and make them detested and disliked by him. Allah said:

"But when you ore invited, enter, and when you have taken your mea;, *disperse without sitting for a talk. Verily, such (behaviour) annoys the Prophet, and he is shy of (asking) you (to go); but Allah is not shy of (telling you) the truth."* (33:53)

In short, the *Taib,* perfume, was one of the dearest objects to the Prophet of Allah sfe. It In addition has a good effect on preserving good health and removing many ailments because it arouses the power of the body.

2. Teen (Clay or Argil)

Several invented *Ahadith* were mentioned regarding the benefits of clay. We should state that every *Hadith* that talks about the benefit of clay is untrue and must not be related from the Messenger of Allah. Clay is harmful and causes clogs in the veins, and it is cold, dry and a strong drying agent. In addition, clay prevents diarrhea and causes hemorrhages and sours in the mouth.

3. *Talh* (Banana or Acacia)

Allah said:

"And among Talh (banana-trees) with fruits piled one above another." (56:29)

The majority of the scholars said that *Talh* means bananas, as they grow in piles one over the other just as the comb's teeth. It was said that the *Talh* is the tree that has thorns and which get replaced by fruits, each in the place of a thorn, just like what occurs on banana trees. This is the best opinion about the meaning of *Talh*. Hence, the So/of (righteous predecessors) who said that the *Talh* means banana trees are just using the banana tree as an example to explain the meaning of the word *Talh,* not that it only means banana trees. Allah has the best knowledge.

Bananas are hot and wet. The best type of bananas is ripe and sweet.

Bananas help against the roughness of the chest and lung, relieve coughing and help against the ulcers of the kidney and prostate. Bananas In addition produce urine (diuretic), stimulate semen production, soften the stomach and arouse the sexual drive; and they should be eaten before meals. Bananas harm the stomach and aggravate the bile and the phlegm, but eating them with sugar and honey reduces their harmful side effects.

4. To/' (Shoots or Clusters of dates)

﴿ وَٱلنَّخْلَ بَاسِقَٰتٍ لَّهَا طَلْعٌ نَّضِيدٌ ﴾ ق (١٠) .

Allah said: **"And tall date-palms, with ranged clusters."** (5O:1O) And He said:

"And green crops *(field) and date-palms with soft spadix."*

(26:148) The *Tal'* of the date trees is the fruit when it is still young.

There are two types of *Tal'* (clusters): male and female. The reproduction process of date trees requires transferring pollen, which resembles the male organ and which looks like a fine powder, and placing it on the female organ. This process is called *Ta'bir.*

Muslim narrated in his *Sahih* that Talhah bin 'Ubaidullah said:

"I and the Messenger of Allah as passed by some date trees and found some people doing *Ta'bir.* The

Prophet sn; asked about what they we.e doing and they said that they were removing the maie sex ual organ and placing it in the female sexual organ. The Prophet *yss,* said, '] do not think that this process will be of much help.' When they heard what the Prophet ^ said, they abandoned what they were doing and the trees did not reproduce. The Prophet s& then said, 'It was only a guess on my part. If (the *Ta'bir)* does help, then do it. I am only human just like you and my guess is either correct or incorrect. But, whatever I inform you from Allah (is true), I will never utter a lie on Allah."

The *Tal'* stimulates semen production and strengthens the sexual drive. When a woman takes the powder of the *Tal'* before having sex, it will help her get pregnant. The clusters of date trees are cold and dry in the second degree, strengthen the stomach and dry it out, and calm irritated blood, but are hard to digest.

Only those who have hot temperament can tolerate eating the *Tal'*. In addition, those who eat the To;' regularly should In addition eat hot sweets with it. The *Tal'* constipates and strengthens the intestines, just as theJummor, fresh dates and Busr that we mentioned before. Eating the *Tal'* in excessive amounts harms the stomach and the chest and might cause painful constipation, while taking it with butter and sweets helps reduce these side effects.

The Letter 'Ayn

1. '/nob (Grapes)

The Messenger of Allah ^ was reported to have liked eating grapes and watermelon. In addition, Allah has mentioned grapes in six instances in the Qura'an while listing the various bounties that He has bestowed on His slaves in this and the Next Life. Grapes are among the best and most beneficial fruits, and they are eaten fresh, dried, green and ripe. Further, Grapes are a type of fruit and nutritious food, along with their benefits as a remedy and a drink. Wetness and hotness are among the characteristics of grapes just as other grains. The best type of grapes is the big grapes that are full of juice, while white grapes are better than the black grapes when both are equal in sweetness. In addition, eating fresh grapes two or three days after harvest is better than eating them immediately otherwise they cause diarrhea and flatulence. The grapes are left on their hanging grapevines until their skin becomes thin. They are a source of good nutrition, just like raisins and figs, and In addition strengthen the body.

When the seeds of the grapes are removed, the grapes become a more effective laxative. Eating grapes excessively causes headache, unless one In addition eats sour pomegranate. Grapes in general are a good laxative and provide a good source of nutrition. The best types of fruits are three: grapes, dates and figs.

2. *'Asal* (Honey)

We mentioned the benefits of honey before.

Ibn Jurayj said that Az-Zuhri said, "Eat honey because it is good for the memory." The best type of honey is the white, pure, light and sweet honey. In addition, the honey that is collected from trees and mountains is better than the honey that is grown in cells. Further, the quality of the honey varies according to the area where the bees collected their food.

3. *'Ajwah* (Pressed, Dried Dates)

Sa'd bin Abu Waqqas narrated that the Prophet a& said:

"Whoever eats seven dates of 'Ajwah in the morning will not be harmed by poison or magic the rest of that day."

In addition, An-Nasa'y and Ibn Majah narrated that the Prophet s& said:

***"The* 'Ajwah is from Paradise, and it is an antidote against poison. The Kamab (truffles) is a type of Manna and its water (extract) cures the eye."**

There is an opinion that this *Hadith* is talking about the *'Ajwah* of Al-Madinah in particular, which is one the best types of dates in the area of Hijaz. The *'Ajwah*, pressed dried dates, is a good type of dates, has firm skin and is one of the softest and most delicious types of dates.

We mentioned the various benefits of the dates and the Tomr when we talked about the letter Too. We In addition mentioned the benefits of the *'Ajwah* in treating poison and fending off the harm of magic.

4. *'Anbar* (Ambergris; Whale)

We mentioned the *Hadith* that is narrated in the Two *Sahihs* about Abu "Ubaydah and the Muslim army finding a huge fish, or whale, and that they ate from it for a half a month. They In addition took some of its meat with them to Al-Madinah and gave the Prophet ﷺ some of it. This *Hadith* indicates that it is allowed for Muslims to eat whatever comes from the sea even when it is dead.

Some people who [disagree with what we stated above] said that the whale was thrown on the shore while still alive and that when the water receded it died. Therefore, they say, the whale died because of the lack of water not naturally.

This opinion is incorrect, because the companions

found the whale dead at the seashore. They did not see it alive and then the water receded causing its death as claimed. Further, if the whale were still alive, the sea would not have thrown it on the shore, since the sea usually throws dead animals and dead fish on the shore.

Furthermore, even if what they claimed had happened to the whale, it will not affect the ruling of permissibility [to eat dead marine creatures]. The Prophet sis disallowed eating game if one finds it dead in the water because there is a doubt if it had died from drowning and not from his weapon. So, if what the opponents say were true, then the fact that there is a doubt concerning how the whale died would disallow eating it [i.e. if their suggestion that the whale died because of lack of air and that dead marine creatures are disallowed dead were both true].

As for Al-'Anbar, amber, which is a type of *Tatb* (perfume), it is one of the best types of perfume after *Musk*. Some people mistakenly preferred *'Anbar* to *Misk*. However, the Prophet ^e described *Musk:*

"It is the best TaJb (perfume)."

Soon afterwards, we will mention the benefits and characteristics of Musk, which is the *Tatb* of Paradise. In addition, the seats in Paradise that belong to the truthful believers are made of A Lusk not *'Anbar*.

Those who thought that *'Anbar* is better than *Musk* were deceived by the fact that the *'Anbar* does not spoil, just like gold. This fact alone does not indicate that the *'Anbar* is better than A/lusk.

There are several types of *'Anbar:* white, gray, red, yellow, green, blue, black and multicolored. The best type of the *'Anbar* is gray, then the blue and then the yellow in color, while the black *'Anbar* is the worst type.

People have conflicting opinions regarding the origin of *'Anbar,* where some people said that it is a plant that grows on the seabed and which sea reptiles eat and then discard to later be thrown on the seashore. Some people say that *'Anbar* is the waste of sea creatures that looks like cow manure. Some people even said that it is a type of foam that the sea discards on the shore. The author of the 'Qanoon' discounted the last two opinions but said that the amber might originate from an undersea spring.

'Anbar is hot and dry and strengthens the heart, the mind and the senses. It In addition strengthens the body and helps relieve facial paralysis, hemiplegia (paralysis), phlegmy ailments, stomach and flatulence. *'Anbar* In addition helps open various clogs if it is used as an ointment or as a drink. When it is inhaled, *'Anbar* will relieve cold symptoms, headaches and migraines.

5. *'Ud* (Indian Aloe Tree)

The Indian *'Ud* comes in two types. One type is used for medicinal purposes, which is called Al-Kust and some people called it Al-Qust. We will mention this type under the letter *Qaf.* The second type of 'Ud is called Aluwwah, aoe wood, which is used as perfume.

Imam Muslim narrated in his *Sahih* that Ibn "Umar used to bum dry aloe wood along with some *Kafur* (camphor), and states that the Messenger of Allah used to do the same. In addition, the Messenger of Allah has described the bounties that the people of Paradise will be enjoying, such as having the aloe wood.

The 'Ud is hot and dry in the third degree, opens the clogs and does away with gas. In addition, 'Ud dries unnecessary moisture while strengthening the intestines and brings relief and comfort to the heart. 'Ud In addition helps the mind, sharpens the senses, constipates and helps relieve the enuresis, bed wetting that result from coldness of the prostate.

Ibn Samjun said, "There are several kinds of 'Ud, and they all carry the general name of Aluwwah. 'Ud is used in and out of the body and is burned alone or with other substances. There is a medicinal significance when the 'Ud is mixed with *Kafur* (camphor), as each of them makes the other milder. In addition, burning the 'Ud helps cleanse the air, which is one of the six necessary elements for the body's well-being."

6. *'Adas* (Lentils)

It was reported that the 'Ados (lentils) was described as the lust of the Jews that they preferred over Manna and quails.

The 'Ados is the companion of garlic and onions. It is cold and dry and has two opposing effects, one that constipates and one that works as a laxative. The skin of the 'Ados is hot and dry in the third degree and In addition works as a laxative. The benefit in the lentils is concentrated in the peelings, and this is why whole lentils are more beneficial than ground lentils, less heavy on the stomach and less harmful.

Lentils cause black bile and harm the melancholy profoundly, along with having a negative effect on the nerves and the eyesight.

'Adas produces thick blood; and those who suffer from black bile should avoid eating it, for when they eat lentils excessively, the lentils will beget obsession, leprosy, quartran fever (a fever that occurs on every fourth day), and other ailments. However, eating lentils with chard and large amounts of grease will lessen their negative side effects. In addition, one should avoid eating lentils with sweets, because lentils could cause clogs in the liver in this case. Further, eating 'Ados on a regular basis causes harm to the eyesight because they are very dry. Lentils In addition cause urine retention, cold swellings and excessive flatulence. The best type of 'Ados is the fat, white 'Ados that digests faster.

Some ignorant people claimed that Prophet Ibrahim used to cook lentils for his guests. However, the Qura'an mentioned that he hosted his guests with a fat roasted calf.

The Letter Ghayn

1. *Gbayth* (Rain)

The *Ghaith* is mentioned in the Qura'an in many instances. The word *Ghaith* is soft on the ear and delightful for the body and the soul. The ears like to hear the word *Ghaith*, while the hearts enjoy its falling.

Rainwater is the best type of water there is and the softest, most beneficial and most blessed. This is especially the case when the rainfall is accompanied by lightning and thunder and is then collected in mountainous areas.

Rainwater is lighter than the other types of water because it is fresh and did not remain on the ground for a long time, in which case it would acquire some of the earth's dryness and hard substances. This is why rainwater gets spoiled quickly because it is pure and light.

There are two opinions regarding which is softer and lighter: rainwater that falls in the spring or winter.

Those who prefer winter rainwater say that in winter, the sun's heat is less and it thus evaporates the softest parts of the seawater. In addition, the air then would be clean and void of dust, and consequently, would not be polluted. Hence, rainwater will not dissolve any pollutants while falling, and this is why rainwater is the softest and the lightest.

Those who prefer spring rainwater say that the hot sun then evaporates heavy substances in the air and makes the air itself lighter and cleaner. In this case, rainwater will be the lightest and the softest, at a time when the plants, the trees and the air become ready to receive rainfall.

Ash-Shafey narrated • that Anas bin Malik said, "Once, we were with the Prophet sg when the rain fell. The Prophet b removed his outer garment (until the rain fell on him) saying:

***It has* just come from its Lord."**

We mentioned the Prophet's guidance in invoking Allah for rain and stated that he used to seek the blessings [that Allah endows] in the rain when it falls.

The Letter Foo

1. Fatihah *Al-Kitab* (the First Chapter in the Qur'an)

Fatihah is the mother of the Qura'an, the seven frequently recited Versus that the Prophet ste was given and the ultimate cure and beneficial remedy that contains the prefect *Ruqiah,* Islamic prayer formula. The *Fatihah* is the key to acquiring the richness, success and strength. The *Fatihah* In addition removes sadness, depression, anguish and fear. Only those who appreciate the value of the *Fatihah* and give it its due consideration, reciting it as it should be recited and knowing the secret of its value as a medicine and as a cure, will acquire such bounties.

One of the Companions unveiled a few of the secrets of the *Fatihah* when he used it as a *Ruqyah for* scorpion stings. The affected person was instantly cured and the Prophet sn asked the Companion:

"How did you know it is a cure?"

They are successful ones who uncover some of the secrets of the *Fatihah* and what it contains of *Tawhid,* knowing Allah and His Names, Attributes, Actions and

Decisions. Those who acquire knowledge of what the Fot/hoh contains of affirming the religion, Predestination, Resurrection, Allah's Oneness in worship and in Lordship and trusting and depending on He Who owns all affairs, the praise and all pure things and to Whom everything must return. Those who acquire the habit of showing meekness to Allah seeking correct guidance which is the basis of the ultimate happiness in this and the Next Life. Those who acquire knowledge in the connection between the meanings contained in the *Fatihah* and acquiring the good and fending off the harm of both lives. Those who understand that their ultimate well-being and receiving the perfect Favor of Allah are all linked to implementing these meanings. It is they who will be able to substitute the *Fatihah* in place of many medicines and use it as an Islamic prayer formula *{Ruqiah)*, and will use it to open the doors of goodness and drive away the elements of evil.

Understanding this subject requires a new nature, a new heart and a new type of Faith. By Allah! You will not find any evil statement, nor misguiding innovation, but the *Fatihah* will contain what nullifies and refutes it with the best, most correct and most direct manner. In addition, you will not find a door that leads to acquiring divine knowledge, correct guidance of the heart and the remedy of the soul against its ills, but that the *Fatihah* will possess its key and the method to best use it. Finally, you will not find a path on which those who seek the Lord of the Worlds are passing, but you will find the *Fatihah* in its beginning and end.

By Allah! The *Fatihah* is much more important than what we have emphasized. The slave who holds fast to the *Fatihah,* comprehends it in the proper manner, relies on it as a perfect remedy, a shield, immunity, and as a light of guidance. He understands its implications as they should be understood. It is he who will not fall into an innovation, or Shirk, or catch an ailment in the heart except briefly!

The *Fatihah* is the ultimate key for the treasures of the earth and Paradise, as well. But not every person knows how to use this key so as to have access to these treasures. If those who seek these treasures were able to uncover the secrets of this chapter [in the Qura'an] and acquire knowledge of its implications, they would add teeth to the key and would have easy access to these treasures.

We are certain of the statements that we have asserted herein because they are true. Allah has Perfect Wisdom in hiding the secrets [of *Al-Fatihah'}* from the hearts of the majority of humankind, just as He has a perfect Wisdom in hiding the treasures of the earth from them.

The hidden treasures of the earth are surrounded by the devils that stand between humankind and these treasures. Only the good souls will be able to defeat these devils with True Faith, which is the weapon that the devils cannot withstand. However, the majority of the souls of mankind are not of this type (are not truly faithful). Therefore, they cannot resist the evil or defeat them to acquire their possessions for, "Whoever kills a combatant will have his possessions."

2. *Faghiyah* (Henna Blossom)

Faghiyah, henna blossom, is one of the best kinds of perfumes, *Faghiyah* is mild in its hotness and dryness and constipates mildly. When Faghiyah is placed between folded wool clothes it protects them from mold and mites. In addition, *Faghiyah* is used in ointments against facial paralysis and aneurysm (dilatation of a portion of the wall of an artery), while its oil helps the organs and relaxes the nerves.

3. *Fiddah* (Silver)

There is an authentic narration that states:

"The Messenger of Allah had a silver ring with a silver face. In addition, the grip of his sword was made from silver."

Unlike disallowing drinking in silver containers, there are no authentic narrations that disallow wearing silver. The category of containers for food and drink is more specific than the category of clothes and adornments. For instance, women are allowed to wear all types of clothes and adornments, while there are specific containers for food and drink that are not allowed to be used (i.e., gold and silver containers). Therefore, the fact that Muslims are not allowed to use some types of containers does not necessarily apply to clothes and adornments [which are a wider category as we have stated]. In the Sunan it is narrated that the Prophet ^e said:

"As *for silver, play with it as you like."*

Furthermore, disallowing wearing silver adornments needs a specific Text (Qura'an or *Sunnah)* or a consensus (of the scholars) for the heart to accept it with certainty. Once, the Prophet ^ held some gold in one hand and some silk in the other hand and said:

"These two are not allowed for the males of my nation and allowed for the females among them."

Silver is one of the wonders that Allah has created on the earth. It is the key to acquiring ones needs and high positions among the people of the earth. Those who have silver are honorable in the eyes of the people and respected in their hearts, allowing them to sit at the head of various meetings and opening all doors in front of them. In addition, the people do not feel bored by sitting next to owners of silver, nor will their presence be heavy. Fingers point at them, while eyes look at them [in admiration]. If they speak, people listen and if they intervene, their mediation will be accepted. If they present their witness, their testimony will be accepted and if they give a speech, they will not be blamed for being incompetent; and even the white hair that they have will be considered more youthful than youth itself!

Silver is one of the remedies that bring joy to the hearts and drive away sadness, depression, and weakness in the heart and its heartbeat. In addition, silver is used in some of the best kinds of ointments and helps extract the harmful substances or conditions of the heart, especially when blended with pure honey and saffron.

Silver is originally cold and dry but In addition produces hotness and wetness.

There are four types of gardens that Allah has prepared for His loyal saves when they meet Him: two made of gold and two made of silver, including all their containers, adornments and whatever is in them.

In the *Sahih* it is narrated that the Prophet s| said:

"*Those who* drink from golden or silver bowls are

only pushing the Fire ofjahannam down into their stomachs."

He In addition said, as narrated in the Saheeh (the sound book)

"Neither drink from golden or silver bowls nor eat on golden on silver plates. It is for them (the disbelievers) in the life of this world and for you in the Next Life."

Some people said that the wisdom behind disallowing using golden and silver containers is to tighten the money supply. They say that if people use silver and gold as containers, then the interests of humankind will not be served well. In addition, some people said that they are disallowed so that whoever uses them does not become arrogant and proud, or so that the poor persons do not become humbled when they see such items, and so forth. These opinions are not sound.

For instance, tightening the money supply should In addition include disallowing wearing golden and silver adornments and canes [not only golden and silver containers]. Further, pride and arrogance are not allowed regarding anything. In addition, making the poor feel humbled is not a precise subject that we can define, for they could In addition feel humbled when they see luxurious homes, spacious gardens and lavish means of transportation, clothes and delicious foods. All these items are allowed for people.

What we think is the valid reason for this prohibition, and Allah has the best knowledge, is that using gold and silver in this manner affects the heart in such a way that contradicts true slavery to Allah. This is why the Prophet gte said that it is for the disbelievers in this life, because the disbelievers do not have a share in the true slavery [to Allah] that will give them the rewards of the Next Life. The slaves of Allah should not use these items in this manner, because only those who do not implement the requirements of their slavery (to Allah) use them in this life, as they prefer the life of this world to the Next Life. Allah has the best knowledge.

The Letter Qaf

1. Qura'an

Allah said:

"And We send down of the Qura'an that which is a healing and a* mercy to those *who believe (in Islamic Monotheism and act on

He In addition said:

﴿ يَـٰٓأَيُّهَا ٱلنَّاسُ قَدْ جَآءَتْكُم مَّوْعِظَةٌ مِّن رَّبِّكُمْ وَشِفَآءٌ لِّمَا فِى ٱلصُّدُورِ وَهُدًى وَرَحْمَةٌ لِّلْمُؤْمِنِينَ ﴿٥٧﴾ ﴾ (٥٧) يونس .

"O mankind! There has come to you a good advice from your Lord (i.e. the Qura'an, enjoining all that is good and forbidding all that is evil), and a healing for that which is in your breasts..." (1O:57)

The Qura'an is the ultimate cure from all types of illnesses and sicknesses that attack the body and the heart and from all the calamities of life and death. Yet, not everyone is suitable or guided to successfully seek the Qura'an as a cure.

When the ill person successfully uses the cure contained in the Qura'an and applies it on his ailment with faith, sincerity, complete acceptance and trust, all the while observing the necessary guidelines in this regard, no illness can resist the cure,

How can any ailment resist [the Book that contains] the Words of the Lord of the earth and heaven, which if it were revealed to a mountain, it would cause it to humble itself and render it asunder. Further, if the Qura'an were revealed to the earth, it would tear it apart. No ailment that attacks the body or the heart, but the Qura'an contains its remedy and cure and would provide immunity against it, that is, for whomever Allah has endowed with the bounty of comprehending His Book.

We stated before that the Qura'an contains the major aspects and basis of the knowledge of medicine: preserving health, diet and extracting of harmful substances. As for the ills that attack the heart, the Qura'an mentions them in detail and directs the people to the cures and remedies to treat them. Allah said:

﴿ مَن كَانَ يَرْجُوا۟ لِقَآءَ ٱللَّهِ فَإِنَّ أَجَلَ ٱللَّهِ لَـَٔاتٍ ۚ وَهُوَ ٱلسَّمِيعُ ٱلْعَلِيمُ ﴾ (٥) العنكبوت .

"Is it not sufficient for them that we have sent down to you the Book (the Qura'an) which is recited to them?" (29:5)

May Allah never cure those whom the Qura'an does not cure, nor suffice for those for whom Allah is not sufficient as a Helper.

2. *Qith-tha'* (Wild Cucumber)

In the *Sunan* it is narrated that Abdullah bin Ja'far said:

"The Prophet b used to eat Qith-tha' with ripe dates." [At-Tirmidhi].

Qith-tha' is cool and wet in the second degree and it cools the hotness in the stomach, it does not spoil quickly and helps relieve prostate pain. In addition, *Qith-tha'* helps relieve nausea while its seeds are a diuretic. When *Qith-tha'* leaves are used as a bandage, they help against dog bites.

Qith-tha' does not digest easily and its coolness sometimes hurts some parts of the stomach. Hence, one should eat *Qith-tha'* with what would make its coolness and wetness milder, just as the Prophet did by eating ripe dates with it. In addition, eating it with raisins or honey makes it milder on the stomach,

3. Qust, or Kust (Costus)

In the *Sahihain* it is narrated that Anas related from the Prophet **b**, that he said:

"Cupping and marine costus are the best of your remedies."

In addition, Imam Ahmad narrated that the Prophet *m,* said:

"Use this Indian wood, because ft contains seven *types of* cures, among them a cure for pleurisy."

There are two kinds of Qust, the white kind that is

called seo-Qust and the *Indian Qust,* which is the hottest among them while the white type is the mildest. Both kinds have many benefits.

Both kinds of Qust are hot and dry in the third degree, and they dry out the phlegm and colds. When they are taken as a drink, they help weak liver and stomach and the colds associated with such cases, Costus In addition helps against victular and quartan fever (fever that comes on every fourth day), the pain on the side of the body and poisons. When the face is anointed with Qust that is kneaded with water and honey, they heal the spots that appear on the face. Galinus said that the costus, "Heals tetanus, the pain in the sides and kills spots (which he called the seeds of the pumpkin),"

Some ignorant doctors are unaware of and deny the Qust as an effective remedy against the pain in the sides of the body. If these ignorant doctors become aware of what Galinus has stated about the Quest, they will quickly embrace it as if it was a divine text. Moreover, many doctors have In addition stated that Qust helps against the pain in the flank that is accompanied by phlegm, as Al-Khattabi related from Muhammad bin Al-Jahm.

We stated before that the difference between the remedies contained in the Prophetic medicine and the remedies of regular doctors is much larger than the difference between folk medicine as compared to regular medicine. We In addition stated that what is sent down of the divine revelation, as compared to what is proven by experimentation, compares to the difference between the noble master and the commoner.

In addition, if any of the ignorant doctors [who ignore the Prophetic medicine] were able to discover a remedy that the Jews, the Christians and the polytheist doctors have prescribed, they would embrace it and would certainly prescribe it.

We do not deny that habits have a role in making the cure work or fail. Those who are used to certain foods and medicines would benefit from such items more than those who are not used to them and who sometimes would not benefit at all from them.

The statements of the best doctors do not apply in all cases and places. Taking the statements of these doctors as being specific and not general does not lessen the degree of their knowledge. The same ruling applies even more to the statements of the Prophets. Yet, the hearts of mankind have a built-in degree of ignorance and injustice, except for those whom Allah has endowed with the light of correct Faith and enlightened their hearts with true guidance.

4. Qosob As-Sukkar (Sugarcane)

Sugar is a relatively new substance that the people of old did not mention or even have knowledge that it existed. This is why they did not describe its role in various types of drinks or cures. Honey, on the other hand, was extensively used as a drink and as a medicine.

Sugarcane is hot and wet, helps relieve coughing and dissipates the excess moistures in the body, prostate and chest. It is more effective as a laxative than sugar itself. In addition, sugarcane induces vomit. is diuretic and stimulates semen production.

Affan bin Muslim As-Saggar said, "Those who suck on sugarcane after eating their meal, will find comfort for the rest of his day." When sugarcane is broiled, it relieves the roughness in the throat and chest. Yet, it causes the accumulation of gasses that would be pacified when sugarcane is peeled and washed in hot water.

Sugar is hot and wet. The best type of sugar is white crystalline, especially when it is old. When sugar is boiled and skimmed, it quenches the thirst and relieves coughing. Sugarcane is not good for the stomach that suffers from bile. The side effects of sugarcane could be pacified by mixing it with lemon water (juice), Naranj (bitter orange) and peeled pomegranate.

Some people prefer sugarcane to honey because it is not as hot as honey and because it is milder on the stomach. This is not fair for honey, which is much more profitable than sugarcane. In addition, Allah has made honey both a cure and a type of sweet. So how can anyone compare the benefits of honey and the benefits of sugarcane? Honey strengthens the stomach, soothes the natural process, strengthens the eyesight and heals diphtheria when gargled, facial paralysis and hemiplegia (paralysis affecting only one side of the body). It In addition helps against all types of cold illnesses that occur in the body because of excess moistures. Honey extracts and pulls excess moistures from the body, preserves the health, increases semen production, cleanses and decomposes the contents of the stomach. In addition, honey cleanses the intestines, fights worms and prevents septic repletion (over eating). Further, honey is a good type of food and favorable for those who suffer from phlegm and for old people. In short, no substance is more beneficial for the body as a food, as a remedy and as an ingredient and a preserver of medications, which In addition strengthens the stomach, than honey. There are many more benefits for honey. So how can anyone compare it to sugarcane, which does not have even a fraction of the benefits contained in honey?

The Letter K'aff

Kitab (Books or Writings)

This chapter contains books or writings of divine remedies, Islamic prayer formulas, as Islamic amulets (prayer formulas written down and worn for a specific purpose).*

1. An Amulet for Fever

Al-Mirwazi said, "Abu Abdullah (Imam Ahmad) was informed that was suffering from fever and he wrote to me a supplication for fever that reads like this, 'In the Name of Allah, the Most Gracious, the Most Beneficent. In the Name of Allah, and depending on Allah.

"We *(Allah) said: 'O fire! Be you coolness and safety for IbrahJm (Abraham)! And they wanted to harm him, but We made them the worst losers.* (21:69,70)

O Allah, the Lord of (angels) Gabriel, Michael and Israfil: cure this person with this supplication by Your Power, Strength and Might, O Lord of the creation. *Ameen.'"*

In addition, Al-Mirwazi said that Abu Ja'far, Muhammad bin Ali was asked about wearing [a written] *Ruqyah* (divine remedy, Islamic prayer formula or amulet). He said, "If it was from the Book of Allah or a *Hadith* [correctly] related from the Prophet, then wear it and use it as a remedy as much as possible." Abu Abdullah was listening to this narration and

In addition, Imam Ahmad did not object when he was asked about wearing a *Ruqyah* amulet after an illness or a calamity strikes. Al-Khallal In addition narrated that Abdullah bin Ahmad told him that his father used to write some supplication in a *Ruqyah* amulet for those who have a certain fear and for fever after it strikes.

An Amulet for Difficult Pregnancies

In addition, Al-Khallal narrated that Abdullah bin Ahmad said that his father wrote a *Ruqyah,* Islamic prayer formula, as an Islamic amulet, on a pure object for women who suffered from difficult pregnancies. In the, amulet, Ahmad wrote the *Hadith* narrated by Ibn Abbas, "There is no deity worthy of worship except Allah, the Most Forbearing, the Most Generous. All praise is due to Allah, the Lord of the Mighty Throne.

"All the praises and thanks are to Allah the Lord of the 'Alamin (mankind, jinn and all that exists)"

"The Day they see it, (it will be) as if they had not tarried (in this world) except an afternoon or a morning." *(79:46)*

﴿ فَٱصْبِرْ كَمَا صَبَرَ أُوْلُواْ ٱلْعَزْمِ مِنَ ٱلرُّسُلِ وَلَا تَسْتَعْجِل لَّهُمْ ۚ كَأَنَّهُمْ يَوْمَ يَرَوْنَ مَا يُوعَدُونَ لَمْ يَلْبَثُوٓاْ إِلَّا سَاعَةً مِّن نَّهَارٍ ۚ بَلَـٰغٌ ۚ فَهَلْ يُهْلَكُ إِلَّا ٱلْقَوْمُ ٱلْفَـٰسِقُونَ ﴾ (٣٥) الأحقاف .

"On the Day when they will see that (torment) with which they are promised (i.e. threatened, it will be) as if they had not stayed more than an hour in a single day. (O mankind! this Qur'an is sufficient as) a clear Message (or proclamation to save yourself from destruction). But shall any be destroyed except the people who are Al-Fasiqun (rebellious against Allah's Command. disobedient to Allah)?" (46:35)

Al-Khallal said that a man came to Abu Abdullah and asked him to write a Islamic prayer formula as an Islamic amulet for a woman who had gone into labor for two days. Imam Ahmad asked the man to bring a wide cup with some Saffron [and wrote the amulet for the man's wife]. He In addition narrated that Imam Ahmad wrote the same amulet for several other people.

It was reported that 'Ikrimah narrated that Ibn Abbas said, "Jesus, the Messenger of Allah **b** once passed by a cow that was suffering from hard labor. The cow said [to Jesus], 'O, Word of Allah (be and he was)! Ask Allah to relieve me from what I am suffering from.'

He said, "O Creator of the soul from another soul, who brings to life a soul from within another soul, relieves her.' The cow then gave birth and soon started to smell her newly born." Ibn Abbas then said, "Therefore, when the woman is suffering from hard labor, write [and recite] this supplication for her."

The types of Islamic prayer formulas as Islamic amulets that we mentioned are beneficial, Allah willing. Further, several scholars among the Salaf have allowed writing the Qura'an and drinking its water as a cure.

Another Amulet for Pregnant Women

One should write the following *Ayah* in a pure pot:

﴿ إِذَا ٱلسَّمَآءُ ٱنشَقَّتۡ ۝١ وَأَذِنَتۡ لِرَبِّهَا وَحُقَّتۡ ۝٢ وَإِذَا ٱلۡأَرۡضُ مُدَّتۡ ۝٣ وَأَلۡقَتۡ مَا فِيهَا وَتَخَلَّتۡ ۝٤ ﴾ (١:٤) الانشقاق .

"When the heaven is split asunder. In addition, listens to and obeys its Lord and it must do so. And when the earth is stretched forth, and has cast out all *that was in it and became empty."* (84:1 - 4)

Then the pregnant woman should drink from this pot and pour some of it on her stomach.

An Amulet for Nosebleeds

Ibn Taymiyyah used to write the following *Ayah* on his forehead:

"And it was said: 'O earth! Swallow up your water, and O sky! Withhold (your rain). And the water was made to subside and the Decree (of Allah) was fulfilled (i.e. the destruction of the people (Noah). "(I :44)

I In addition heard him say, "I wrote [this A/oh] for several people and they were cured." He In addition said [about the Ayah], "It is not allowed to write it with the blood of the nosebleed as some ignorant people do, because blood is impure and one is not allowed to use it to write Allah's Speech."

Another Amulet for nose bleeds

It was reported that Prophet Musa .*Once* went out wearing an outer garment and then suffered from nosebleed and covered [his nose].

An Amulet for fungus

One should write [the following for it:}

"...then *it is struck with a fiery whirlwind, so that it is burnt...?"*

Another Amulet for fungus

When the sun becomes yellow, one should write [the Ayah],

﴿ يَٰٓأَيُّهَا ٱلَّذِينَ ءَامَنُوا ٱتَّقُوا ٱللَّهَ وَءَامِنُوا بِرَسُولِهِۦ يُؤْتِكُمْ كِفْلَيْنِ مِن رَّحْمَتِهِۦ وَيَجْعَل لَّكُمْ نُورًا تَمْشُونَ بِهِۦ وَيَغْفِرْ لَكُمْ ۚ وَٱللَّهُ غَفُورٌ رَّحِيمٌ ﴿٢٨﴾ ﴾ (٢٨) الحديد .

"O you who believe [in Musa fMoses) (i.e. Jews) and Musd (Jesus) (i.e.. Christians)]! Fear Allah, and believe in His Messenger (Muhammad gg) He will give you a double portion of His Mercy. and He will give you a light by which you shall walk (straight). And He will forgive you. And Allah is Oft-Forgiving. Most Merciful." (57:28)

An Amulet for three-day Fever

One should write on three separate papers, "In the Name of Allah it is running away. In the Name of Allah it has subsided. In the Name of Allah it has decreased."

Every day [that the fever lasts], one should swallow the paper with some water. **An Amulet for sciatica**

One should write, "In the Name of Allah. O Allah, Lord of everything, Owner of everything and Creator of everything! You have created the sciatic nerve and me. Do not give it power over me, nor allow me to cut it. Heal me completely and eradicate the illness. There is none who can heal except You."

An Amulet for bleeding veins

At-Tirmidhi narrated that Ibn Abbas said that the Messenger of Allah **b** used to teach them to recite [the following Ruqyoh], against fever and various pains, 'In the Name of Allah, the Most Great, I seek refuge with Allah, the All-Mighty, from the evil of bleeding veins and from the evil of the fire's heat,"

An Amulet for Toothache

One should write on the cheek that is closer to the pain, "In the Name of Allah, Most Gracious, Most Merciful.

﴿ وَهُوَ ٱلَّذِىٓ أَنشَأَ لَكُمُ ٱلسَّمْعَ وَٱلْأَبْصَـٰرَ وَٱلْأَفْـِٔدَةَ ۚ قَلِيلًا مَّا تَشْكُرُونَ ﴿٧٨﴾ ﴾ (٧٨) المؤمنون .

"It is He Who has created for you (the sense of) hearing (ears), eyes (sight), and hearts (understanding). Little thanks you give." (23:78)

Or,

﴿ ۞ وَلَهُۥ مَا سَكَنَ فِي ٱلَّيۡلِ وَٱلنَّهَارِۚ وَهُوَ ٱلسَّمِيعُ ٱلۡعَلِيمُ ﴿١٣﴾ ﴾

(١٣) الأنعام

"And to Him belongs whatsoever exists in the night and the day, and He is the All-Hearing, the All-Knowing." (6:13)

An Amulet for abscess

One should write [this amulet and place it] on the abscess,

﴿ وَيَسۡـَٔلُونَكَ عَنِ ٱلۡجِبَالِ فَقُلۡ يَنسِفُهَا رَبِّي نَسۡفٗا ﴿١٠٥﴾ فَيَذَرُهَا قَاعٗا صَفۡصَفٗا ﴿١٠٦﴾ ﴾

(١٠٥: ١٠٦) طه

"And they ask you concerning the mountains: say, "My Lord will blast them and scatter them as particles of dust. Then He shall leave them as a level smooth plain." (2O:1O5,106)

2. *Kamah* (Truffles)

In the *Sahihain* it is narrated that the Prophet said:

"The *Kamah is among the Manna and its water (extract or juice) cures the eye."*

The *Kamah* grows wild underground, and it is called *Kamah* because it grows hidden beneath the earth. The *Kamah* does not have leaves or stems.

The essence of the *Kamah* is partly earthly and partly steamy and remains concealed underground during winter and then starts to grow above the ground with spring rainfall. This is why it is called the smallpox of the land, for it is similar to smallpox, which is caused by moistures clogged with blood that get aggravated during the early childhood years when the body starts to gain strength.

Kamah {truffles) grow in the spring and are eaten raw or cooked. The Arabs used to call *truffles* 'the plant of the thunder, because they grow in the aftermath of thunderstorms. The nomads in the desert use mushrooms in their regular diet. Further, the best type of *truffles* grow on sandy dry land. There are several types of *Kamah*, among which is a poisonous plant which is reddish in color and which causes asphyxiation.

The *Kamah* is cold and wet in the third degree, and it is not favorable for the stomach and not easily digested. Eating *Kamah* on a regular basis causes constipation, gastric pain, facial paralysis, stomachache and dysuna (painful urination). Humid kinds of mushrooms are less harmful than dry ones. Therefore, those who wish to eat *Kamah* should bury them in a muddy area and then boil them in water, add salt and mint, and then eat them with oil and spices. This is because the *Kamah* has a heavy, earthly essence, although it contains a fair amount of water in its essence that makes it a little light. In addition, using the *Kamah* as kohl helps in cases of bad eyesight and ophthalmia (conjunctivitis).

Some of the best doctors have agreed that truffle water or juice helps strengthen the eyesight.

There are two opinions regarding the meaning of what the Prophet **b** said:

4- Hurf (Cress)

Cress seed are used in remedies and are called Ath'uf which Prophet **b** mentioned.

The messenger of Allah **b** said:

What a cure do the two bitter remedies carry: the Ath'uf'a and aloe.

Cress is hot and dry in the third degree and it heats and relaxes the stomach.

5: Hilb'ah (Fenugreek)

The prophet **b** was reported to have visited Sa'ad bin Aby Waq'ass once when he was ill while in Mecca and he asked that a doctor be brought to examine him. They brought Al Harith bin Kaladah who examined him and said: There is no harm with him, just cook some fenugreek with dates and let him eat them, Saad was reported to have done that and then healed.

Helb'ah In addition relieves urine retention and works as a laxative. When it is placed on the erratic nail, it will heal it.

Letter Kh'aa

1- Kh'obz (brea)

in the sound book it is narrated that Prophet **b** said:

On the Day Resurrection, the earth will look like one piece of beard which the Most Mighty would prepare with His Hand as a residence for the people of Paradise.

Khal (vinegar)

Muslim narrated that the messenger of Allah **b** asked his wife for food and she said that she had vinegar. He **b** said: What an excellent food is vinegar (he **b** ate it with bread.)

Khilal (toothpick)

Toothpicks are helpful for the gingival and teeth and preserve their health.

Letter d'al

1- Dohn (Fat)

fat closes the pores of the body and prevents the skin from decomposing. When it is used after one take a bath with hot water. It will humidify the body and polish it.

The letter Z'al

1- Thareerah (Hemarthria - Arum)

in the two sound books it is narrated that the messenger of Allah **b** in the farewell Haj A'esha perfumed him with Thareerah.

2- Zobab (flies))

we mentioned the Hadith by Hurayrah about the prophet's command to dip the housefly in the food or drink when it falls in it to get the antidote that its wing carries.

3-Z'ahab (Gold)

Gold is the joy of the life of this world and the precious material. When gold is buried in the ground, sand does not effect on it. It cures weak hearts when it is used in certain remedies. Gold is such a beloved object to the hearts that when they acquire it, it will be sufficient for the people to forget the other beloved objects of this earthy life.

The letter R'aa

Rotab (Ripe dates)

Allah said to Mary:

And shake the trunk of date palm towards you.

4. *Hurf* (Cress)

Abu Hanifah Ad-Daynoory said, "Cress seeds are used in remedies and are In addition called Ath-Thuffaa, which the Prophet *s&,* mentioned. Its plant is called Al-Hurf while Rashad seeds is its popular name." In addition, Abu Ubayd said that Ath-Thuffaa is the Hurf.

The *Hadith* that Abu Hanifah referred to is what Abu Ubay and other scholars have related from Ibn Abbas that the Prophet **b** was reported to have said:

"What a cure do the two bitter *remedies carry: the Thuffaa and aloe."*

Cress is hot and dry in the third degree, and it heats and relaxes the stomach, removes different types of worms, decomposes the spleen tumors, excites the sexual drive and heals the ulcers of mange and herpes.

When the cress is used as a bandage along with honey, it will decompose spleen tumors. When it is cooked with henna, it will extract harmful accumulations in the chest, while taking it as a drink helps against venomous bites and stings.

When it is burned, its smoke repulses venomous beasts and prevents the hair form falling. In addition, when it is mixed with barley flour and vinegar and used as a bandage it helps against decomposes hot tumors.

Further, when it is used as a bandage with water, it brings the pustules to maturity and helps against flabbiness in various organs, strengthens the sexual drive and works as an appetite stimulant. It In addition helps against asthma, hard breathing, relieves the thickness in the spleen, purifies the chest and increases the menstrual flow. It In addition helps against sciatic nerve and the cavity of the hip, due to the extraction power of the cress when one drinks it or is injected with it. It In addition purifies the chest and the lungs from phlegm.

When cress is crushed and taken in a drink with warm water, it will work as a laxative, decomposes flatulence and helps against the pain caused by constipation. Further, cress In addition helps against leprosy when it is crushed and used in a drink.

In addition, when the cress is blended with vinegar and used as an ointment on leprous skin and on white pigmentation disorder, it helps relieve these conditions. It a so relieves headaches that are caused by colds and by phlegm accumulation. When it is fried and drunk (with water), it constipates, especially when it is not crushed, as its consistency will be softened when it is fried.

Galinus said that the strength of the cress, "Is similar to the effectiveness of mustard grains. Hence it could be used to heat the pain in the hip, which is known as Noso and headaches, as each of these symptoms requires heat, similar to mustard seed. Sometimes, cress is mixed with other remedies and used to treat asthma, as it is known that it dissolves thick mixtures, again just as mustard seed does. It is similar to mustard seed in every respect."

5. *'Hulba* (Fenugreek)

The Prophet *s* was reported to have visited Sa'd bin Abi Waqqas **b** .mi once when he was ill while in Makkah and he asked that a doctor be brought to examine him. They brought Al-Harith bin Kaladah who examined him and said, "There is no harm with him, just cook some fenugreek with dates and let him eat them." Sa'd was reported to have done that and was then healed.

Hulbah is hot in the second degree and dry in the first degree.

When the fenugreek is cooked in water, it will soften the throat, chest and the stomach. It In addition relieves coughing, dryness, asthma, hard breathing and increases the sexual drive. It In addition relieves flatulence, phlegm, piles and the various accumulations in the intestines. It In addition dissolves the phlegm from the chest and helps against gastric ulcer and lung diseases. *'Hulbah* is used to heal the intestines, mixed with some ghee and fanith.

When five measures of fenugreek is taken in a drink, it will increase the flow of menstruation, and when it is cooked and the hair is washed with it, it will make it curly and will combat dandruff.

When the flour of the fenugreek is blended with some vinegar and natron and used as a bandage on the tumor of the spleen, it will dissolve it. In addition, the woman who suffers from pain in the vagina due to a tumor will benefit if she sits in the water in which the fenugreek was cooked.

When it is used as a bandage and placed on hard, cold tumors, it will help dissolve these tumors. In addition, when its water is drunk, it will help against the pain in the stomach that results from accumulating gaseous materials and will cleanse the intestines.

When one eats the *Hulbah* cooked in honey, dates or figs on an empty stomach, it will dissolve the phlegm that accumulates in the chest and stomach, and will help against coughing that accompanies such ailments.

Hulbah In addition relieves urine retention and works as a laxative. When it is placed on the erratic nail, it will heal it, while its oil helps against cracked skin due to extreme cold, when it is mixed with wax. There are many other benefits for the *Hulbah* (fenugreek).

Some doctors stated, "If the people had knowledge of its benefits, they would buy it with its weight worth of gold."

The Letter k'aff

1. Khubz (Bread)

In the *Sahih* it is narrated that the Prophet ^s said:

"On the Day of Resurrection, the earth will look like one piece of bread which the Most Mighty would prepare with His Hand as a residence for the people of

Paradise."

A fake Hadith disallows cutting bread with a knife. In addition another fake Hadith disallows cutting meat with a knife. Muhanna said that he asked Imam Ahmad about the *Hadith* related from A'esha that narrates that the Prophet as disallowed using a knife to cut meat, because it is an act of non-Arabs. Imam Ahmad said that it is not correct and that it contradicts the *Hadith* narrated by 'Amr bin Umayyah and Al-Mughirah. The *Hadith* that he referred to is what 'Amr bin Umayyah related that the Prophet sag used to cut some pieces of ewe meat with a blade. In addition, Al-Mughirah narrated that when he asked the Prophet ^ to be his guest, he ordered that a piece of meat be broiled and he then started cutting the meat with a blade.

The best type of bread is yeasty and kneaded

The next best is furnace bread, then oven baked bread, then bread cooked under hot ashes, using fresh flour.

The most nutritious kind of bread is semolina bread, because it digests slowly and because it does not have excessive amounts of bran, then chalky bread and lastly black bread.

The best time to eat the bread is in the last part of

the day when it is baked. In addition, unlike dry bread, soft bread is lighter, more nutritious, humidifying and digests faster.

Wheat bread is hot in the second degree and is mild concerning wetness and dryness, unless dried by fire.

Wheat bread In addition fattens the body rapidly. The Qatayif (similar to pancakes) cause a thick condition, while breadcrumbs provoke swelling in the stomach and digests with difficulty. Further, bread made with milk causes clogs and is difficult to digest, although it is nutritious.

Barley bread is cold and dry in the first degree and it not as nutritious as wheat bread.

2. *Kh'al* (Vinegar)

Muslim narrated in his *Sahih* that Jabir bin 'Abdullah said, "The Messenger of Allah b asked his wife for food and she said that I have vinegar. He asked for some of it and started eating from it while saying:

" *"What an excellent food is vinegar." (He ate it with bread.)*

Khall is a substance that is both hot and cold, although coldness is usually more apparent. It is In addition dry in the third degree and a strong drying agent.

Vinegar In addition soothes the body and softens the nature,

Wine vinegar helps against gastric inflammation and bile and prevents the harm of toxic medications. It In addition decomposes milk and the blood when coagulated, and helps the spleen, coats the stomach, constipates, quenches the thirst and prevents tumors from occurring. It In addition helps the digestion process, works against phlegm, softens thick foods and softens the consistency of the blood.

When vinegar is drunk with salt, it will help against poisonous mushrooms. When vinegar is sipped, it will dissolve the clogs that occur in the blood in the lower jaw. When one rinses his mouth with warm vinegar, it relieves toothache and strengthens the gingival.

Vinegar In addition helps against a septic finger when it is anointed with it, and relieves pustules, hot tumors and fire burns. Vinegar is an appetite stimulant, softens the stomach, and favorable for young people and for those who live in warm areas.

3. *Khilal* (Toothpick)

Toothpicks are helpful for the gingival and teeth and preserve their health, and help keep the breath fresh. One of the best types of toothpicks are those made from olive wood. It is not advised to use reed, myrtle, or basil to pick the teeth.

The Letter D'al

1. Duhn (Fat or Grease)

Fat closes the pores of the body and prevents the skin from decomposing. When it is used after one takes a bath with hot water, it will humidify the body and polish it. When the hair is anointed with grease, it will beautify it and make it longer. It In addition helps against measles and most other ailments that could affect the hair.

At-Tirmidhi narrated that Abu Hurairah related from the Prophet afe that he said:

"Use grease *in your food and as an ointment."*

In the warm areas, such as Hijaz, grease works as one of the best preservers of health and as a remedy, making it necessary for the residents of such areas. As for those who live in cold areas, it is not as necessary for them. We should mention that using grease on the head on a regular basis causes harm to the sight.

The most beneficial simple kinds of grease are regular oil, then fat and then sesame oil.

As for the compound greases, some kinds are wet

and cold, such as the essence of violet, which helps against hot headaches and brings sleep to the eye. It In addition moisturizes the brain, helps against cracks (or fractures) and excessive dryness of the skin. It is a so a beneficial ointment against mange and dry rashes, along with helping the joints be flexible. It is In addition suitable for those who tend to be hot during the summer.

Some types of compound greases are hot and wet, such as ben-tree grease, which is the extract of white seeds that look like dusty pistachio and which is greasy and fatty. This type of grease relaxes the nerves and helps against spots and lack of pigment in certain areas of the skin. It In addition draws thick phlegm, softens dry ligaments and heats the nerves. It In addition cleans the teeth, makes them shiny and helps them against corrosion. In addition whoever anoints his head and face with ben-tree grease will not come down with measles or cracks. Anointing the sexual organs and groins with it In addition helps against the coldness of the kidneys and dripping urine.

The Letter Thal

1. *Tharirah* (Hemarthria/Arum)

In the *Sahihain* it is narrated that A'esha said that during the Farewell *Hajj,* she perfumed the Messenger of Allah **b** with *Tharirah* for his *Ihram* and otherwise.

We mentioned the *Tharirah* and its benefits before.

2. *Zubab* (Flies)

We mentioned the *Hadith* by Abu Hurairah *ιs* ın the *Sahihain* about the Prophet's command to dip the housefly in the food or drink when it falls in it to get the antidote that its wing carries. This antidote works as the antidote of the poison that the fly carries on the other wing. We In addition mentioned the benefits of the flies before.

3. *Zahab* (Gold)

Abu Dawud and At-Tirmidhi narrated that the Prophet s& allowed Arfajah bin As'ad, who lost his nose during the battle of Kulab and had to use a nose made of silver that later rotted, to wear a nose made of gold. Arfajah is only mentioned in this one *Hadith*.

Gold is the joy of the life of this world and the precious material possession of this existence that brings joy to the hearts and strength to the back. It is In addition Allah's secret on His earth. Gold's condition is suitable in all types of environments and has a soft hotness that is used in various light and soothing remedies. It is In addition the most mild of all minerals.

When gold is buried in the ground, sand does not affect it adversely. When gold is used in certain remedies, it helps cure weak hearts and the fibrillation that accompanies black bile. It In addition helps against obsession, sadness, depression, fear and love. It brings fatness to the body, dissipates pallor and lightens the color. It In addition helps against leprosy and the various other ailments including black bile. Drunk or used as an ointment, gold is an effective ingredient in the remedies for treating alopecia (a skin disease characterized by loss of hair, partial or total), and viper stings. It In addition clears the eye and strengthens it, and helps against several ailments while brining strength to the various organs of the body.

Foul breath would dissipate if one holds some gold in his mouth. In addition, those who have a disease that requires cauterization and use gold for this purpose it will heal quickly and the wound would not be covered with blisters. In addition, when gold is used as kohl, it purifies and strengthens the eyes. Further, when a golden ring is heated and applied on pigeon wings, the pigeons will be accustomed to their homes and will not abandon them.

Gold is especially effective in strengthening the hearts and this is why it was allowed in times of war and in times of peace, except when there is proof to the contrary. At-Tirmidhi narrated that Buraydah Al-'Asri said, "The Messenger of Allah si entered (Mecca) the Day of *Al-Fath* (conquering of Mecca) with gold and silver on his sword."

Gold is such a beloved object to the hearts that when they acquire it, it will be sufficient for the people to forget the other beloved objects of this earthly life.

Allah said:

﴿ زُيِّنَ لِلنَّاسِ حُبُّ ٱلشَّهَوَٰتِ مِنَ ٱلنِّسَآءِ وَٱلْبَنِينَ وَٱلْقَنَٰطِيرِ ٱلْمُقَنطَرَةِ مِنَ ٱلذَّهَبِ وَٱلْفِضَّةِ وَٱلْخَيْلِ ٱلْمُسَوَّمَةِ وَٱلْأَنْعَٰمِ وَٱلْحَرْثِ ۗ ذَٰلِكَ مَتَٰعُ ٱلْحَيَوٰةِ ٱلدُّنْيَا ۖ وَٱللَّهُ عِندَهُۥ حُسْنُ ٱلْمَـَٔابِ ﴿١٤﴾ ﴾ (١٤) آل عمران .

"Beautified for men is the love of things they covet; women, children, much of gold and silver (wealth), branded beautiful horses, cattle and well-tilled land." (3:14)

In addition, in the *to sound books* is narrated that the Prophet **b** said:

"If the son of Adam had a valley of gold, he would seek a second. If he bad two, he would seek a third.

Nothing fills the stomach of the son of Adam except dirt, and Allah forgives those who repent."

Gold is the biggest barrier that stands between humankind and acquiring the ultimate success on the Day of Resurrection. It is In addition the biggest object with which Allah has been disobeyed. Because of gold, relations of the womb were severed, blood was shed, prohibitions were violated, rights were unjustly taken and slaves committed injustice against each other. Gold is the reason behind liking the life of this world and its shortness, and the cause behind disliking the Next Life and what Allah has prepared in it for His loyal supporters. With gold, so many truths were and are buried, so much falsehood was and is brought to life, so many unjust people were and are given support and so many innocent people were and are being dealt with unjustly.

The Letter R'aa

1. Rutab (Ripe Dates)

Allah said to Mary:

﴿ وَهُزِّىٓ إِلَيْكِ بِجِذْعِ ٱلنَّخْلَةِ تُسَـٰقِطْ عَلَيْكِ رُطَبًا جَنِيًّا ﴿٢٥﴾ فَكُلِى وَٱشْرَبِى وَقَرِّى عَيْنًا ۖ فَإِمَّا تَرَيِنَّ مِنَ ٱلْبَشَرِ أَحَدًا فَقُولِىٓ إِنِّى نَذَرْتُ لِلرَّحْمَـٰنِ صَوْمًا فَلَنْ أُكَلِّمَ ٱلْيَوْمَ إِنسِيًّا ﴿٢٦﴾ ﴾ (٢٥:٢٦) مريم .

"And shake the trunk of date palm towards you. it will let fall fresh ripe dates upon you. So eat, drink, and be glad. Moreover, if you see any human being, say: 'Verily, I have vowed a fast unto

The Most Gracious (Allah) so I shall not speak to any human being this day." (19: 25, 26)

In addition, in the *Sahihain* it is narrated that Abdullah bin Ja'far said:

I saw the Messenger of Allah b eating cucumbers with ripe dates."

Abu Dawud In addition narrated in his *Sunan* that Anas said:

"The Messenger of Allah b used to break his fast on some ripe dates, and if he did not have any, on dry dates. Otherwise, if be did not have dry dates, he would have several sips of water."

Ripe dates are just like water, hot and wet, and they are favorable for and strengthen the cold stomach, increase the production of semen and fertility, are suitable for cold temperaments and are very nutritious.

Ripe dates are the best types of fruit for the people of Al-Medina specifically and for all others in general where ripe dates grow. It is In addition a very beneficial fruit for the body, although ripe dates spoil quickly in the stomach of those who are not used to eating them and thus produce putrid blood. In addition, eating excessive amounts of ripe dates cause headaches and black bile and harms the teeth. Oxymel (Sakanjabin) helps neutralize the irritants that accompany eating ripe dates.

When the Prophet **b** used to break his fast, he used to eat first ripe or dry dates, or would drink some water. This is a wise decision, because fasting empties the stomach of food. Thus the liver would not find any sufficient energy that it could transfer to the various organs. Sweets are the fastest food to reach the liver and are favored by the liver, especially when one eats ripe dates, in which case the liver accepts it even more favorably, benefits from it and then transfers the benefit to the rest of the organs of the body. If there are no ripe dates available, one should eat dried dates because they are sweet and nutritious. Otherwise, some sips of water would extinguish the heat of the stomach and the Fast. The stomach's appetite would then increase and become ready to accept (and digest) food.

2. Roihon (Myrtle / Basil)

Allah said:

﴿ فَأَمَّآ إِن كَانَ مِنَ ٱلْمُقَرَّبِينَ ﴿٨٨﴾ فَرَوْحٌ وَرَيْحَانٌ وَجَنَّتُ نَعِيمٍ ﴾

(٨٨:٨٩) الواقعة .

"Then, if he (the dying person) be of the Muqarrabun (those brought near to Allah), (There is for him) rest and provision, and a Garden of Delights (Paradise)." (56:88,89)

And He said:

﴿ وَٱلْحَبُّ ذُو ٱلْعَصْفِ وَٱلرَّيْحَانُ ﴿١٢﴾ ﴾ (١٢) الرحمن .

"And In addition corn, with (its) leaves and stalk for fodder, and sweet-scented plants." (55:12) Muslim narrated that the Prophet **b** said:

"Whoever was presented with Rayhan should not refuse it, because it is easy to wear and has a good scent."

Ibn Majah narrated in his Sunon that Usamah related from the Prophet **b** that he said:

"Is there anyone who is ready to enter Paradise, for Paradise is all good (and pure). It is, by the Lord of the Ka'bah, a shining light, a twinkling Raihan, a luxurious palace, a running river, a ripe date, and a beautiful, pretty wife. It has many suits, eternal residence in a good place of dwelling, fruits, vegetables, comfort and bounty in an exalted, comfortable dwelling."

They said, " 'Yes, O Messenger of Allah **b** We are ready for it!' He said, 'Say, by Allah's Leave.' They said, By Allah's Leave.' "

Every plant that has good scent is called *'Raihan* . Therefore, every area gives a certain plant that name. For instance, the people to the west, as well as, the Arabs call the aromatic plants *Raihan.* The people in Iraq and Sham call the Hibk (a type of mint) a *Raihan.*

Raihan or myrtle is cold in the first degree and dry in the second degree. Yet, it is a compound of several qualities, most of which consist of earthly cold essence. Myrtle In addition consists of a soft hot substance. Myrtle dries the head nicely and is effective as a constipating agent.

Myrtle prevents bile diarrhea and dissipates hot and wet vapor when one smells its scent. Its scent In addition brings relief to the heart and prevents various ailments, especially when the plant is spread around the house.

In addition, myrtle heals the tumors that occur in the two ureters when it is coated on them. When fresh myrtle leaves are ground, blended with vinegar, and then placed on the head, they will stop nose bleeding. When dried myrtle leaves are crushed and the powder is sprinkled on wet ulcers it will heal them and will help weak organs when used as a bandage, relieve septic finger and heal spots and the ulcers on the hands and feet,

When myrtle is used to rub the body, it eliminates sweat, dries the excess wetness and dissipates underarm odor. When one sits in the water that myrtle was cooked in, it will help against infections on the buttocks and vagina and will heal weak joints and broken bones, when it is poured on the wound.

In addition, myrtle helps eliminate dandruff, the wet ulcers, and the spots that appear on the head. It In addition helps the hair against falling and gives it a black color. When myrtle leaves are ground with a little water and then blended with some oil or rose grease and then used as a bandage, it will be suitable against fresh (or humid) ulcers, canker sores, erysipelas (skin infection), acute tumors, urticaria (hives) and hemorrhoids.

Myrtle seeds In addition help against hemoptysis (spiting up blood) of the chest and lungs. It In addition coats the stomach, does not harm the chest or the stomach, and cleanses them. It In addition helps against diarrhea and coughing, and this is a special quality for myrtle that is rarely found in other medications. Myrtle seeds In addition help urine production and heal vesica (bladder) infections, spider bites and scorpion stings. Using myrtle roots to clean between the teeth is harmful, though.

Persian *Raihan,* which is In addition called *Hibq,* is hot, and when its scent is smelled, it helps against hot headaches when water is sprinkled on the *Hibq* and then is allowed to cool down. It is In addition said that this kind of myrtle is cold, but it looks like it has some of the four types of temperament. It In addition helps bring sleep to the eye.

The seeds of Persian myrtle relieve diarrhea of the bile, stomach, strengthen the heart and help against black bile ailments.

3. *Rumman* (Pomegranate)

Allah said:

﴿ فِيهِمَا فَٰكِهَةٌ وَنَخْلٌ وَرُمَّانٌ ﴿٦٨﴾ ﴾ (٦٨) الرحمن .

"In them (both) will be fruits, and date palms and pomegranates." (55:68)

In addition, "Ali was reported to have said: "Eat *Rumman* with its pulp, because it coats the stomach."

Sweet pomegranate is hot and wet, good for the stomach, and strengthens it because of its being a mild constipating agent. It is In addition good for the throat, chest and lungs, along with relieving coughing. The water (or juice) in the pomegranate softens the stomach and is a nutrient for the body. It In addition digests quickly because it is light and produces heat along with some air in the stomach. It helps increase the semen production and is not favorable for those who have fever. Pomegranate has a special quality, that is, when one eats bread with it, it prevents it from being spoiled.

Bitter pomegranate is cold and dry and constipates mildly. It is In addition good for overheated stomach and helps produce more urine than the other types of pomegranate. It In addition softens bile symptoms, relieves diarrhea, prevents vomiting and is slightly tarry. It In addition stops the heat in the liver, strengthens the organs, helps against bilious shaking, heartaches and the ache of the tip of the stomach. It. In addition helps the stomach, rids it of excrements, extinguishes the bile, and benefits the blood.

When pomegranate's juice is extracted and is cooked with some honey until it becomes like an ointment and used as eye drops, it will clear the yellow color from the eye and will dissipate the thick wetness. When it is placed on the gingival (gums), it will help against the rashes that appear on the gingival. In addition, pomegranate juice extracted with the rind will work as a laxative and will rid the body from septic bilious moistures, along with helping against short-term fever.

As for sour pomegranate, its qualities are in the middle between the two other kinds we mentioned, although this kind leans more towards being sour. Pomegranate seeds that are mixed with honey will alleviate septic finger and malignant ulcers. Pomegranate flowers In addition help heal wounds. It is said that if one swallows three pomegranate flowers each year, he will be immune from ophthalmia (conjunctivitis) for an entire year.

The Letter Zal

2 - Zait (Olive Oil)

Allah the Glorified said:

"Lit from a blessed tree, an olive, neither of the east (i.e. neither it gets sun-rays only in the morning) nor of the west (i.e. nor it gets sun-rays only in the afternoon, but it is exposed to the sun all day long), whose oil would almost glow forth (of itself), though no fire touched it." (24:35)

At-Tirmidhi and Ibn Majah narrated that Abu Hurairah related from the Prophet **b** that he said:

"Eat the Zait and use it as an ointment, because it is produced by a blessed tree."

Al-Bayhaqi and Ibn Majah In addition narrated that 'Abdullah bin 'Umar said that the Messenger of Allah **b** said:

"Eat oil and use it as an ointment because it is from *a blessed tree (olive tree)."*

Zait is hot and wet in the first degree. In addition, the quality of the oil depends on the tree that produces it. For instance, the best type of olive oil is that squeezed from ripe olives, while oil from unripe olives is cold and dry. Red olives produce oil that is between these while black olives produce hot and wet oil. Olive oil helps against poisons, works as a laxative and rids the body of worms. Old olive oil leans more towards being hot and decomposing. When the oil is blended with water, it becomes less hot, milder, and thus more beneficial. All kinds of olive oil soften the skin and slow the aging process. The salty water blended with oil helps burned skin against blistering. It In addition strengthens the gingival.

2. *Zubd* (Butter)

Abu Dawood narrated in his *Sunan* that the two children of Busr said, "The Messenger of Allah **b** came by us and we offered him some butter and dried dates, as he used to like eating butter and dried dates."

Butter is hot and wet and has many benefits, such as maturing the mixtures (bodily wastes) and decomposing them, along with relieving the tumors that appear next to the ears and ureters (tubes leading from the kidney to the bladder). When butter is used, alone it In addition heals mouth cankers and the various other types of tumors that attack children and women. When one licks butter, it will help against lung hemoptysis (spitting up blood) and will mature the tumors of the lungs.

Butter softens the nature, the nerves and the hard tumors that result from black bile and phlegm and relieves the dryness in the body. When butter is laid on the place where children's' teeth emerge, it will help the teeth grow. Butter In addition soothes the coughing that accompanies colds and dryness. It In addition heals herpes and the roughness in the body and works as a laxative. Yet, butter reduces the appetite and the sweetness of honey and dates.

The wisdom behind the Prophet sag eating dried dates with butter is that they would neutralize the effect of each other.

3. *Zabib* (Raisins)

The best type of *Zabib* is the largest in size, the fattest and that has thin skin and small seeds, especially when the seeds are removed before eating them. Raisins are hot and wet in the first degree, while their seeds are cold and dry.

Raisins are similar to the type of grape they are made of, as sweet raisins are hot, sour raisins are cold and constipating and white raisins are more effective constipating agents. Raisin pulp is suitable for the windpipe and relieves coughing, liver, and prostate pain. It In addition strengthens the stomach and soothes the intestinal cavity.

Sweet raisin pulps are more nutritious than grapes, but less nutritious than dried figs. In addition, raisin pulps possess maturing qualities and mildly constipate. In general, raisins strengthen the stomach, the spleen and the liver and benefit tile throat, chest, liver and prostate.

The best way to have raisins is to eat them without the seeds. Raisins provide good nutrition arid do not cause clogs like dates do. Eating raisins with their seeds I increase the nutritious intake and will benefit the stomach, liver and spleen. When one is suffering from loose nails and places raisin pulps on them, they will! Remove the nails quickly. Sweet, seedless raisins benefit for who suffer from excessive wetness and phlegm and help the liver.

Raisins In addition help memo-y power, as Az-Zuhri said, "Those who seek to memorize the *Hadith*: should eat raisins," In addition, it was reported that Abdullah Ibn 'Abbas described the raisins that, "Their seeds are an ailment while their pulp is cure.

4. *Zanjabil* (Ginger)

Allah said:

﴿ يُوفُونَ بِٱلنَّذْرِ وَيَخَافُونَ يَوْمًا كَانَ شَرُّهُۥ مُسْتَطِيرًا ٧ ﴾

(٧) الإنسان .

"And they will be give) to drink there of a cup (of wine) mixed with anjabtl (ginger)." (76: 7)

Abu Nu'aym In addition narrated in his book on the Prophetic medicine that Abu Sa'id Al-Khudri said:

Ginger is hot in the second degree and wet in the first degree. It heats the body, helps the ingestion process, softens the stomach mildly, helps open the clogs of the liver that are caused by coldness and wetness and helps against the wetness that causes sight impairment, when it is eaten or used as kohl. Ginger In addition strengthens the sexual power and decomposes the thick gases accumulating in the intestines and the stomach.

In general, ginger is good for the cold temperament of the liver and the stomach. When one takes some ginger along with two measures of sugar and some hot water, it will work as a laxative and will rid the body of harmful excrements. Ginger is an effective ingredient in the ointments that dissolve the phlegm.

Sour ginger is hot and dry and it excites the sexual drive, increases semen production, heats the stomach and the liver, helps the digestion process, dries the phlegm that prevails in the body and increases the memory power. It is In addition suitable for the coldness in the liver and stomach and washes the harmful effect of eating fruit. It In addition makes the scent better and fends off the harm of thick, cold foods.

The Letter Seen

1. Senna

We mentioned Senna before and stated that it is In addition called Sanut. There are seven opinions regarding what the word Senna means.

Senna is said to mean honey, the thick juice that appears on the surface of the butter and which looks like black stripes, cumin like seeds, Persian cumin, dill, dried dates or fennel.

2. *Safarjal* (Quince)

Quince is cold and dry, constipates and benefits the stomach. Sweet quince is cold and dry and is somewhat mild. Sour quince constipates more than sweet quince and is colder and drier. All types of *Safarjal* quench the thirst, stop vomiting, help produce urine and constipate. *Safarjal* In addition helps against stomach ulcers, hemoptysis (spitting up blood), diarrhea and nausea. *Safarjal* In addition prevents the ascending of gaseous material when one eats it after the meal. In addition, the ashes of washed *Safarjal* leaves and stems are similar to zinc in benefit.

Consuming Safarjal before the meal constipates, while consuming it after the meals softens the stool and helps the digestion process. Eating excessive amounts of *Safarjal* harms the nerves and causes painful constipation. *Safarjal* helps extinguish the yellow bile of the stomach.

When the quince is broiled, it will become softer and milder. When one removes the pips of. the quince, stuffs them with honey, dips them in a paste and then broil them under hot ashes, they will become very beneficial.

The best way to eat the quince is broiled or cooked in honey. The seeds of *Safarjal* In addition help against dryness in the throat, the windpipe and several other ailments. Its oil stops sweating and strengthens the stomach. *Safarjal* jam In addition strengthens the stomach and the liver and relieves the heart and the soul.

3. *Siwak*

In the *Sahihain* it is narrated that the Prophet **b** said:

"If it was not for the fact that my nation would not be able to bear it, I would have ordered them to use Siwak before every prayer."

In addition, in the *Sahihain* it is narrated that:

"Whenever the *Prophet* as *would wake up at night, he would clean his mouth with Siwak."*

***Al-Kukhari In addition narrated that ;he Prophet* b said:**

"*Siwak* cleans the mouth and pleases the Lord." Further, Muslim r.arrated that:

"Whenever the *Prophet* b *would enter his house, he would first use the Siwak."*

There are many other *Ahadith* on this subject.

An authentic *Hadith* In addition stated that just before he died, the Prophet **b** used the *Siwak*. The Prophet **b** said:

I have *troubled you by frequently stressing using*

***the** Siwak."* The best type of *Siwak* is made from Arak trees. Further, one should not use an unknown tree for *Siwak* for it might be poisonous. In addition, *Siwak* should be used moderately, because it might cause the coating of the teeth to wear away and thus the teeth will be susceptible to the hot vapors or gasses that ascend from the stomach and to all kinds of dirt. When the *Siwak* is used moderately, it will polish the teeth, strengthen the roots of the teeth, help the tongue, prevent plaque, perfume the breath, clear the mind and strengthen the appetite.

The best way to use the *Swak* is by soaking it in rose water. In addition, the best type of *Siwak* is made from walnut stems. The author of At-Taysir said, "It was said that when one uses the *Siwak* once every five days, it will clear the head, sharpen the senses and alert the mind."

Siwak is beneficial for many reasons, such as perfuming the breath, strengthening the gingiva, clearing the phlegm and the sight and preventing cavities. It In addition preserves the health of the stomach, clears the voice, helps the digestion process, helps make the speech clear and encourages one to recite the Qura'an, remember Allah and pray. *Siwak* In addition fights sleepiness, pleases the Lord, delights the angels and increases the number of the good deeds.

Siwak is preferred at any time, especially before the prayer, ablution, when waking up and when the mouth emits foul odor. It is In addition preferred for those who are fasting and all other people at all times. There are *Ahadith* that allow this practice for those who are fasting, because it is beneficial for them and pleases the Lord. Pleasing the Lord when one is fasting is even more desired than at other times. In addition the *Siwak* cleans the mouth, and cleanliness for the fasting person is one of his best deeds.

In the *Sunan* it is narrated that 'Amir bin RabT'ah said: "I saw the Messenger of Allah **b** on numerous occasion using the *Siwak* when he was fasting."

Al-Bukhari In addition said that Ibn 'Umar said that the Prophet sg used the *Siwak* at the two ends of the day.

There is a consensus that the fasting person rinses his mouth while performing ablution, and rinsing the mouth is an obligation or a more preferred act than using the Siwak. In addition, Allah does not have a use for the people to worship him while their mouths are emitting foul odor, nor is it an act of worship. When the Prophet mentioned that the odor that the mouth of the fasting person emits is better in His Sight than the scent of *Musk*, he meant to encourage the practice of fasting, not the practice of allowing the mouth to emit foul odor. Hence, the fasting person needs the *Siwak* more than anyone else. In addition, Allah's Pleasure is much better than His preferring the odor that the mouth of the fasting person emits.

Further, Allah prefers using the Siwak more than for the odor that comes out of the mouth of the fasting person to remain.

In addition, using *Siwak* does not prevent the good scent that Allah creates in the fasting person's mouth on the Day of Resurrection. Rather, the mouth of the fasting person will smell better than Musk on the Day of Resurrection as a sign of his observing the Fast, even if the Siwak removed the odor that used to come from his mouth. Similarly, whoever suffers a wound [for the sake of Allah] in this life is commanded to remove the blood from his body in this life, but his wound would still have the color of blood on the Day of Resurrection.

Furthermore, the *Siwak* does not completely remove the odor of the mouth for the fasting person because its reason still remains, that is, the stomach being empty of food. Only the effect of this fact will be lessened from the teeth and gums.

The Prophet **b** taught his nation the preferred and the disliked acts of the Fast. He did not mention the *Siwak* among the disliked acts although he knew they were using it. Rather, he encouraged them in general to use the *Siwak* and they saw him using it himself at innumerable times, knowing that they would imitate him. Never did he discourage them from using the *Siwak* in the afternoon (when they are fasting). It is a fact that the Prophet ^g is required to offer the religious ruling when it is needed.

4. Somn (Shortening)

There is a weak *Hadith* that narrates that the Prophet as encouraged the Muslim to drink cow milk, because it is a remedy and because the butter of that milk is a cure, while stating that cow meat is an ailment, The chain of narrators for this *Hadith* is not authentic.

Somn is hot and wet in the first degree, it is mild, and helps eliminate the various tumors that attack the soft parts of the body. Somn is stronger than butter as a maturing agent, Galinus said that he used shortening to cure the tumors that occur in the ear and the tip of the nose. In addition, when the base of the teeth is anointed with shortening, the teeth will emerge faster.

When shortening is blended with honey and bitter almonds, it will clear the chest and the lungs and will dissipate various ailments; Shortening is harmful for the stomach, especially if the person has a mucus condition.

When the shortening made of cow and goat milk is mixed with honey, it helps against toxic materials and snake and scorpion stings. Ibn As-Sunni mentioned that 'Ali said that the people never use a better remedy than shortening.

5. *Samok* (Fish)

Imam Ahmad and Ibn Majah narrated that 'Abdullah Ibn 'Umar said that the Prophet **b** said:

"We were *allowed two dead animals and two bloods: fish and locust, and liver and spleen."*

There are many kinds offish, the best of which is the most delicious, the best scented, moderate in size, which has fine scales, the softest meat, which live in fresh water that flows on pebbles and which eat plants and not organic waste. The best areas for the fish to live are those with the freshest water that runs through rocks, then the areas that have sandy ground void of filth or wastes and which are mildly calm and exposed to the sun and wind,

Sea fish are In addition soft and delicious. The meat of sea fish that has soft skin is cold and wet, difficult to digest and produces excessive amounts of phlegm, but In addition produce acceptable temperament, increase semen production and fertility and suit hot conditions.

The best kind of salted fish is the most recently salted. Salted fish is hot and dry, and the older they get the hotter and drier they become. Silurid (similar to catfish) is very viscous, and the Jews do not eat this type of fish. Yet, soft Silurid meat softens the stomach, and when it is salted, kept and then eaten, it will clear the windpipe and make the voice finer. When it is ground and used as an external ointment, it will extract the wastes that accumulate inside the body, as it has the quality of extracting such substances,

Sitting in the salty water of Silurid relives the effects of newly formed ulcers and extracts the harmful substances to the surface. Salty water of Silurid In addition relieves sciatic nerve ailment when one is injected with it.

The best part of fish meat is closer to the tail, and the soft and fatty fish meat produces fatness and flesh.

In the *Sahihain* it is In addition narrated that Jabir bin Abdullah said, "The Prophet **b** sent us with three hundred riders under the leadership of Abu 'Ubaidah bin Al-Jarrah. We went by the seashore and were soon very hungry until we ate tree leaves. The sea then threw out a whale that is called 'Anbar. We ate from it for a half a month and In addition used its fat in our food. Abu Ubaidah then took a rib of the fish and asked a man to ride on his camel and then pass under the rib, which he easily did."

6. Silqh (Chard)

At-Tirmidhi and Abu Dawud narrated that Umm Al-Munthir said, "The Messenger of Allah b came by along with Ali when he was still recovering from an illness. Then, we had some hanging clusters of dates. The Messenger of Allah b started eating from it, and he (Ali) joined him. The Messenger of Allah b then said to him:

"You are still recuperating, until 'Ali stopped eating.' I then made some barley with chard and brought it to them. The Prophet b *said, to* 'Ali 'Eat from this: this more beneficial for you.'"

Silqh is hot and dry in the first degree and has a soothing coofness in it. Chard In addition decomposes and opens the clogs. The *black chard* constipates and helps against alopecia (A skin disease characterized by loss of hair, partial or total), spots, *dandruff and warts if* its water is used as ointment. It In addition kills lice and is used as ointment when blended with honey to cure herpes. *Silqh* In addition opens the clogs in the liver and spleen.

The black chard constipates as we have stated, especially when taken with lentils, both of which are not suitable for the stomach. However, white chard with lentils softens the stomach and is used as a laxative and is used to treat hemiplegia (Paralysis affecting only one side of the body), when blended with food aliments and condiments. Yet, it is not nutritious, produces harmful mixtures and burns the blood. Eating it with vinegar and mustard helps neutralize these side effects. Finally, eating it excessively causes constipation and flatulence.

The Letter Shin

1. *Shuneiz* (The Black Seed)

We talked about the Black Seed before under the letter 'Hoo.

2. *Shubrum* (Euphorb)

At-Tirmidhi and Ibn Majah narrated that the Messenger of Allah **b** asked Asma' bint 'Umais

"How do you treat *constipation? She said. 'with Shubrum'. The Prophet* its said, 'Hot and too strong of a *laxative."*

Shubrum is a small tree that sometimes grows to be as tall as a man. The *Shubrum* has red branches with some whiteness, while the tips of its branches end with a cluster of leaves, *Shubrum* flowers are small and yellowish with some whiteness. When its flowers they fall small stems that have small grains and which look like terebinth replace them. The color of these stems is reddish and has red peels that cover its ribs. The parts of the *Shubrum* that are used are its peels, ribs and stem extract,

Shubrum is hot and dry in the fourth degree and drives away the black bile, yellow water and phlegm. It In addition causes nausea and distress. Using it in excessive amounts might even case death. When intending to use the *Shubrum,* it should first be soaked in milk for a day and a night, and the milk should be changed twice or thrice during the day. Then, the *Shubrum* should be dried in the shadow, blended with roses, tragacanth (In addition known as goats' horn), and then consumed with honey water or grape juice.

Two to four small measures of the *Shubrum* constitute one dose. We should state that Hunain said, "As for *Shubrum* milk, I do not see any goodness in it and thus do not recommend it. Common doctors have killed many people with it."

3. Sho'fr (Barley)

Ibn Majah narrated that "Aishah said: "When a member of the family of the Messenger of Allah **b** would fall sick, he would order that barley soup is made and then the ill person would be commanded to have some of it. He used to say, 'It strengthens the heart of the sad person and relieves the heart of the ill person, just as one of you would wash the dirt off of her face with water.' "

We mentioned that the remedy mentioned in this *Hadith* entails boiled barley water which is more nutritious than its flour. Barley water helps against coughing and throat roughness, relieves the irritant excess excrement, produces more urine, cleanses the stomach, quenches the thirst and extinguishes heat. It In addition provides comfort and has a decomposing quality.

This remedy entails preparing a portion of a good type of barley and five times as much water, placing them in a clean pot and cooking them under moderate temperature until only two fifths of the mixture remains in the pot. The resulting soup is then purified and used as much as needed.

4. Shown (Roasted Meat)

Allah said that when Prophet Ibrahim had the honorable guests:

"And he hastened to entertain them with a roasted calf." (I 1:69) Ibrahim had roasted the calf on heated stones.

At-Tirmidhi narrated that Umm Salamah said that she once brought the Prophet s& a roasted piece of meat and that he ate from it and then stood up to pray without repeating the ablution. At-Tirmidhi then commented that this *Hadith* is authentic. At-Tirmidhi In addition narrated that Abdullah bin Al-Harith said, "We ate some roasted meat with the Messenger of Allah as inside the mosque." Further, At-Tirmidhi narrated that Al-Mughirah bin Shu'bah said, "I was a guest of the Messenger of Allah b one night and he ordered that a piece of meat be roasted and then took the blade and started to cut pieces of it for me. Then, Bilâl came to make the call to prayer and the Prophet s& dropped the blade and said, 'What is the matter with him?"

The best type of roast is the meat of a one-year old sheep, then a fat sheep. This type of food is hot and wet, produces black bile, but is one of the most nutritious foods for healthy, ill and recovering persons alike. Cooked meat is better, lighter on the stomach and has more wetness. Fried meat is less beneficial while meat dried in the sun is the worst kind. In addition, roasting meat on burning stones is better than flame broiled meats.

5. *Sha'hm* (Fat or Grease)

In Al-Musnad it is narrated that Anas said that a Jewish man asked the Prophet ste to be his guest and that he offered him some barley bread and melted grease.

In the *Sahih* it is In addition narrated that

Abdullah bin Mughaffal said, "On the Day of Khaibar, a bag full of grease was lowered and I took possession of it and said, 'By Allah! I will not give anyone any of it!' When I turned around I found that the Messenger of Allah ^ was laughing and did not comment.' "

The best type of grease is that taken from a grown animal. Grease is hot and wet but less wet than clarified butter. This is why when both grease and clarified butter are melted, grease hardens faster.

Grease helps against throat roughness, it represses and causes rotting. To neutralize the harmful effects of grease, one should use lemon, salt and ginger. In addition, goat grease constipates more than any other type of grease, while Billy goat grease is more decomposing and helps against stomach ulcers. Goat grease helps against stomach ulcers and is used as an injection to relieve excoriation (the rubbing away of skin from injury or disease), and (spasms of the bladder or anus).

The Letter Sod

1. The So/at (The Formal Prayer)

Allah said:

﴿ وَٱسْتَعِينُوا۟ بِٱلصَّبْرِ وَٱلصَّلَوٰةِ ۚ وَإِنَّهَا لَكَبِيرَةٌ إِلَّا عَلَى ٱلْخَـٰشِعِينَ ﴾

(٤٥) البقرة .

"And seek help in patience and As-Salat (the prayer) and truly, it is extremely heavy and hard except for Al-Khashi'un [i.e. the true believers in Allah - those who obey Allah with full submission, fear much from His punishment, and believe in His Promise (Paradise) and in His Warnings (Hell)]." (2:45)

And:

﴿ يَـٰٓأَيُّهَا ٱلَّذِينَ ءَامَنُوا۟ ٱسْتَعِينُوا۟ بِٱلصَّبْرِ وَٱلصَّلَوٰةِ ۚ إِنَّ ٱللَّهَ مَعَ ٱلصَّـٰبِرِينَ ﴿١٥٣﴾ ﴾

(١٥٣) البقرة .

"O you who believe! Seek help in patience and As-Salat (the prayer). Truly, Allah is with As-Sabirun (the patient)." (2:153)

In addition, Allah said,

﴿ وَأْمُرْ أَهْلَكَ بِالصَّلَوٰةِ وَاصْطَبِرْ عَلَيْهَا ۖ لَا نَسْـَٔلُكَ رِزْقًا ۖ نَّحْنُ نَرْزُقُكَ ۗ وَالْعَـٰقِبَةُ لِلتَّقْوَىٰ ﴾ (١٣٢) طه .

"And enjoin As-Salat (the prayer) on your family, and be patient in offering them [i.e. the Salat (prayers)]. We ask not of you a provision (i.e. to give Us something: money): We provide for you. And the good end (i.e. Paradise) is for the Muttaqun (the pious)." (20:132)

Furthermore, in the Sunon it is narrated;

"Whenever the Messenger of Allah would be concerned about a matter, he would turn to prayer."

We In addition mentioned using the prayer as a cure for various types of illnesses before these illnesses progress.

The prayer brings about sustenance, preserves the health, discards harm, eradicates illness, strengthens the heart, radiates the face with light, brings joy to the soul and dissipates laziness. In addition, the prayer energizes the limbs, sustains power, opens the chest, nourishes the soul, brings light to the heart, protects the bounty, shields from the anger (of Allah), brings about blessings, takes one away from Satan and draws him closer to the Most Beneficent.

In general, the prayer has a profound effect in preserving the health of the body and the heart. The prayer In addition discards harmful substances. No two persons would catch a type of disease or suffer an affliction, but whoever prays among them would suffer the minimal effects of the illness or the affliction.

The prayer has a profoundly wonderful effect in repelling the evils of this life, especially when the prayer is given its due right inwardly and outwardly. Certainly, the evils of this life and the Next Life would be most effectively repelled while their good would be most effectively brought forth through prayer. The secret in this is that the prayer is the connection with Allah. The closer the connection is between the slave and his Lord, the more open the doors of all types of good will be for him, while closing the ways to evil. In this case, the tools of success will descend on the slave from his Lord, along with good health, many bounties and riches, comfort, delight, joy, happiness and the good things of life,

2. Sabr (Patience)

Sabr, patience, is one half of Faith, which is half patience and half praise and thankfulness. Some of the

So/of said, "Iman has two halves, one half patience and one half praise (and appreciation)." Allah said:

﴿ فَقَالُوا رَبَّنَا بَاعِدْ بَيْنَ أَسْفَارِنَا وَظَلَمُوا أَنفُسَهُمْ فَجَعَلْنَاهُمْ أَحَادِيثَ وَمَزَّقْنَاهُمْ كُلَّ مُمَزَّقٍ إِنَّ فِي ذَٰلِكَ لَآيَاتٍ لِّكُلِّ صَبَّارٍ شَكُورٍ ﴾ (١٩) سبأ .

"Verily, in this are indeed signs for every steadfast, grateful (person)." (34:19)

To Faith, *Sabr* is just like the head to the body. There are three types of Sabr. First, there is the Sabr while performing Allah's Commands, so that one does not ignore [or get bored with] them. There is a Sabr with shunning the prohibitions, so that one does not violate them. There is In addition a Sabr with the appointed destiny and decisions of Allah, so that one is not enraged because of them. When one acquires all three types of Sabr, his Sabr will be complete and the delight of this and the Next Life will be whole, along with gaining and winning in both lives. No person shall achieve these great prizes except by passing on the bridge of Sabr, just as no person will reach Paradise except by passing over the Sfrot (the bridge over hell). Umar said, "We achieve the best living by Sabr."

When one thinks about the grades of perfection achieved in this life, he will realize that all of them are connected to *Sabr*. On the other hand, when one thinks about the blame worthy types of failure that one can and should avoid, he will realize that they are all connected to impatience. For instance, courage, honor, generosity and preferring others with good things are patience for a short time only (meaning this life is short).

Much of the illnesses and the sicknesses that attack the body and the heart are a result of impatience. In addition, *Sabr* is the best preserver for the health of the heart, the body and the soul, as it is the great distinction and the biggest cure. If *Sabr* only carries the reward of Allah being with the patient slaves and His love for them, it would be sufficient. Allah loves *Sabr* and supports its people:

"Certainly, victory comes with patience"

In addition, patience is good for its people.

﴿ وَإِنْ عَاقَبْتُمْ فَعَاقِبُوا۟ بِمِثْلِ مَا عُوقِبْتُم بِهِۦ ۖ وَلَئِن صَبَرْتُمْ لَهُوَ خَيْرٌ لِّلصَّـٰبِرِينَ ﴿١٢٦﴾ ﴾ (١٢٦) النحل .

"But if you endure patiently, verily, it is better for As-Sabirun (the patient)." (16:126)

Further, patience is the tool to achieve success.

﴿ يَٰٓأَيُّهَا ٱلَّذِينَ ءَامَنُوا۟ ٱصْبِرُوا۟ وَصَابِرُوا۟ وَرَابِطُوا۟ وَٱتَّقُوا۟ ٱللَّهَ لَعَلَّكُمْ تُفْلِحُونَ ۝٢٠٠ ﴾ (٢٠٠) آل عمران .

"O you who believe! Endure and be more patient (than your enemy), and guard your territory by stationing army units permanently at the places from where the enemy can attack you, and fear Allah, so that you may be successful." (3:2OO)

3. Sobir (Aloe)

Sabir has many benefits, especially the Indian *Sabir,* as it rids the body of bilious excrements in the brain and the optic nerves. When the *Sabir* is used as an ointment on the forehead and the cheeks, after blending it with rose oil, it helps relieve headaches. It In addition helps relieve the sores and cankers that appear in the mouth and nose and helps against black bile and depression.

The Persian *Sabir* sharpens the mind and brings firmness to the heart, and In addition releases from the body bilious mixtures and the phlegm that accumulates in the stomach, when one takes two spoons of *Sabir* mixed with water.

Caution: drinking *Sabir* in cold weather might cause diarrhea with blood.

4. *Sawm* (Fasting)

Fasting is a shield from many illnesses of the soul, the heart and the body and has tremendous benefits. Fasting In addition preserves the health and rids the body of harmful substances while preventing it from consuming what might harm it, especially when one fasts in the best times that the religion states or when the body needs it. Fasting relieves the muscles and the rest of the body and ensures regenerating its strength. Fasting In addition has a characteristic that should make one eagerly prefer it, that is, bringing joy and relief to the heart sooner or later (i.e. on the Last Day). Fasting is the best resort for those suffering from excess bodily moistures and substances and In addition protects and preserves their health.

Fasting is a type of spiritual and physical remedy. When the fasting person observes various rulings and guidelines regarding the Fast, his heart and body will benefit from the Fast the most. In addition, the body will get rid of the harmful foreign substances that his body is susceptible to receive, along with getting rid of the harmful substances that have already penetrated the body. The Fast In addition helps the fasting person to stay away from what he is supposed to avoid and to implement and seek the goals behind the Fast and what it is supposed to achieve for him. Fasting does not only entail abstaining from food and drink. There is another goal that fasting seeks to achieve which made it an act that Allah will specify its reward [only on the Day of Judgment]. The Fast is In addition a shield between the slave and what might harm his body and soul sooner or later, and this is why Allah said,

﴿ يَـٰٓأَيُّهَا ٱلَّذِينَ ءَامَنُوا۟ كُتِبَ عَلَيْكُمُ ٱلصِّيَامُ كَمَا كُتِبَ عَلَى ٱلَّذِينَ مِن قَبْلِكُمْ لَعَلَّكُمْ تَتَّقُونَ ﴿١٨٣﴾ ﴾ (١٨٣) البقرة .

"O you who believe! Observing As-Saum (the fasting) is prescribed for you as it was prescribed for those before you, that you may become Al-Muttaqun (the pious)." (2:183)

Fasting is a shield and a protection making it a type of tremendously beneficial diet. Another goal that the Fast seeks to achieve is the heart being busy with Allah, thus enlisting and recruiting the various powers of the body to implement what Allah loves and the requirements of worshiping Him. We mentioned some of the secrets of the Fast when we mentioned the Prophet's guidance on this subject.

The Letter Dhad

1. *Dhabb* (Lizards)

In the *Sahihain* it is narrated that Ibn 'Abbas said that the Messenger of Allah ^ was asked if eating the Dhabb was disallowed, because he did not eat from it when it was presented to him. The Prophet $s replied:

"No. But this food is not found in my *people's land and I do not have the appetite to eat it."*

The *Dhabb* was then eaten in the presence of the Prophet **b** In addition, the *Sahihain* it is narrated that Ibn 'Umar related from the Prophet sg that he said:

"/ neither allow it nor disallow it."

The meat of the *Dhabb* is hot and dry and strengthens the sexual drive. When it is ground and placed on a thorn that pierced someone's skin, it will extract the thorn.

2. Dhifdi' (Frog)

Imam Ahmad said, "(Killing) frogs is not allowed for medicinal purposes, because the Messenger of Allah s® has disallowed killing them." Ahmad was referring to the *Hadith* that he narrated in his *Musnad* in which

Uthman bin Abdur-Rahman said that a doctor mentioned using frogs for medicinal purposes, and the Messenger disallowed killing them.

The author of 'Al-Qanoon said, "Eating the meat or the blood of the frog might cause swellings in the body, pale color and [uncontrollable] ejaculation until death. This is why the doctors hesitate to use it formedicinal purpose because of its harm." There are two types of frogs, land and water frogs. Some of the land frogs are POISONED.

The Letter To'

1. *TaJb* (Perfume)

The Messenger of Allah b said:

"From your world, women and Tatb (perfume) were made beloved to me and the comfort of my eye is the prayer."

The Messenger of Allah ^ used to frequently use *Tatb* and did not like foul odors.

Taib (perfume) is the fuel of the soul, which is the engine of the powers of the body. Therefore, various strengths and powers in the body are nurtured in the presence of *Taib.* Similarly, the powers of the body are nurtured by consuming food and drink, feeling comfort and elation, being close to loved ones, receiving good news and by the absence of hateful, disliked persons whose presence is heavy on the heart. Indeed, associating with disliked persons weakens the strength and causes sadness and depression, just as the effects that fever and foul odor have on the body. This is why the companions of the Messengers were disallowed from acquiring the characteristics that would bother the Prophet and make them detested and disliked by him. Allah said:

"But when you ore invited, enter, and when you have taken your mea;, *disperse without sitting for a talk. Verily, such (behaviour) annoys the Prophet, and he is shy of (asking) you (to go); but Allah is not shy of (telling you) the truth."* (33:53)

In short, the *Taib,* perfume, was one of the dearest objects to the Prophet of Allah sfe. It In addition has a good effect on preserving good health and removing many ailments because it arouses the power of the body.

2. *Teen* (Clay or Argil)

Several invented *Ahadith* were mentioned regarding the benefits of clay. We should state that every *Hadith* that talks about the benefit of clay is untrue and must not be related from the Messenger of Allah. Clay is harmful and causes clogs in the veins, and it is cold, dry and a strong drying agent. In addition, clay prevents diarrhea and causes hemorrhages and sours in the mouth.

3. *Talh* (Banana or Acacia)

Allah said:

"And among Talh (banana-trees) with fruits piled one above another." (56:2^)

The majority of the scholars said that *Talh* means bananas, as they grow in piles one over the other just as the comb's teeth. It was said that the *Talh* is the tree that has thorns and which get replaced by fruits, each in the place of a thorn, just like what occurs on banana trees. This is the best opinion about the meaning of *Talh.* Hence, the So/of (righteous predecessors) who said that the *Talh* means banana trees are just using the banana tree as an example to explain the meaning of the word *Talh,* not that it only means banana trees. Allah has the best knowledge.

Bananas are hot and wet. The best type of bananas is ripe and sweet.

Bananas help against the roughness of the chest and lung, relieve coughing and help against the ulcers of the kidney and prostate. Bananas In addition produce urine (diuretic), stimulate semen production, soften the stomach and arouse the sexual drive; and they should be eaten before meals. Bananas harm the stomach and aggravate the bile and the phlegm, but eating them with sugar and honey reduces their harmful side effects.

4. To/' (Shoots or Clusters of dates)

Allah said: **"And *tall date-palms, with ranged clusters.*"** (5O:1O) And He said:

"And green crops *(field) and date-palms with soft spadix."*

(26:148) The *Tal'* of the date trees is the fruit when it is still young.

There are two types of *Tal'* (clusters): male and female. The reproduction process of date trees requires transferring pollen, which resembles the male organ and which looks like a fine powder, and placing it on the female organ. This process is called *Ta'bir.*

Muslim narrated in his *Sahih* that Talhah bin 'Ubaidullah said:

"I and the Messenger of Allah as passed by some date trees and found some people doing *Ta'bir.* The Prophet sn; asked about what they were doing and they said that they were removing the male sexual organ and placing it in the female sexual organ. The Prophet *yss,* said, '] do not think that this process will be of much help.' When they heard what the Prophet ^ said, they abandoned what they were doing and the trees did not reproduce. The Prophet s& then said, 'It was only a guess on my part. If (the *Ta'bir)* does help, then do it. I am only human just like you and my guess is either correct or incorrect. But, whatever I inform you from Allah (is true), I will never utter a lie on Allah."

The *Tal'* stimulates semen production and strengthens the sexual drive. When a woman takes the powder of the *Tal'* before having sex, it will help her get pregnant. The clusters of date trees are cold and dry in the second degree, strengthen the stomach and dry it out, and calm irritated blood, but are hard to digest.

Only those who have hot temperament can tolerate eating the *Tal'*. In addition, those who eat the To;' regularly should In addition eat hot sweets with it. The *Tal'* constipates and strengthens the intestines, just as theJummor, fresh dates and Busr that we mentioned before. Eating the *Tal'* in excessive amounts harms the stomach and the chest and might cause painful constipation, while taking it with butter and sweets helps reduce these side effects.

The Letter 'Ayn

1. '/nob (Grapes)

The Messenger of Allah ^ was reported to have liked eating grapes and watermelon. In addition, Allah has mentioned grapes in six instances in the Qura'an while listing the various bounties that He has bestowed on His slaves in this and the Next Life. Grapes are among the best and most beneficial fruits, and they are eaten fresh, dried, green and ripe. Further, Grapes are a type of fruit and nutritious food, along with their benefits as a remedy and a drink. Wetness and hotness are among the characteristics of grapes just as other grains. The best type of grapes is the big grapes that are full of juice, while white grapes are better than the black grapes when both are equal in sweetness. In addition, eating fresh grapes two or three days after harvest is better than eating them immediately otherwise they cause diarrhea and flatulence. The grapes are left on their hanging grapevines until their skin becomes thin. They are a source of good nutrition, just like raisins and figs, and In addition strengthen the body.

When the seeds of the grapes are removed, the grapes become a more effective laxative. Eating grapes excessively causes headache, unless one In addition eats sour pomegranate. Grapes in general are a good laxative ınd provide a good source of nutritior. The best types of ruits are three: grapes, dates and figs.

:. *'Asal* (Honey)

We mentioned the benefits of honey before.

Ibn Jurayj said that Az-Zuhri said, "Eat honey because it is good for the memory." The best type of honey is the white, pure, light and sweet honey. In addition, the honey that is collected from trees and mountains is better than the honey that is grown in cells. Further, the quality of the honey varies according to the area where the bees collected their food.

3. *'Ajwah* (Pressed, Dried Dates)

Sa'd bin Abu Waqqas narrated that the Prophet a& said:

"Whoever eats seven dates of 'Ajwah in the morning will not be harmed by poison or magic the rest of that day."

In addition, An-Nasa'y and Ibn Majah narrated that the Prophet s& said:

***"The* 'Ajwah is from Paradise, and it is an**

antidote against poison. The Kamab (truffles) is a type of Manna and its water (extract) cures the eye."

There is an opinion that this *Hadith* is talking about the *'Ajwah* of Al-Madinah in particular, which is one the best types of dates in the area of Hijaz. The *'Ajwah,* pressed dried dates, is a good type of dates, has firm skin and is one of the softest and most delicious types of dates.

We mentioned the various benefits of the dates and the Tomr when we talked about the letter Too. We In addition mentioned the benefits of the *'Ajwah* in treating poison and fending off the harm of magic.

4. *'Anbar* (Ambergris; Whale)

We mentioned the *Hadith* that is narrated in the Two *Sahihs* about Abu "Ubaydah and the Muslim army finding a huge fish, or whale, and that they ate from it for a half a month. They In addition took some of its meat with them to Al-Madinah and gave the Prophet **b** some of it. This *Hadith* indicates that it is allowed for Muslims to eat whatever comes from the sea even when it is dead.

Some people who [disagree with what we stated above] said that the whale was thrown on the shore while still alive and that when the water receded it died. Therefore, they say, the whale died because of the lack of water not naturally.

This opinion is incorrect, because the companions found the whale dead at the seashore. They did not see it alive and then the water receded causing its death as claimed. Further, if the whale were still alive, the sea would not have thrown it on the shore, since the sea usually throws dead animals and dead fish on the shore.

Furthermore, even if what they claimed had happened to the whale, it will not affect the ruling of permissibility [to eat dead marine creatures]. The Prophet sis disallowed eating game if one finds it dead in the water because there is a doubt if it had died from drowning and not from his weapon. So, if what the opponents say were true, then the fact that there is a doubt concerning how the whale died would disallow eating it [i.e. if their suggestion that the whale died because of lack of air and that dead marine creatures are disallowed dead were both true].

As for Al-'Anbar, amber, which is a type of *Tatb* (perfume), it is one of the best types of perfume after *Musk.* Some people mistakenly preferred *'Anbar* to *Misk.* However, the Prophet ^e described *Musk:*

"It is the best TaJb (perfume)."

Soon afterwards, we will mention the benefits and

characteristics of Musk, which is the *Tatb* of Paradise. In addition, the seats in Paradise that belong to the truthful believers are made of A Lusk not *'Anbar*.

Those who thought that *'Anbar* is better than *Musk* were deceived by the fact that the *'Anbar* does not spoil, just like gold. This fact alone does not indicate that the *'Anbar* is better than A/lusk.

There are several types of *'Anbar:* white, gray, red, yellow, green, blue, black and multicolored. The best type of the *'Anbar* is gray, then the blue and then the yellow in color, while the black *'Anbar* is the worst type.

People have conflicting opinions regarding the origin of *'Anbar,* where some people said that it is a plant that grows on the seabed and which sea reptiles eat and then discard to later be thrown on the seashore. Some people say that *'Anbar* is the waste of sea creatures that looks like cow manure. Some people even said that it is a type of foam that the sea discards on the shore. The author of the 'Qanoon' discounted the last two opinions but said that the amber might originate from an undersea spring.

'Anbar is hot and dry and strengthens the heart, the mind and the senses. It In addition strengthens the body and helps relieve facial paralysis, hemiplegia (paralysis), phlegmy ailments, stomach and flatulence. *'Anbar* In addition helps open various clogs if it is used as an

ointment or as a drink. When it is inhaled, *'Anbar* will relieve cold symp'oms, headaches and migraines.

5. *'Ud* (Indian Aloe Tree)

The Indian *'Ud* comes in two types. One type is used for medicinal purposes, which is called Al-Kust and some people called it Al-Qust. We will mention this type under the letter *Qaf*. The second type of 'Ud is called Aluwwah, aoe wood, which is used as perfume.

Imam Muslim narrated in his *Sahih* that Ibn "Umar used to bum dry aloe wood along with some *Kafur* (camphor), and states that the Messenger of Allah used to do the same. In addition, the Messenger of Allah has described the bounties that the people of Paradise will be enjoying, such as having the aloe wood.

The 'Ud is hot and dry in the third degree, opens the clogs and does away with gas. In addition, 'Ud dries unnecessary moisture while strengthening the intestines and brings relief and comfort to the heart. 'Ud In addition helps the mind, sharpens the senses, constipates and helps relieve the enuresis, bed wetting that result from coldness of the prostate.

Ibn Samjun said, "There are several kinds of 'Ud, and they all carry the general name of Aluwwah. 'Ud is used in and out of the body and is burned alone or with other substances. There is a medicinal significance when the 'Ud is mixed with *Kafur* (camphor), as each of them makes the other milder. In addition, burning the 'Ud helps cleanse the air, which is one of the six necessary elements for the body's well-being."

6. 'Adas (Lentils)

It was reported that the 'Ados (lentils) was described as the lust of the Jews that they preferred over Manna and quails.

The 'Ados is the companion of garlic and onions. It is cold and dry and has two opposing effects, one that constipates and one that works as a laxative. The skin of the 'Ados is hot and dry in the third degree and In addition works as a laxative. The benefit in the lentils is concentrated in the peelings, and this is why whole lentils are more beneficial than ground lentils, less heavy on the stomach and less harmful.

Lentils cause black bile and harm the melancholy profoundly, along with having a negative effect on the nerves and the eyesight.

'Adas produces thick blood; and those who suffer from black bile should avoid eating it, for when they eat lentils excessively, the lentils will beget obsession, leprosy, quartran fever (a fever that occurs on every fourth day), and other ailments. However, eating lentils with chard and large amounts of grease will lessen their negative side effects. In addition, one should avoid eating lentils with sweets, because lentils could cause clogs in the liver in this case. Further, eating 'Ados on a regular basis causes harm to the eyesight because they are very dry. Lentils In addition cause urine retention, cold swellings and excessive flatulence. The best type of 'Ados is the fat, white 'Ados that digests faster.

Some ignorant people claimed that Prophet Ibrahim used to cook lentils for his guests. However, the Qura'an mentioned that he hosted his guests with a fat roasted calf.

The Letter Ghayn

1. *Gbayth* (Rain)

The *Ghaith* is mentioned in the Qura'an in many instances. The word *Ghaith* is soft on the ear and delightful for the body and the soul. The ears like to hear the word *Ghaith,* while the hearts enjoy its falling.

Rainwater is the best type of water there is and the softest, most beneficial and most blessed. This is especially the case when the rainfall is accompanied by lightning and thunder and is then collected in mountainous areas.

Rainwater is lighter than the other types of water because it is fresh and did not remain on the ground for a long time, in which case it would acquire some of the earth's dryness and hard substances. This is why rainwater gets spoiled quickly because it is pure and light.

There are two opinions regarding which is softer and lighter: rainwater that falls in the spring or winter.

Those who prefer winter rainwater say that in winter, the sun's heat is less and it thus evaporates the softest parts of the seawater. In addition, the air then would be clean and void of dust, and consequently, would not be polluted. Hence, rainwater will not dissolve any pollutants while falling, and this is why rainwater is the softest and the lightest.

Those who prefer spring rainwater say that the hot sun then evaporates heavy substances in the air and makes the air itself lighter and cleaner. In this case, rainwater will be the lightest and the softest, at a time when the plants, the trees and the air become ready to receive rainfall.

Ash-Shafey narrated • that Anas bin Malik said, "Once, we were with the Prophet sg when the rain fell. The Prophet b removed his outer garment (until the rain fell on him) saying:

"*It has* just come from its Lord."

We mentioned the Prophet's guidance in invoking Allah for rain and stated that he used to seek the blessings [that Allah endows] in the rain when it falls.

The Letter Foo

1. Fatihah *Al-Kitab* (the First Chapter in the Qur'an)

Fatihah is the mother of the Qura'an, the seven frequently recited Versus that the Prophet ste was given and the ultimate cure and beneficial remedy that contains the prefect *Ruqiah,* Islamic prayer formula. The *Fatihah* is the key to acquiring the richness, success and strength. The *Fatihah* In addition removes sadness, depression, anguish and fear. Only those who appreciate the value of the *Fatihah* and give it its due consideration, reciting it as it should be recited and knowing the secret of its value as a medicine and as a cure, will acquire such bounties.

One of the Companions unveiled a few of the secrets of the *Fatihah* when he used it as a *Ruqyah for* scorpion stings. The affected person was instantly cured and the Prophet sn asked the Companion:

"How did you know it is a cure?"

They are successful ones who uncover some of the

secrets of the *Fatihah* and what it contains of *Tawhid*, knowing Allah and His Names, Attributes, Actions and Decisions. Those who acquire knowledge of what the Fot/hoh contains of affirming the religion, Predestination, Resurrection, Allah's Oneness in worship and in Lordship and trusting and depending on He Who owns all affairs, the praise and all pure things and to Whom everything must return. Those who acquire the habit of showing meekness to Allah seeking correct guidance which is the basis of the ultimate happiness in this and the Next Life. Those who acquire knowledge in the connection between the meanings contained in the *Fatihah* and acquiring the good and fending off the harm of both lives. Those who understand that their ultimate well-being and receiving the perfect Favor of Allah are all linked to implementing these meanings. It is they who will be able to substitute the *Fatihah* in place of many medicines and use it as an Islamic prayer formula *(Ruqiah)*, and will use it to open the doors of goodness and drive away the elements of evil.

Understanding this subject requires a new nature, a new heart and a new type of Faith. By Allah! You will not find any evil statement, nor misguiding innovation, but the *Fatihah* will contain what nullifies and refutes it with the best, most correct and most direct manner. In addition, you will not find a door that leads to acquiring divine knowledge, correct guidance of the heart and the remedy of the soul against its ills, but that the *Fatihah* will possess its key and the method to best use it. Finally, you will not find a path on which those who seek the Lord of the Worlds are passing, but you will find the *Fatihah* in its beginning and end.

By Allah! The *Fatihah* is much more important than what we have emphasized. The slave who holds fast to the *Fatihah,* comprehends it in the proper manner, relies on it as a perfect remedy, a shield, immunity, and as a light of guidance. He understands its implications as they should be understood. It is he who will not fall into an innovation, or Shirk, or catch an ailment in the heart except briefly!

The *Fatihah* is the ultimate key for the treasures of the earth and Paradise, as well. But not every person knows how to use this key so as to have access to these treasures. If those who seek these treasures were able to uncover the secrets of this chapter [in the Qura'an] and acquire knowledge of its implications, they would add teeth to the key and would have easy access to these treasures.

We are certain of the statements that we have asserted herein because they are true. Allah has Perfect Wisdom in hiding the secrets [of *Al-Fatihah'}* from the hearts of the majority of humankind, just as He has a perfect Wisdom in hiding the treasures of the earth from them.

The hidden treasures of the earth are surrounded by the devils that stand between humankind and these treasures. Only the good souls will be able to defeat these devils with True Faith, which is the weapon that the devils cannot withstand. However, the majority of the souls of mankind are not of this type (are not truly faithful). Therefore, they cannot resist the evil or defeat them to acquire their possessions for, "Whoever kills a combatant will have his possessions."

2. *Faghiyah* (Henna Blossom)

Faghiyah, henna blossom, is one of the best kinds of perfumes, *Faghiyah* is mild in its hotness and dryness and constipates mildly. When Faghiyah is placed between folded wool clothes it protects them from mold and mites. In addition, *Faghiyah* is used in ointments against facial paralysis and aneurysm (dilatation of a portion of the wall of an artery), while its oil helps the organs and relaxes the nerves.

3. *Fiddah* (Silver)

There is an authentic narration that states:

***"The Messenger* of Allah had a silver ring with**

a silver face. In addition, the grip of his sword was made from silver."

Unlike disallowing drinking in silver containers, there are no authentic narrations that disallow wearing silver. The category of containers for food and drink is more specific than the category of clothes and adornments. For instance, women are allowed to wear all types of clothes and adornments, while there are specific containers for food and drink that are not allowed to be used (i.e., gold and silver containers). Therefore, the fact that Muslims are not allowed to use some types of containers does not necessarily apply to clothes and adornments [which are a wider category as we have stated]. In the Sunan it is narrated that the Prophet ^e said:

"As *for silver, play with it as you like."*

Furthermore, disallowing wearing silver adornments needs a specific Text (Qura'an or *Sunnah)* or a consensus (of the scholars) for the heart to accept it with certainty. Once, the Prophet ^ held some gold in one hand and some silk in the other hand and said:

"These two are not allowed for the males of my nation and allowed for the females among them."

Silver is one of the wonders that Allah has created on the earth. It is the key to acquiring ones needs and high positions among the people of the earth. Those who have silver are honorable in the eyes of the people and respected in their hearts, allowing them to sit at the head of various meetings and opening all doors in front of them. In addition, the people do not feel bored by sitting next to owners of silver, nor will their presence be heavy. Fingers point at them, while eyes look at them [in admiration]. If they speak, people listen and if they intervene, their mediation will be accepted. If they present their witness, their testimony will be accepted and if they give a speech, they will not be blamed for being incompetent; and even the white hair that they have will be considered more youthful than youth itself!

Silver is one of the remedies that bring joy to the hearts and drive away sadness, depression, and weakness in the heart and its heartbeat. In addition, silver is used in some of the best kinds of ointments and helps extract the harmful substances or conditions of the heart, especially when blended with pure honey and saffron.

Silver is originally cold and dry but In addition produces hotness and wetness.

There are four types of gardens that Allah has prepared for His loyal saves when they meet Him: two made of gold and two made of silver, including all their containers, adornments and whatever is in them.

In the *Sahih* it is narrated that the Prophet s| said:

"Those who drink from golden or silver bowls are only pushing the Fire ofjahannam down into their stomachs."

He In addition said, as narrated in the Sohi'h:

"Neither drink from golden or silver bowls nor eat on golden on silver plates. It is for them (the disbelievers) in the life of this world and for you in the Next Life."

Some people said that the wisdom behind disallowing using golden and silver containers is to tighten the money supply. They say that if people use silver and gold as containers, then the interests of mankind will not be served well. In addition, some people said that they are disallowed so that whoever uses them does not become arrogant and proud, or so that the poor persons do not become humbled when they see such items, and so forth. These opinions are not sound.

For instance, tightening the money supply should In addition include disallowing wearing golden and silver adornments and canes [not only golden and silver containers]. Further, pride and arrogance are not allowed regarding anything. In addition, making the poor feel humbled is not a precise subject that we can define, for they could In addition feel humbled when they see luxurious homes, spacious gardens and lavish means of transportation, clothes and delicious foods. All these items are allowed for people.

What we think is the valid reason for this prohibition, and Allah has the best knowledge, is that using gold and silver in this manner affects the heart in such a way that contradicts true slavery to Allah. This is why the Prophet gte said that it is for the disbelievers in this life, because the disbelievers do not have a share in the true slavery [to Allah] that will give them the rewards of the Next Life. The slaves of Allah should not use these items in this manner, because only those who do not implement the requirements of their slavery (to Allah) use them in this life, as they prefer the life of this world to the Next Life. Allah has the best knowledge.

The Letter Qaf

1. Qura'an

Allah said:

"And We send down of the Qura'an that which is a healing and a* mercy to those *who believe (in Islamic Monotheism and act on

He In addition said:

﴿ يَٰٓأَيُّهَا ٱلنَّاسُ قَدْ جَآءَتْكُم مَّوْعِظَةٌ مِّن رَّبِّكُمْ وَشِفَآءٌ لِّمَا فِى ٱلصُّدُورِ وَهُدًى وَرَحْمَةٌ لِّلْمُؤْمِنِينَ ﴿٥٧﴾ ﴾ (٥٧) يونس .

"O mankind! There has come to you a good advice from your Lord (i.e. the Qura'an, enjoining all that is good and forbidding all that is evil), and a healing for that which is in your breasts..." (1O:57)

The Qura'an is the ultimate cure from all types of illnesses and sicknesses that attack the body and the heart and from all the calamities of life and death. Yet, not everyone is suitable or guided to successfully seek the Qura'an as a cure.

When the ill person successfully uses the cure contained in the Qura'an and applies it on his ailment with faith, sincerity, complete acceptance and trust, all the while observing the necessary guidelines in this regard, no illness can resist the cure,

How can any ailment resist [the Book that contains] the Words of the Lord of the earth and heaven, which if it were revealed to a mountain, it would cause it to humble itself and render it asunder. Further, if the Qura'an were revealed to the earth, it would tear it apart. No ailment that attacks the body or the heart, but the Qura'an contains its remedy and cure and would provide immunity against it, that is, for whomever Allah has endowed with the bounty of comprehending His Book.

We stated before that the Qura'an contains the major aspects and basis of the knowledge of medicine: preserving health, diet and extracting of harmful substances. As for the ills that attack the heart, the Qura'an mentions them in detail and directs the people to the cures and remedies to treat them. Allah said:

﴿ مَن كَانَ يَرْجُوا۟ لِقَآءَ ٱللَّهِ فَإِنَّ أَجَلَ ٱللَّهِ لَءَاتٍ ۚ وَهُوَ ٱلسَّمِيعُ ٱلْعَلِيمُ ﴾ (٥) العنكبوت .

"Is it not sufficient for them that We have sent down to you the Book (the Qura'an) which is recited to them?" (29:5)

May Allah never cure those whom the Qura'an does not cure, nor suffice for those for whom Allah is not sufficient as a Helper.

2. Qith-tha' (Wild Cucumber)

In the *Sunan* it is narrated that Abdullah bin Ja'far said:

"The Prophet b ***used to eat Qith-tha' with ripe dates."*** **[At-Tirmidhi].**

Qith-tha' is cool and wet in the second degree and it cools the hotness in the stomach, it does not spoil quickly and helps relieve prostate pain. In addition, *Qith-tha'* helps relieve nausea while its seeds are a diuretic. When *Qith-tha'* leaves are used as a bandage, they help against dog bites.

Qith-tha' does not digest easily and its coolness sometimes hurts some parts of the stomach. Hence, one should eat *Qith-tha'* with what would make its coolness and wetness milder, just as the Prophet did by eating ripe dates with it. In addition, eating it with raisins or honey makes it milder on the stomach,

3. Qust, or Kust (Costus)

In the *Sahihain* it is narrated that Anas related from the Prophet **b**, that he said:

"Cupping and marine costus are the best of your remedies."

In addition, Imam Ahmad narrated that the Prophet *m,* said:

"Use this Indian wood, because ft contains seven types *of cures, among them a cure for pleurisy."*

There are two kinds of Qust, the white kind that is

called seo-Qust and the *Indian Qust,* which is the hottest among them while the white type is the mildest. Both kinds have many benefits.

Both kinds of Qust are hot and dry in the third degree, and they dry out the phlegm and colds. When they are taken as a drink, they help weak liver and stomach and the colds associated with such cases, Costus In addition helps against victular and quartan fever (fever that comes on every fourth day), the pain on the side of the body and poisons. When the face is anointed with Qust that is kneaded with water and honey, they heal the spots that appear on the face. Galinus said that the costus, "Heals tetanus, the pain in the sides and kills spots (which he called the seeds of the pumpkin),"

Some ignorant doctors are unaware of and deny the Qust as an effective remedy against the pain in the sides of the body. If these ignorant doctors become aware of what Galinus has stated about the Quest, they will quickly embrace it as if it was a divine text. Moreover, many doctors have In addition stated that Qust helps against the pain in the flank that is accompanied by phlegm, as Al-Khattabi related from Muhammad bin Al-Jahm.

We stated before that the difference between the remedies contained in the Prophetic medicine and the remedies of regular doctors, is much larger than the difference between folk medicine as compared to regular medicine. We In addition stated that what is sent down of the divine revelation, as compared to what is proven by experimentation, compares to the difference between the noble master and the commoner.

In addition, if any of the ignorant doctors [who ignore the Prophetic medicine] were able to discover a remedy that the Jews, the Christians and the polytheist doctors have prescribed, they would embrace it and would certainly prescribe it.

We do not deny that habits have a role in making the cure work or fail. Those who are used to certain foods and medicines would benefit from such items more than those who are not used to them and who sometimes would not benefit at all from them.

The statements of the best doctors do not apply in all cases and places. Taking the statements of these doctors as being specific and not general does not lessen the degree of their knowledge. The same ruling applies even more to the statements of the Prophets. Yet, the hearts of mankind have a built-in degree of ignorance and injustice, except for those whom Allah has endowed with the light of correct Faith and enlightened their hearts with true guidance.

4. Qasab As-Sukkar (Sugarcane)

Sugar is a relatively new substance that the people of old did not mention or even have knowledge that it existed. This is why they did not describe its role in various types of drinks or cures. Honey, on the other hand, was extensively used as a drink and as a medicine.

Sugarcane is hot and wet, helps relieve coughing and dissipates the excess moistures in the body, prostate and chest. It is more effective as a laxative than sugar itself. In addition, sugarcane induces vomit. is diuretic and stimulates semen production.

Affan bin Muslim As-Saggar said, "Those who suck on sugarcane after eating their meal, will find comfort for the rest of his day." When sugarcane is broiled, it relieves the roughness in the throat and chest. Yet, it causes the accumulation of gasses that would be pacified when sugarcane is peeled and washed in hot water.

Sugar is hot and wet. The best type of sugar is white crystalline, especially when it is old. When sugar is boiled and skimmed, it quenches the thirst and relieves coughing. Sugarcane is not good for the stomach that suffers from bile. The side effects of sugarcane could be pacified by mixing it with lemon water (juice), Naranj (bitter orange) and peeled pomegranate.

Some people prefer sugarcane to honey because it is not as hot as honey and because it is milder on the stomach. This is not fair for honey, which is much more profitable than sugarcane. In addition, Allah has made honey both a cure and a type of sweet. So how can anyone compare the benefits of honey and the benefits of sugarcane? Honey strengthens the stomach, soothes the natural process, strengthens the eyesight and heals diphtheria when gargled, facial paralysis and hemiplegia (paralysis affecting only one side of the body). It In addition helps against all types of cold illnesses that occur in the body because of excess moistures. Honey extracts and pulls excess moistures from the body, preserves the health, increases semen production, cleanses and decomposes the contents of the stomach. In addition, honey cleanses the intestines, fights worms and prevents septic repletion (over eating). Further, honey is a good type of food and favorable for those who suffer from phlegm and for old people. In short, no substance is more beneficial for the body as a food, as a remedy and as an ingredient and a preserver of medications, which In addition strengthens the stomach, than honey. There are many more benefits for honey. So how can anyone compare it to sugarcane, which does not have even a fraction of the benefits contained in honey?

The Letter Kaff

Kitab (Books or Writings)

This chapter contains books or writings of divine remedies, Islamic prayer formulas, as Islamic amulets (prayer formulas written down and worn for a specific purpose).*

1. An Amulet for Fever

Al-Mirwazi said, "Abu Abdullah (Imam Ahmad) was informed that was suffering from fever and he wrote to me a supplication for fever that reads like this, 'In the Name of Allah, the Most Gracious, the Most Beneficent. In the Name of Allah, and depending on Allah.

﴿ قُلْنَا يَـٰنَارُ كُونِى بَرْدًا وَسَلَـٰمًا عَلَىٰٓ إِبْرَٰهِيمَ ﴿٦٩﴾ وَأَرَادُوا۟ بِهِۦ كَيْدًا فَجَعَلْنَـٰهُمُ ٱلْأَخْسَرِينَ ﴿٧٠﴾ ﴾ (٦٩:٧٠) الأنبياء .

"We (Allah) said: 'O fire! Be you coolness and safety for IbrahJm (Abraham)! And they wanted to harm him, but We made them the worst losers. (21:69,7O)

O Allah, the Lord of (angels) Gabriel, Michael and Israfil: cure this person with this supplication by Your

Power, Strength and Might, O Lord of the creation. *Ameen.*'"

In addition, Al-Mirwazi said that Abu Ja'far. Muhammad bin Ali was asked about wearing [a written] *Ruqyah* (divine remedy, Islamic prayer formula or amulet). He said, "If it was from the Book of Allah or a *Hadith* [correctly] related from the Prophet, then wear it and use it as a remedy as much as possible." Abu Abdullah was listening to this narration and

In addition, Imam Ahmad did not object when he was asked about wearing a *Ruqyah* amulet after an illness or a calamity strikes. Al-Khallal In addition narrated that Abdullah bin Ahmad told him that his father used to write some supplication in a *Ruqyah* amulet for those who have a certain fear and for fever after it strikes.

An Amulet for Difficult Pregnancies

In addition, Al-Khallal narrated that Abdullah bin Ahmad said that his father wrote a *Ruqyah,* Islamic prayer formula, as an Islamic amulet, on a pure object for women who suffered from difficult pregnancies. In the, amulet, Ahmad wrote the *Hadith* narrated by Ibn Abbas, "There is no deity worthy of worship except Allah, the Most Forbearing, the Most Generous. All praise is due to Allah, the Lord of the Mighty Throne.

"All the praises and thanks are to Allah the Lord of the 'Alamin (mankind, jinn and all that exists)"

﴿ كَأَنَّهُمْ يَوْمَ يَرَوْنَهَا لَمْ يَلْبَثُوٓاْ إِلَّا عَشِيَّةً أَوْ ضُحَىٰهَا ﴿٤٦﴾ ﴾

(٤٦) النازعات .

"The Day they see it, (it will be) as if they had not tarried (in this world) except an afternoon or a morning." *(79:46)*

﴿ فَٱصْبِرْ كَمَا صَبَرَ أُوْلُواْ ٱلْعَزْمِ مِنَ ٱلرُّسُلِ وَلَا تَسْتَعْجِل لَّهُمْ ۚ كَأَنَّهُمْ يَوْمَ يَرَوْنَ مَا يُوعَدُونَ لَمْ يَلْبَثُوٓاْ إِلَّا سَاعَةً مِّن نَّهَارٍ ۚ بَلَٰغٌ ۚ فَهَلْ يُهْلَكُ إِلَّا ٱلْقَوْمُ ٱلْفَٰسِقُونَ ﴿٣٥﴾ ﴾ (٣٥) الأحقاف .

"On the Day when they will see that (torment) with which they are promised (i.e. threatened, it will be) as if they had not stayed more than an hour in a single day. (O mankind! this Qur'an is sufficient as) a clear Message (or proclamation to save yourself from destruction). But shall any be destroyed except the people who are Al-Fasiqun (rebellious against Allah's Command. disobedient to Allah)?" (46:35)

Al-Khallal said that a man came to Abu Abdullah and asked him to write a Islamic prayer formula as an Islamic amulet for a woman who had gone into labor for two days. Imam Ahmad asked the man to bring a wide cup with some Saffron [and wrote the amulet for the man's wife]. He In addition narrated that Imam Ahmad wrote the same amulet for several other people.

It was reported that 'Ikrimah narrated that Ibn Abbas said, "Jesus, the Messenger of Allah **b** once passed by a cow that was suffering from hard labor. The cow said [to Jesus], 'O, Word of Allah (be and he was)! Ask Allah to relieve me from what I am suffering from.' He said, "O Creator of the soul from another soul, who brings to life a soul from within another soul, relieves her.' The cow then gave birth and soon started to smell her newly born." Ibn Abbas then said, "Therefore, when the woman is suffering from hard labor, write [and recite] this supplication for her."

The types of Islamic prayer formulas as Islamic amulets that we mentioned are beneficial, Allah willing. Further, several scholars among the Salaf have allowed writing the Qura'an and drinking its water as a cure.

Another Amulet for Pregnant Women

One should write the following *Ayah* in a pure pot:

﴿ إِذَا ٱلسَّمَآءُ ٱنشَقَّتۡ ۝١ وَأَذِنَتۡ لِرَبِّهَا وَحُقَّتۡ ۝٢ وَإِذَا ٱلۡأَرۡضُ مُدَّتۡ ۝٣ وَأَلۡقَتۡ مَا فِيهَا وَتَخَلَّتۡ ۝٤ ﴾ (١:٤) الانشقاق .

"When the heaven is split asunder. In addition, listens to and obeys its Lord and it must do so. And when the earth is stretched forth, and has cast out all that was in it and became empty." (84:1 -4)

Then the pregnant woman should drink from this pot and pour some of it on her stomach.

An Amulet for Nosebleeds

Ibn Taymiyyah used to write the following *Ayah* on his forehead:

"And it was said: 'O earth! Swallow up your water, and O sky! Withhold (your rain). And the water was made to subside and the Decree (of Allah) was fulfilled (i.e. the destruction of the people (Noah). "(I :44)

I In addition heard him say, "I wrote [this A/oh] for several people and they were cured." He In addition said [about the Ayah], "It is not allowed to write it with the blood of the nosebleed as some ignorant people do, because blood is impure and one is not allowed to use it to write Allah's Speech."

Another Amulet for nose bleeds

It was reported that Prophet Musa .*Once* went out wearing an outer garment and then suffered from nosebleed and covered [his nose].

An Amulet for fungus

One should write [the following for it:]

"...then it is struck with a fiery whirlwind, so that it is burnt...?"

)(By Allah's Will and Power. **Another Amulet for fungus**

When the sun becomes yellow, one should write [the Ayah],

﴿ يَٰٓأَيُّهَا ٱلَّذِينَ ءَامَنُوا۟ ٱتَّقُوا۟ ٱللَّهَ وَءَامِنُوا۟ بِرَسُولِهِۦ يُؤْتِكُمْ كِفْلَيْنِ مِن رَّحْمَتِهِۦ وَيَجْعَل لَّكُمْ نُورًا تَمْشُونَ بِهِۦ وَيَغْفِرْ لَكُمْ ۚ وَٱللَّهُ غَفُورٌ رَّحِيمٌ ﴿٢٨﴾ ﴾ (٢٨) الحديد .

"O you who believe [in Musa (Moses) (i.e. Jews) and Musd (Jesus) (i.e.. Christians)]! Fear Allah, and believe in His Messenger (Muhammad gg) He will give you a double portion of His Mercy. and He will give you a light by which you shall walk (straight). And He will forgive you. And Allah is Oft-Forgiving. Most Merciful." (57:28)

An Amulet for three-day Fever

One should write on three separate papers, "In the Name of Allah it is running away. In the Name of Allah it has subsided. In the Name of Allah it has decreased."

Every day [that the fever lasts], one should swallow the paper with some water. **An Amulet for sciatica**

One should write, "In the Name of Allah. O Allah, Lord of everything, Owner of everything and Creator of everything! You have created the sciatic nerve and me. Do not give it power over me, nor allow me to cut it. Heal me completely and eradicate the illness. There is none who can heal except You."

An Amulet for bleeding veins

At-Tirmidhi narrated that Ibn Abbas said that the Messenger of Allah **b** used to teach them to recite [the following Ruqyoh], against fever and various pains, 'In the Name of Allah, the Most Great, I seek refuge with Allah, the All-Mighty, from the evil of bleeding veins and from the evil of the fire's heat,"

An Amulet for Toothache

One should write on the cheek that is closer to the pain, "In the Name of Allah, Most Gracious, Most Merciful.

﴿ وَهُوَ ٱلَّذِىٓ أَنشَأَ لَكُمُ ٱلسَّمْعَ وَٱلْأَبْصَـٰرَ وَٱلْأَفْـِٔدَةَ ۚ قَلِيلًا مَّا تَشْكُرُونَ ﴿٧٨﴾ ﴾ (٧٨) المؤمنون .

"It is He Who has created for you (the sense of) hearing (ears), eyes (sight), and hearts (understanding). Little thanks you give." (23:78)

Or,

﴿ ۞ وَلَهُۥ مَا سَكَنَ فِى ٱلَّيْلِ وَٱلنَّهَارِ ۚ وَهُوَ ٱلسَّمِيعُ ٱلْعَلِيمُ ﴿١٣﴾ ﴾

(١٣) الأنعام .

"And to Him belongs whatsoever exists in the night and the day, and He is the All-Hearing, the All-Knowing." (6:13)

An Amulet for abscess

One should write [this amulet and place it] on the abscess,

﴿ وَيَسْـَٔلُونَكَ عَنِ ٱلْجِبَالِ فَقُلْ يَنسِفُهَا رَبِّى نَسْفًا ﴿١٠٥﴾ فَيَذَرُهَا قَاعًا صَفْصَفًا ﴿١٠٦﴾ ﴾ (١٠٥:١٠٦) طه .

"And they ask you concerning the mountains: say, "My Lord will blast them and scatter them as particles of dust. Then He shall leave them as a level smooth plain." (2O:1O5,1O6)

2. *Kamah* (Truffles)

In the *Sahihain* it is narrated that the Prophet said:

"The *Kamah is among the Manna and its water (extract or juice) cures the eye."*

The *Kamah* grows wild underground, and it is called *Kamah* because it grows hidden beneath the earth. The *Kamah* does not have leaves or stems.

The essence of the *Kamah* is partly earthly and partly steamy and remains concealed underground during winter and then starts to grow above the ground with spring rainfall. This is why it is called the smallpox of the land, for it is similar to smallpox, which is caused by moistures clogged with blood that get aggravated during the early childhood years when the body starts to gain strength.

Kamah (truffles) grow in the spring and are eaten raw or cooked. The Arabs used to call *truffles* 'the plant of the thunder, because they grow in the aftermath of thunderstorms. The nomads in the desert use mushrooms in their regular diet. Further, the best type of *truffles* grow on sandy dry land. There are several types of *Kamah,* among which is a poisonous plant which is reddish in color and which causes asphyxiation.

The *Kamah* is cold and wet in the third degree, and it is not favorable for the stomach and not easily digested Eating *Kamah* on a regular basis causes constipation, gastric pain, facial paralysis, stomachache and dysuna (painful urination). Humid kinds of mushrooms are less harmful than dry ones. Therefore, those who wish to eat *Kamah* should bury them in a muddy area and then boil them in water, add salt and mint, and then eat them with oil and spices. This is because the *Kamah* has a heavy, earthly essence, although it contains a fair amount of water in its essence that makes it a little light. In addition, using the *Kamah* as kohl helps in cases of bad eyesight and ophthalmia (conjunctivitis).

Some of the best doctors have agreed that truffle water or juice helps strengthen the eyesight.

2. Kamah (Truffles)

In the Sahihain it is narrated that the Prophet said:

"The Kamah is among the Manna and its water (extract or juice) cures the eye."

The Kamah grows wild underground, and it is called Kamah because it grows hidden beneath the earth. The Kamah does not have leaves or stems.

The essence of the Kamah is partly earthly and partly steamy and remains concealed underground during winter and then starts to grow above the ground with spring rainfall. This is why it is called the smallpox of the land, for it is similar to smallpox, which is caused by moistures clogged with blood that get aggravated during the early childhood years when the body starts to gain strength

Kamah (truffles) grow in the spring and are eaten raw or cooked. The Arabs used to call truffles 'the plant of the thunder, because they grow in the aftermath of thunderstorms. The nomads in the desert use mushrooms in their regular diet. Further, the best type of truffles grow on sandy dry land. There are several types of Kamah, among which is a poisonous plant which is reddish in color and which causes asphyxiation.

The Kamah is cold and wet in the third degree, and it is not favorable for the stomach and not easily digested. Eating Kamah on a regular basis causes constipation, gastric pain, facial paralysis, stomachache and dysuria (painful urination). Humid kinds of mushrooms are less harmful than dry ones. Therefore, those who wish to eat Kamah should bury them in a muddy area and then boil them in water, add salt and mint, and then eat them with oil and spices. This is because the Kamah has a heavy earthly essence, although it contains a fair amount of water in its essence that makes it a little light. In addition, using the Kamah as kohl helps in cases of bad eyesight and ophthalmia (conjunctivitis).

Some of the best doctors have agreed that truffle water or juice helps strengthen the eyesight.

There are two opinions regarding the meaning of what the Prophet **b** said: "The Kamah is among the Manna."

Some people said, 'the Manna that Allah has sent down to the Children of Israel was not only the sweetmeat that we know, but In addition several other plants that grow in the wild without effort or planting on the people's part to grow. The Manna, in their opinion, means the

Favor, and thus, every type of plant or bounty that Allah grants to mankind without effort on their part is called Manna. All of Allah's bounties that He grants to mankind are a Favor from Him. Yet, Allah specifically mentioned the types of His Favors concerning which the slave does not make any effort, whether in growing or producing them, and called these Favors, Manna.

During the years of wandering in the earth with which Allah tested the Children of Israel, they used to sustain themselves on truffles that sufficed for bread. In addition, Allah gave them quails that sufficed as meat, and made their sweet the Manna that descends from trees. Therefore, their diet was complete.

Further, the Prophet's statement:

"The Kamah is a type of the Manna that Allah has sent down on the Children of Israel."

Some considered that the Kamah is a type of Manna, although the word 'Manna is usually used to describe the dew that descends on trees, which is originally called Taranjabin.

The second opinion states that the Kamah was called Manna because it resembles the Manna that descends on trees, in that it is collected without effort to plant or water.

If one asks, this is the case with Kamah, then what about the harm that it contains?

Know that Allah created everything in a perfect shape and essence. What Allah created is free from defects and harm and is beneficial for mankind. The various types of ailments occur later on when what Allah creates becomes spoiled somehow by being mixed or polluted by other substances, and so forth. If what Allah creates is left in its original shape that Allah has created, it does not contain any harm.

Those who have knowledge of the world and of the creation realize that all types of evil or harm in the air, land, plants and various creations occur after they are created. In addition, ever since mankind started disobeying their Prophets, all types of general and private evil occurred, that which causes them pain, illnesses, diseases, plagues, famines and loss of blessings in the land and in what it produces. The fruits and plants have thus lost their value and benefit gradually.

If one does not comprehend these facts, the following Ayah should be enough for him to understand.

﴿ ظَهَرَ ٱلْفَسَادُ فِى ٱلْبَرِّ وَٱلْبَحْرِ بِمَا كَسَبَتْ أَيْدِى ٱلنَّاسِ لِيُذِيقَهُم
بَعْضَ ٱلَّذِى عَمِلُوا۟ لَعَلَّهُمْ يَرْجِعُونَ ﴿٤١﴾ ﴾ (٤١) الروم .

"Evil (sins and disobedience to Allah) has appeared on land and sea because of what the hands of men have earned (by oppression and evil deeds)." (30:41)

One should apply this Ayah to what occurs in this world and compare them together.

Further, the people notice how various illnesses and sicknesses occur in plants, animals and fruits. These illnesses only produce other types of illnesses and diseases. The more mankind starts a new type of evil and sin, the more illnesses and diseases Allah brings to their foods, fruits, air, water sources, bodies, shapes and outer appearance. In addition, the people's behavior suffers a type of harm or alteration that is compatible with what their bodies commit of injustice and sin.

Before this time, the crops and grains used to be larger in size than at the present time, for the blessings in such items was bigger than at the present time. Imam Ahmad narrated, "A bundle that contained some wheat seeds as big as date seeds was found in a safe that belonged to members of the Umayyad dynasty. On it, these words were written, This used to grow during the times when justice prevailed.' "Imam Ahmad mentioned this story after narrating one of the Prophet's Ahadeeth.

The majority of the diseases and illnesses are the

remnant of the torments that were inflicted on the nations that lived before our time. These illnesses and diseases remained for those who followed their lead and imitated the previously tormented nations. This is a just judgment that the Prophet b mentioned when he stated that the Plague:

"It is the remnant of an affliction that Allah has sent on the Children of Israel."

In addition, Allah sent the wind on the people of 'Ad for seven nights and eight days. Allah has left some of this strong wind for the people who came after them to serve as a reminder [of what happened to Ad].

Allah made the works of the righteous and the sinning people as reasons behind much of what has happened in this world. For instance, when the people do not work righteousness or give in charity, the rain does not fall on them, and thus famine occurs. In addition, when the meek and powerless people are dealt with unjustly, when the people cheat in weights, and when the strong transgress the rights of the weak, the injustice committed by the [tyrant] rulers intensifies as a consequence. Such unjust rulers do not grant mercy if they are asked for mercy, nor are they kind when they are called on to be kind. In reality, what the rulers do and commit is a mere reflection of what their subjects do and commit. Allah, with His Wisdom and Just Decisions, makes people's work appear to them in various forms that are compatible to their works. Sometimes Allah strikes mankind with famines, sometimes with an enemy, sometimes with unjust rulers, sometimes with diseases, and sometimes with depression and sadness that will remain with them. Sometimes Allah strikes mankind with preventing the blessings from descending on them and by allowing the devils to have power over them, and leading them to what is certain torment. In this case, mankind will revert to what they were created for [either Paradise or the Fire].

The wise person thinks about the world and seeks the areas where Allah exerts His Justice and Wisdom, Then he will realize that the Prophets and their followers are passing on the path of safety, while the rest of mankind are leading themselves to the path of destruction and the land of failure. Allah will certainly bring His judgement and command to a successful conclusion, none can avert His decisions or commands. All success comes from Allah.

There are three opinions regarding the meaning of the Prophet's statement:

"And its water cures the eye."

First: that the K'ama'a water is an ingredient in the

remedies for eye ailments, not that it is used alone.

Second: that K'ama'a is used alone after broiling it and extracting its juice, The fire matures and softens the truffles, thus dissolving the harmful wetness and excrements that the K'ama'a contains and leaving the beneficial ingredients.

Third: that the meaning of 'its water' entails the rain that makes the mushroom grow and which is the first patch of rain that falls. In this case, the Hadith will be talking about the rain not the mushrooms themselves. Ibn Al-Jawzi mentioned this opinion, which is the weakest among the three opinions mentioned herewith.

Other people said that this portion of the Hadith entails using K.amah water to cool the eye. Hence its water alone is a cure, while the other parts are used as ingredients in compound remedies.

Al-Ghafiqi said, "The K'ama'a water (juice) is the best remedy for the eye when kneaded with the Ithmid (antimony type of Kohl) and then used as kohl (i.e. eyeliner). It In addition strengthens the eyelid and the eyesight and prevents many illnesses from attacking the eye."

3. Kabath (Arak Tree Fruit)

In the Sahihain it is narrated that Jabir bin Abdullah said, "We were with the Messenger of Allah ^ collecting Kabath when he said, "Collect the blaçk type of Kabath because it is the best type."

The Kabath is the fruit that grows on the plant called Arak which grow in the area of Hijaz [and whose branches are used for Siwak as we have stated]. It is hot and dry and carries the same benefits as the Arak tree: strengthening the stomach, helping the digestion, dissolving phlegm and relieving back pain and several other illnesses. Ibn Juljul said, "Drinking its soup produces urine as a diuretic, and cleanses the prostate." In addition, Ibn Radhwan said, "[The Kabath] strengthens the stomach and constipates (mildly)."

4. Katam (Plants Used to Dye the Hair Black)

Al-Bokhary narrated that Uthman bin Abdullah bin Mawhab said, "We came to Umm Salamah and she took out some of the

Messenger's hair that was dyed with henna and Katam." In addition in the four books of Sunan (Abu Dawood, At-Termezey, An-Nas'ay and Ibn Majah) it is narrated that the Prophet b said:

"Henna and Katam are the best of what you use to change (the color of) white hair."

In additi•n, in the Sahihain it is narrated that Anas said, "Abu Bakr once dyed (his hair) with henna and Katam." Further, Abu Dawood narrated that Ibn Ab'ass said, "A man who tinted (his hair) with henna passed by the Prophet s, who said, 'How good this is.' Then another man who tinted (his hair) with both henna and Katam passed by and the Prophet sag said, 'This is even better.' Then another man who tinted with Sufrah (a black dye) passed by and the Prophet **b** said, 'This is the best of all.'"

Al-Ghafiqi said, "Katam is a plant that grows in valleys and its leaves are similar to olive-leaves and grows higher than a (man's) shoulders. Its fruit grows to the size of peppers and have seeds in the middle. When the seeds are crushed, they turn black and when the leaves are squeezed and one drinks a small measure [of the extract], it causes vomiting. Katam In addition benefits against dog bites. When the stem is boiled in water, it is used as ink." Al-Kindi In addition stated that, "If one uses the Katam's seed as Kohl (i.e., eyeliner), it will clear the eye from the water that accumulates in it."

Some people thought that Katam is the Wasmah or the Nile-Leaves. This is not true, because Wasmah is a different plant. The author of the Sahih said, "Katam, which is used to dye the hair, is a plant that is mistakenly taken for Wasmah." The Wasmah has long leaves that are bluish in coor and which are larger than the Khilaf (Chalef) leaves and are similar to pea leaves but larger in size. Further, Wasmah is collected in Hijaz and Yemen.

If someone asks, "In the Sahih it is narrated that the Prophet s& did not dye (his hair)." We answer that Imam Ahmad said that other Companions have narrated that the Prophet s*l dyed (his hair). Those who were witnesses to an act are not like those who did not witness it. Hence, Imam Ahmad affirmed that the Prophet sg; had indeed used Khid'ab (dyed the hair), although Imam Malik denied it.

If someone says that in Sahih Muslim it is narrated the Hadith that disallows dying the hair black, when Abu Bakr's father was brought to the Prophet b with all his hair being white. The Prophet b said at that time:

"Change this white hair but avoid the black color."

Katam changes the color of the hair to black. There are two ways to answer this argument.

First, the Prophet b disallowed dying the hair black. But if the black color is mixed with henna and Katam, there is no harm in it. Katam and henna dye the hair between red and black colors, unlike Wasmah, which turns the hair black. This is the most plausible answer to the argument.

The second answer is that dying the hair black sometimes occurs for the purpose of deceiving others, such as when an old woman dyes her hair black to deceive the husband or other people, or when an old man dyes his hair black to deceive a woman. This is a type of cheating that is disallowed. On the other hand, if dying the hair black does not entail deceit, it is allowed. There are authentic narrations that Al-Hasan and Al-Husayn used to dye their hair black, as Ibn Jarir has reported. He In addition reported that this is the opinion of Uthman bin 'Affan, Abdullah bin Ja'far, Sad bin Abu Waqqas, "Uqbah bin 'Amir, Al-Mughirah bin Shu'bah, Jarir bin Abdullah and Amr bin Al-'Aas. He In addition related this opinion to several of the Tabi'in, the second generation of Islam, such as Amr bin Uthman, Ali bin Abdullah Ibn Ab'ass, Abu Salamah bin Abdur-Rahman, Abdur-Rahman bin Al-Aswad, Musa bin Talhah, Az-Zuhri, Ayyub and Isma'il bin M'ad Yakrib. Ibn Al-Jawzi In addition related this opinion to Mu'harib bin Dithar, Yazid, Ibn Jurayj, Abu Yusuf, Abu Is'haq, Ibn Abu Layla, Ziyad bin 'Alaqah, Ghaylan bin Jami', Nafi' bin Jubayr, 'Amr bin 'Ali Al-Muqaddami and Al-Qasim bin Sallam.

5. Karm, which is the grapevine

It is not preferred that one calls the grapevine Karm, as Muslim narrated that the Prophet b said:

"None of you should call the grapevine Karm, for Al-Karm is the Muslim man."

In another narration the Prophet b said:

"The Karm is the beli'ever's heart."

In addition another narration states:

"Do not say (for grapes) Al-Karm, rather say 'Inob (grape), and Hablah (grapevine)."

This Hadith entails two meanings that the Arabs used to call the grapevine Al-Karm because of its tremendous benefits. This is why the Prophet as disliked calling it Karm because this exotic name drives the heart to like it and to later like what it is used to produce: alcohol, which is the mother of all impure things. The Prophet s& disliked calling what is used to produce alcohol with one of the best names.

The second, this Hadith is similar to the Ahadeeth,

"The strong person is not one who overpowers others physically."

And

"The Miskin (poor) is not one who keeps wandering in the land."

In this case, the Hadith (about Al-Karm) means, "You call the grapevine Karm because of its many benefits, while the believing heart or the Muslim person deserves this good name even more, for indeed, the believer is all pure and beneficial." The Hadith then draws the attention to what the believer's heart has of goodness, generosity, faith, enlightenment, guidance, fear from Allah and the rest of the good characteristics because of which the believer deserves the name Karm more than the grapevine.

The grapevine is cool and dry, while its leaves are cool in the first degree. When the grape leaves are crushed and their powder is used as a bandage for headache, they relieve the pain and In addition relieve swelling and stomach infections.

When one drinks the juice of grapevine stems, it will get rid of nausea sensation and will constipate the stomach, and when its hearts are chewed wet, they In addition produce the same benefits. In addition, the extract of grapevine leaves helps relieve stomach ulcers, hemoptysis (spitting up blood), vomit and stomach ache in general.

The sap contained in hanging grapevine stems acts just like gum extracts if one drinks it, as it dissipates stones. Further, when it is used as ointment, it will bring relief to the hearts and will heal the open sores caused by mange, but it is better to wash the affected wound beforehand with water and Natron, When one uses it as an ointment along with oil, it will remove the hair effectively.

The ashes of grapevine stems are In addition used as a bandage, blended with vinegar, rose oil and rue, to relieve spleen swellings. In addition, just as rose oil (or essence), the oil of vine blossoms constipates the stomach and has many other benefits. In general, grapevines have as much benefit as the date tree.

6. Karfas (Celery)

Karfas has a good aroma and when it is hung under the neck, it relieves toothache.

Karfas is hot and dry, and it opens the clogs of the liver and the spleen. Wet celery leaves helps the stomach and the cold liver, causes urine as a diuretic, menstrual flow, and dissolves stones. Celery grains are more effective in this regard. Karfas In addition stimulates semen production and relieves offensive breath. Ar-Razi said, "One should avoid eating it if he fears he might suffer a scorpion sting."

7. Kurrath (Leek)

There are two types of Kurrath, a Nabatean type and a Shami (Syrian) type. People eat the Nabatean type, which is a vegetable, while the Syrian type has many heads. Kurrath is hot and dry and causes headaches. When Kurrath is cooked, one could eat it or drink its water to help against cold hemorrhages. When its seeds are crushed and kneaded with some tar and then applied on decaying teeth, they will cleanse the rotted teeth and will relieve the pain. Further, the smoke of burnt Kurrath seeds helps dry out hemorrhages. All these benefits are for the Nabatean Kurrath.

Yet, the Kurrath is harmful for the teeth and the gums, causes headaches and nightmares and brings darkness to the sight. In addition, it provokes offensive breath, is diuretic, stimulates menstruation flow and semen production, and is not easily digested.

The Letter Lam

1. Lahm (Meat)

Allah said:

﴿ وَأَمْدَدْنَٰهُم بِفَٰكِهَةٍ وَلَحْمٍ مِّمَّا يَشْتَهُونَ ﴿٢٢﴾ ﴾ (٢٢) الطور .

"And We shall provide them with fruit and

meat such as they desire." (52:22)

﴿ وَلَحْمِ طَيْرٍ مِّمَّا يَشْتَهُونَ ۝ ﴾ (٢١) الواقعة .

"And with the flesh of fowls that they desire." (56:21) In the Sahih it is In addition narrated that the Prophet **b** said:

"The virtue of 'A'esha compared to the rest of the women is like the virtue of the Tharid as compared to the rest of the foods." (Tharid means bread and meat).

Az-Zuhri said, "Eating meat brings about strength in seventy different ways." In addition, Muhammad bin Wasi' said, "Eating meat strengthens the sight." In addition, Ali was reported to have said, "Eat meat, because it makes the skin's color lighter, the stomach firmer and the behavior better. "Ibn 'Umar used to eat meat frequently when Ramadan started and when traveling." Finally, All was reported to have said, "Whoever refrains from eating meat for forty days will acquire bad behavior."

There are different types of meat that we will mention, describe briefly and elaborate on their benefit or harm.

Sheep Meat (Mutton)

Mutton is warm in the second degree and wet in the first degree. The best type of mutton comes from the one-year old animal, which generates good blood if digested properly. This type of meat is suitable for those who have hot or cold temperaments and for those who practice sports activity in cold areas and cold weather. It is In addition beneficial for those who suffer from black bile, and it In addition strengthens the mind and the memory. However, the mutton of old, thin animals is not good, as is the ewe's meat.

The best type of mutton is the dark meat of the male animal, for it is lighter, tastier and more beneficial. The mutton of castrated sheep is even better and more beneficial. The red meat of fat sheep is lighter and more nutritious, while the chest of the goat is less nutritious and floats in the stomach.

The best parts of mutton meat are the meat that covers the bones, the right side, which is lighter and tastier than the left side, and the front parts rather than the back parts. The best part of sheep meat to the Prophet **b**, was the front part, which is closer to the head, but not the head itself. The front part is lighter and tastier. Once, Al-Farazdaq gave a man some money to buy meat for him, saying, "Buy the front parts and avoid the head and the intestines, because that is where disease resides."

The meat on the neck is In addition tasty and easy to digest. The meat that covers the arm is the lightest meat, the tastiest, the healthiest and the easiest to digest. In the Sahihain it is narrated that the Messenger of Allah ;§& used to like eating the meat of the sheep arm. Furthermore, the meat on the back of the sheep is nutritious and produces sanitary blood.

Goat Meat

It is cold and dry, and the mixtures that goat meat produces are harmful. Goat meat is not digested easily and is not significant nutrition-wise. The meat of billy goats is not beneficial, because it is rather dry, heavy on the stomach and produces black bile.

Al-Jahith once said, "A skilled doctor once said to me, 'O Abu Uthman! Avoid goat meat because it causes depression, causes black bile, forgettulness, and spoils the blood. By Allah! It In addition drives children wild.'"

Some doctors say that the goat meat that is not preferred is the meat of old goats, especially for old people. They In addition say that goat meat is not bad for whoever is used to eating it.

When the doctors state that goat meat is not beneficial, they specifically mean those who have weak stomachs and those who are not used to eating it, such as the people who live in luxury in cities and who are used to the better types of foods. But this is not the majority.

The meat of young - but not very young - goats is milder, especially when the goat is still nursing. This type of goat meat is digested faster, because it still possesses the strength of its mother's milk. The meat of young goats is In addition milder for most people and lighter than camel meat. In addition, young goat's meat produces moderate blood.

Cow Meat

Cow Meat is cold and dry, heavy on the stomach and produces black, bilious blood that is only suitable for hard workers. Eating cow meat excessively for those who are not used to it causes such black bilious illnesses as vitiligo (a skin condition of unknown cause, characterized by patchy loss of pigment), mange, herpes, leprosy, elephantiasis, cancer, obsession, quartran fever and various tumors. The harm that this meat causes will be neutralized when one eats it with spices, garlic, ginger and cinnamon. The meat of male cows is colder than female cows' meat, which is less dry.

The meat of fat calves is one of the best, mildest and tastiest types of food. It is warm and wet, and if fully digested, it provides good nutrition.

Horse meat

In the Sahih it is narrated that Asma said, "We slaughtered a horse during the time of the Messenger of Allah a§ and ate it." In addition, the Prophet b:

"Allowed eating horsemeat but disallowed eating (domesticated) donkey meat." [Al-Bokhary and Muslim].

The fact that Allah mentioned horses along with mules and donkeys [in the Qura'an] does not indicate that the ruling about their meat is identical. Sometimes Allah mentions several similar things together and sometimes mentions several different things together. What Allah said is:

"For you to ride." (16:8)

This does not indicate that horsemeat is not allowed, just as it does not indicate that one is not allowed to benefit from horses except by riding. Rather, the Ayah only mentioned the best benefit and value that the horse represents, which is its being a means of transportation. Furthermore, the two Ahadeeth we mentioned unequivocally indicate that horsemeat is allowed.

Horsemeat is hot, dry, tough and dark. It is In addition harmful for soft stomachs and bodies.

Camel Meat

The difference between the Shiite and the Sunnis and between the Jews and Muslims is that the Muslims eat camel meat. In addition, the Shiites and the Jews neither praise nor eat camel meat. It is well established in the religion that Muslims are allowed to eat camel meat and that the Messenger of Allah **b** and his Companions used to eat it while traveling and otherwise.

Young camel meat is one of the tastiest and most nutritious types of foods, and those who are used to eating it find it as light and beneficial as sheep meat. Some doctors did not like eating camel meat for residents of the cities because they are not used to it. Camel meat is hot and dry, difficult to digest and begets black bile.

Camel meat has an especially strong effect on the body and this is why the Prophet **b** ordered the Muslims to perform ablution after eating it.* We should state here that it is an erroneous method to alter the meaning of the two correct Ahadeeth on this subject so that 'ablution' only means washing the hands, thus altering the true meaning of the word. In addition, the Prophet **b** made a distinction between eating camel meat and sheep meat, as he gave the choice to Muslims if they want to perform ablution after eating sheep meat. Meanwhile, the Prophet m, commanded the Muslims to perform ablution after eating camel meat. If ablution in these Ahadeeth was held to mean just washing the hands, it should In addition apply to what the Prophet b said:

"Whoever touched his sexual organ is obliged to perform ablution."

Furthermore, those who eat camel meat might not touch the meat with their hands. So if 'ablution' in this case means just washing the hands, it would be a senseless act and would alter the true meanings desired by the Ahadeeth. In addition, claiming that the Hadith which states,

"The last ruling that the Prophet b chose is that he abandoned performing ablution from eating what is cooked by fire," includes camel meat is not correct.

First, this Hadith carries a general meaning, while the Hadith about camel meat is specific.

Second, the two Ahadeeth are not talking about the same subject. For instance, one should perform ablution even if he eats dried, cooked or uncooked camel meat. Using fire does not have a bearing on the ruling about camel meat. As for abandoning performing ablution after eating what is cooked by fire, it only indicates that using fire does not require ablution. Therefore, there is a difference between the two Ahadeeth, as one of them orders the Muslims to perform ablution after eating camel meat while the other indicates that performing ablution is not required after eating the food that was cooked by fire.

Third, the Hadith about the Prophet ^ abandoning performing ablution after eating the food that was cooked on fire came after the Prophet **b** had performed ablution from eating such meat earlier. The Hadith states that the Prophet SB was once brought meat and that he ate from it and then performed ablution and prayed. Later on, he was brought meat and he ate from it and then prayed without performing ablution. The Hadith states, the last ruling on this matter is that it is not necessary to perform ablution after eating what was cooked by fire. So there are two rulings regarding the same subject [eating what was touched by fire], one came earlier than the second ruling. Some of the narrators of the Hadith only mentioned the latter incident to make the story short. Therefore, how can anyone use this Hadith to prove that it overrules performing ablution from eating camel meat (when the earlier Hadith that was overruled talks about another subject)? Even if the Ahadeeth in general allow not performing ablution after eating what was cooked on fire, the specific Hadith still stands because it entails a specific ruling [concerning camel meat].

D'abb Meat

We stated before that eating D'abb meat is allowed. This type of meat is hot and dry and excites the sexual drive.

Gazelle meat

Gazelle meat is the best among the meats of wild game. It is hot and dry and beneficial for the healthy body, especially the fawn's meat.

Antelope Meat

Antelope meat is hot and dry in the first degree, dehydrates the body and is beneficial for the humid bodied.

The author of the 'Qanoon' said, "The best type of game meat is the antelope's, although it tends to cause black bile."

Rabbit Meat

Rabbit meat was mentioned in the Sahihain, as Anas said, "We hunted a rabbit after pursuing it for a while. Afterwards, Abu Talhah sent its hip to the Messenger of Allah b who accepted it."

Rabbit meat is mildly hot and dry, and the best

part of it is the hip. The best way to eat rabbit meat is by roasting it. Rabbit meat constipates, produces urine, as a diuretic, and dissolves stones. Eating the rabbit's head benefits against convulsive shaking.

Zebra meat

In the Sahihain it is narrated that Abu Qatadah said that the Companions were once with the Messenger of Allah **b** during an Umrah trip and that he hunted a zebra and the Prophet **b** told them to eat it. They were assuming the state of Ihram then, unlike Abu Qatadah.

Ibn Majah In addition narrated that Jabir 'a <iii ^ said, "During the battle of Khaibar, we ate horsemeat and zebra meat."

Zebra meat is hot and dry, nutritious and produces thick, bilious blood. Its fat is beneficial when mixed with Qust oil to treat toothache and flatulence that weakens the kidneys. Further, when its grease is applied on spots, it will heal them.

In general, all types of wild-game meat produce thick, bilious blood. In addition, the best type of wild—game meat is gazelle then **rabbit meat.**

The meat of animal fetuses is not preferred because the blood is still trapped in it. However, it is still allowed, for the Prophet s, said:

"Slaughtering the fetus is included in slaughtering its mother."

The scholars of Iraq do not allow eating fetus's meat except if one kills it before it dies. They altered the meaning of the last Hadith saying that the fetus should be slaughtered as its mother was slaughtered according to the Hadith, as they claimed.

However, this claim is false. The Hadith states that the Prophet s& was asked, "O Messenger of Allah b . We slaughter a sheep and sometimes find a fetus still in its womb, should we eat it?" The Prophet b, said, "Eat it if you wish, because slaughtering it is included in slaughtering its mother."

In addition, when one studies this matter further, his analysis will In addition demonstrate that it is allowed to eat animal fetuses. The fetus is still a part of the mother, and since slaughtering the mother allows us to eat all of its parts, then the fetus should be included, as well. This is the meaning that the Prophet b meant when he said:

"Slaughtering it is included in slaughtering its mother."

If the authentic Sunnah had not specifically allowed eating the fetus, the correct mind would still guide us that it is allowed.

Eating Dried (Jerked) Meat

It the Sunan **it** is narrated that Thawban said, "I slaughtered a sheep for the Messenger of Allah **b** while we were traveling, and he said to me:

"Dry its meat."

I kept feeding the Prophet as from its meat until we reached Al-Medina."

Dried meat is better than old meat and strengthens the body, although it causes skin rashes sometimes, a side effect that could be neutralized with cold, humid spices. In addition, jerked meat is favorable for hot conditions. Old meat is hot and dry, favorable for hot conditions and the best type of this meat is that which is fat and wet. Finally, old meat constipates unless cooked in milk and grease. Fowl meat

Allah said:

﴿ وَلَحْمِ طَيْرٍ مِّمَّا يَشْتَهُونَ ﴾ (٢١) الواقعة .

"And with the flesh of fowls that they desire." (56:21)

Some types of fowl meats are allowed and some are prohibited. The prohibited types include the birds that have claws, such as the falcon, hawk and peregrine, and those that eat carrion, such as the eagle, vulture, stork, magpie, spotted and black crows. In addition, this list includes the birds that we are not allowed to kill, such as the hoopoe and the shrike, and some of the birds that we are allowed to kill, such as kite and crow.

There are many types of fowl that are allowed, such as chicken meat. In the Sahihain it is narrated by Abu Musa that the Prophet ^ ate chicken meat.

Chicken Meat

Chicken meat is hot and dry in the first degree and it is easy on the stomach and digests quickly. Chicken meat strengthens the mind and increases the production of semen. It a so makes the voice softer, the mind stronger and produces healthy blood. It was said that eating chicken meat on a regular basis causes gout, but this is not confirmed by fact.

The cock' meat, on the other hand, is hotter and less wet. The meat of old cocks helps against constipation, asthma and thick flatulence when cooked with safflower, canella and chabt (Shibit). The castrated cock' meat is nutritious and easy to digest. Pullet meat is easy to digest and mild on the stomach and produces mild blood.

Francolin Meat

Francolin meat is hot and dry in the second degree, soft and light, easy to digest and produces mild blood. Eating this type of meat In addition strengthens the sight.

Partridge meat

This type of meat produces good blood and is easily digested.

Goose Meat

Goose meat is hot and dry and is not healthy if eaten on a regular basis, and it does not produce extensive excrement.

Duck Meat

Duck meat is hot and wet, and it is not suitable for the stomach, difficult to digest and produces excessive excrements.

Bustard Meat

Bustard meat is hot and dry, heavy on the stomach but good for those who perform sports activities and for hard workers.

Crane Meat

This type of meat is dry and light. It produces bilious blood, and it is good for hard workers. It is better to eat the crane's meat one or two days after it is slaughtered.

Bird and Lark Meat

An-Nas'ay narrated in his Sunnan that Abdullah bin Umar said that the Prophet b said:

"No person kills a bird and a larger animal without justification, but will be asked about it on the Day of Resurrection. He was asked, 'O Messenger of Allah! When is it justified?' He said, 'You slaughter it and eat it, but do not cut its head and discard its body (i.e. for sport only).'"

In addition, An-Nas'ay narrated that the Messenger of Allah b said:

"Whoever kills a bird for fun, the bird will complain to Allah, 'O my Lord, Such and such person killed me for fun, not for a useful purpose.'"

Bird meat is hot and dry, constipates and stimulates semen production. Bird meat soup constipates and helps the joints. If one eats birds' brain with ginger and •nion, it excites the sexual desire. The mixtures that bird's produce is not favorable.

Pigeon Meat

Pigeon meat is hot and wet, although the meat of wild pigeons is less wet. The meat of pigeon chicks is more humid, especially the chicks of domesticated pigeons. Young pigeons are less meaty but a better food. The meat of male pigeons is a good cure for numbness, narcosis, apoplexy and convulsive shaking or trembles. Pigeon chick meat is favorable for the sexual drive and the kidneys and produces more blood.

Sand Grouse Meat

This type of meat is dry and causes black bile and constipation. It is not a good food, except that it helps cure dropsy.

Quail Meat

Quail meat is hot and dry and helps the joints. It harms the hot kidney unless it is taken with vinegar and coriander. Eating the meat of the quails that live in filthy areas should be avoided.

Fowl meats are all more easily digested than cattle

meat. The parts of the birds that are the most easily digested are the necks and the wings. In addition, the brains of the fowls are a better food than cattle brains,

Locust Meat

In the Sahihain it is narrated that Abdullah bin Abi Awfa said, "We went to seven battles with the Messenger of Allah during which we used to eat locust." The Musnad In addition narrated that the Messenger of Allah said:

"We were allowed two types of dead animals and two bloods: fish and locust; liver and spleen."

This Hadith is In addition related from Ibn 'Umar .

Locust meat is hot and dry and not very nutritious. In addition, eating locust meat regularly makes the body thin, emaciated. The smoke of burnt locust helps in cases of dysuria (impaired ability to pass urine), especially for women, and is favorable for hemorrhoids. Eating fat wingless locust roasted is a good cure for scorpion stings. In addition, locust meat is not favorable for those suffering from epilepsy and produces septic mixtures in the stomach.

There is a difference on allowing eating locust when it is dead, where the majority of the scholars except Malik allow it. Yet, there is no difference that it is allowed if the locust died because of a reason, such as being burnt or pressed.

It is not good for the health to eat meat on a regular basis because it causes bloody sanguineous illnesses and various types of allergies, Hippocrates once said, "Do not turn your stomachs to a graveyard for animals."

2. Laban (Milk)

Allah said:

﴿ وَإِنَّ لَكُمْ فِي ٱلْأَنْعَٰمِ لَعِبْرَةً نُّسْقِيكُم مِّمَّا فِي بُطُونِهِۦ مِنۢ بَيْنِ فَرْثٍ وَدَمٍ لَّبَنًا خَالِصًا سَآئِغًا لِّلشَّٰرِبِينَ ﴿٦٦﴾ ﴾ (٦٦) النحل .

"And verily, in the cattle, there is a lesson for you. We give you to drink of that which is in their bellies, from between excretions and blood, pure milk; palatable to the drinkers." (16:66)

In addition Allah said, while describing Paradise:

﴿ مَّثَلُ ٱلْجَنَّةِ ٱلَّتِى وُعِدَ ٱلْمُتَّقُونَ ۖ فِيهَآ أَنْهَٰرٌ مِّن مَّآءٍ غَيْرِ ءَاسِنٍ وَأَنْهَٰرٌ
مِّن لَّبَنٍ لَّمْ يَتَغَيَّرْ طَعْمُهُۥ وَأَنْهَٰرٌ مِّنْ خَمْرٍ لَّذَّةٍ لِّلشَّٰرِبِينَ وَأَنْهَٰرٌ مِّنْ
عَسَلٍ مُّصَفًّى ۖ وَلَهُمْ فِيهَا مِن كُلِّ ٱلثَّمَرَٰتِ وَمَغْفِرَةٌ مِّن رَّبِّهِمْ ۖ كَمَنْ
هُوَ خَٰلِدٌ فِى ٱلنَّارِ وَسُقُوا۟ مَآءً حَمِيمًا فَقَطَّعَ أَمْعَآءَهُمْ ﴿١٥﴾ ﴾

(١٥) محمد .

"In it are rivers of water the taste and smell of which are not changed, rivers of milk of which the taste never changes." (47:15)

In the Sunan it is In addition narrated:

\"Whoever Allah gives some type of food, let him supplicate. 'O Allah! Bless it for us and grant us what is better.' Whoever Allah grants some Laban, let him say. 'O Allah! Bless it for us and grant us more of it,' for I do not know of a more complete food or drink than milk.'"

Although milk is a simple type of food, it is very natural to the body as it contains three major substances: cheese, fat and water. Cheese is cold and wet and provides good nutrition. The fat contained in the milk is mild regarding warmth and wetness, and it very beneficial for healthy bodies.

The water part contained in milk is hot and wet, and it softens the stomach and provides the body with beneficial moistures. Laban in general is mild regarding warmth and wetness, although there are other opinions in this regard.

Milk is best when it has just been milked, and its value decreases by the passage of time thereafter. When it is freshly milked, milk is less cold and more humid. Sour milk is the opposite. In addition, milk is better forty days after the animal has given birth. The best type of milk is the most white in color, as it has a good scent, delicious taste, mildly sweet, less fat and light consistency. It is In addition best when young healthy animals are milked, especially those that have less meat and which graze in healthy grazing lands. Milk is good and produces red blood, brings wetness to the body and is In addition a nutritious food. In addition, milk helps relieve depression, obsession and black bile ailments. When milk is drunk with honey, it will help cleanse the insides of septic materials. Drinking milk with sugar makes the color of the skin fairer. Milk helps the body regain its strength after sexual intercourse and is In addition favorable for the chest, the lungs and for those suffering from tuberculosis,

Further, milk is not favorable for the head, the stomach, the liver and the spleen. In addition, drinking milk excessively is harmful for the teeth and the gums, and this is why it is better to rinse the mouth after one drinks it. In the Sahihain it is narrated that the Prophet b once drank some milk and then asked for some water and rinsed his mouth, saying: "It has fat."

Milk is not good for those suffering from fever and headaches and is not favorable for the weakness in the head and the brain. Excessive drinking of milk causes darkness in the sight, sight impairment, gout, kidney clogs and swelling in the stomach and the intestines. These side effects will be neutralized when mixing milk with honey, ginger, and so forth, for those who are not used to drinking it.

Sheep Milk

Sheep milk is the most watery, and it has more fat and bad odor than goat or cow milk. Sheep milk produces phlegm and causes white spots or stains on the skin if one drinks it on a regular basis. This is why it is better that sheep milk is mixed with water so that its concentration becomes less. Sheep milk quenches the thirst quicker and cools the body faster than other milks.

Goat Milk

Goat milk is mild and light, works as a mild laxative, is wet for dry bodies and helps cure mouth cankers, dry cough and epistaxis (nosebleeds).

Milk in general is the most beneficial drink for the body due to its nutritional value and closeness to the nature of the body and to the childhood of mankind. In the Sahihain it is narrated;

"The night of the Isr'aa" (the Prophet's journey from Mecca to Jerusalem and then to heaven), the Messenger of Allah **b** was given two cups, one containing milk and the other wine. The Prophet is, looked at them and then took the cup of milk. Gabriel said, 'You have accepted what is natural, (True Religion i.e. Islam) and if you had taken the wine, your followers would have gone astray.'"

Sour goat milk is not digested quickly and produces unfavorable mixtures. The hot tempered stomach benefits from goat milk, though, and easily digests it.

Cow Milk

Cow milk provides nutrition for the body and is In addition a mild laxative. Cow milk is one of the best milks, between sheep milk and goat milk regarding thickness and fat.

'Abdullah bin Mas'ud narrated that the Prophet **b** once said:

"Drink cow milk because it grazes on all types of trees."

Camel Milk

We mentioned camel milk in the beginning of the chapter, so there is no need to repeat it.

3. Lubon (Frankincense), which is the Kundur:

It was reported that once a man complained to 'Ali ^ AI ^ that he forgets and that 'Ali said to him, "Resort to the Luban, because it strengthens the heart and does away with forgetfulness."

In addition, it was reported that Ibn Ab'ass said, "Drinking Luban with sugar on an empty stomach is favorable for the urine and helps against forgetfulness." In addition, it was reported that Anas said to a man who complained to him of forgetfulness, "Resort to Kundur! Soak it overnight and in the morning take a sip of it on an empty stomach, because it is good against forgetfulness."

There is an apparent reason for this benefit.

Forgetfulness is the result of cold, humid, bad moods that affect the brain in a way that makes the brain not recall the memory easily. In this case, Luban helps. When forgetfulness is a result of other physical causes, refreshing drinks help in that case. The difference between the two cases is that dry substances help one stay up at night and recall old memories rather than current memories. The wet drinks have the opposite effect.

Sometimes forgetfulness occurs because of cupping on the back of the head and excessive eating of wet coriander and sour apples. In addition, depression, sadness, looking at stagnant water for a long time and urinating in it might cause forgetfulness. In addition, looking at crucified people, reading grave commemorations, walking between two tarred camels, eating mice wastes by mistake, all cause forgetfulness.

Luban is hot in the second degree and dry in the first degree. It is In addition a mild constipation agent. It is very beneficial and its side effects are minimal. Among the benefits of the Luban is that it stops and heals bleeding, stomach ache, diarrhea, helps digest the food, gets rid of flatulence, cures eye sores, helps the body grow flesh on most ulcers and strengthens the weak stomach. Luban In addition dries the phlegm and the moistures accumulating in the chest, cures eyesight impairment and prevents malignant sores from progressing.

When Luban is chewed alone or mixed with Persian thyme, it will provoke phlegm, release and relax the tongue muscles and help the mind become sharper. When the Luban is burnt, it helps cure some illnesses and makes the air smell fresh.

The Letter Mim

1. M'aa(Water)

M'aa (Water), is the resource of life, the best drink there is, and one of the pillars of existence. Rather it is the most important pillar of life, as Allah has created every living thing from water.

There is a difference of opinion if water is a source of nutrition for the body, or if it only helps wash down and dissolve the food. Water is a wet, cold substance that removes heat, preserves the body's moisture, restores the moisture that the body has lost, makes the food softer and helps carry it through the blood vessels.

There are ten standards with which we test water's freshness. First, its color should be crystal clear. Second, water should not have any odor at all, Third, water should be sweet and fresh just as the water of the Nile and the

Euphrates. Fourth, water should be light. Fifth, water sources should be pure and not stagnant. Sixth, water is fresher when its source is deeper or farther. Seventh, water should be exposed to the wind and the sun, not hidden under the earth. Eighth, water sources should not be stagnant and should be fast running. Ninth, water should be plentiful which helps purify whatever impurities it might carry. Tenth, water source should be running north to south or west to east.

When all these characteristics are sought together, they will all be found in four rivers, the Nile, the Euphrates, Say'han (or Sayhoun) and Jay'han (or Jayhoun). In the Sahihain it is narrated that Abu Hurayrah related from the Prophet b that he said:

"Sayhan. jayhun, the Nile and the Euphrates are all among the rivers of Paradise."

As for the water being light, there are three methods to verify it. First, water should easily absorb the cold and the heat. Hippocrates said, "The water that becomes hot or cold easily is the lightest water." Second; by weight. Third, when one wets two pieces of cotton, which are exactly the same weight, with water from two different sources, and then both pieces are dried and weighed. The one that has the lightest weight indicates the water it absorbed was the lightest, The environment that the water passes through has a profound effect on the water. For instance, water sources that are located to the north are generally cooler and their water is generally thicker due to the northern wind. In addition, the water that passes through mineral rich rocks is affected by this fact.

Fresh water is beneficial for both the ill and the healthy. Cool or chilled water is the most beneficial and has the best taste. Yet, one should not drink water soon after he wakes up, after sex, taking a bath or eating fruit. There is no harm if one drinks water while eating, but not excessively. Feather, having a few sips of water in this case is better and does not harm the stomach but strengthens it, excites the sexual drive and quenches the thirst.

Warm water, on the other hand, swells the stomach and causes the opposite effects that we mentioned regarding cold water. Old warm water is better than fresh warm water.

Cold water is better than warm water inside the body, as it cleanses the blood and clears the head. In addition, cold water removes rot and is mild and favorable for the teeth, the mood and hot weather. Yet, cold water is not good for those suffering from colds or swelling, since such cases need heat to decompose. Very cold water harms the teeth and drinking it on a regular basis could cause bronchitis and chest pains.

Very hot and very cold waters are very harmful to the nerves and most of the limbs and body organs. One of them decomposes (hot water), while the other concentrates moistures. Warm water relieves hot mixtures, decomposes, matures and extracts excrement and brings wetness and hotness, but does not help the digestion as the food then floats up close to the upper side of the stomach. Warm water In addition does not quench the thirst quickly, weakens the body and causes many harmful illnesses. Yet, warm water is good for old people and those suffering from epilepsy, cold headaches and ophthalmia (inflammation of the eye).

There are no Hadith about sun heated water, nor did any of the renowned doctors of old discourage drinking it. Yet, very hot water dissolves the fat around the kidneys.

We talked about rainwater when we talked about the letter Ghayn.

Water contained in ice and hail.

In the Sahihain it is narrated that the Prophet **b** used to say the following supplication after starting the prayer:

"O Allah! Wash my sins with water (rain), snow and hail." Snow is accumulated due to the moisture in the air. We mentioned the wisdom in asking Allah to wash the sins with snow, as the heart needs the coolness and its strength. We stated before the subject of curing the ills of the heart and treating them with their opposites and neutralizers.

Hail water is sweeter than snow water, while the quality of melted ice water depends on its source.

We should mention that the quality of the snow is affected by the area and the mountains that it falls on.

One should avoid drinking icy water after taking a bath, having sex, sports activity, eating hot foods, when coughing and having chest pains, weak liver and cool tempers.

Water from wells and ground water Well water is not favorable, while underground water is heavy. This is because the first one (well water) rarely escapes rot, while underground water is not exposed to fresh air. Hence, one should not drink such types of water until exposing the water to air for at least a night. The worst type of well or underground water is that which runs through lead-rich stones and unused wells, especially if its soil is not good.

Zamzam Water

Zamzam water is the best, freshest, most beneficial, most beloved and most precious water there is. Further, Zamzam water was dug up by Jibril and the source that Prophet Isma'il ,^LJI ^ drank from.

In the Sahihain it is narrated that the Prophet ^ said to Abu Tharr, who remained at the Ka'bah for forty days without food (or drink) living on Zamzam water: "It is a nutritious food." Muslim added that the Prophet **b** said:

"And a cure from ailment."

Furthermore, Ibn Majah narrated that Jabir bin 'Abdullah related from the Prophet **b** that he said:

"Zamzam water is for whatever was intended behind drinking it."

We were told that Abdullah bin Al-Mubarak once said, "O Allah! Ibn Al-Mu'ammil told us that Muhammad bin Al-Munkadir related from Jabir that your Prophet **b** said:

"The water of Zamzam is for the purpose it is drank for, and I drink it to relieve my thirst on the Day of Resurrection."

This Hadith is of the Hasan (Sound) type.

Many other people and I have tried drinking from Zamzam water for the purpose of being cured from various illnesses, and by the will of Allah, I was indeed cured from several illnesses. I In addition saw some people who lived on Zamzam water for a long time, fifteen days or a little longer without complaining from hunger. Such people would perform Jawaf with other people at a normal pace. Someone even told me that Zamzam water was his only food and drink for forty days and that he still had enough strength to have sex with his wife, fast and perform Jawaf many times.

The Nile

The Nile is one of the rivers of Paradise that flows from deep inside Ethiopia. It is collected from the rainfall and the floods that supply it with water. Then, Allah directs this river that flows with water to dry areas, causing the vegetation, on which people and animals live, to grow and flourish.

The land that the river flows to is dry and does not keep rainwater that falls on it, which is insufficient to grow vegetation anyway. On the other hand, when such a land receives more than the normal rainfall, the houses and life will be destroyed. Allah has caused the rain to fall on far lands and then directed this rain to flow in a huge river in sufficient amounts that would benefit the people and the animals. When the river provides enough water for farming and to grow vegetation, the water level then decreases so that the people are able to tend and harvest the vegetation, The water of the Nile has the ten characteristics that we mentioned before, and this is why it is among the lightest, sweetest and freshest waters.

Seawater

The Prophet **b** said about the sea:

"Its water is pure and its dead is allowed (to eat)."

Allah has made the sea salty for the benefit of the people and the animals of the earth. Seawater is plentiful and has sufficient amounts of animals [and fish] that die but do not get buried in it. If the seawater is fresh and sweet, the animals that would die in it would make it rotten, adversely affecting the quality of the air on the earth. Allah's wisdom has decided that seawater is salty, that even if the entire dead corpses produced on the earth were thrown in it, it would still be fresh until Allah brings this world to its inevitable end. This is one of the reasons why seawater is salty, along with its soil and sand In addition being salty.

Taking a bath ın seawater helps relieve many illnesses and infections that appear on the skin. Drinking seawater is harmful, it causes diarrhea, weakens the body and causes rashes, mange and thirst.

Those who have to drink seawater do so for certain medicinal purposes. In this case, seawater should be boiled in a pot that is covered by wool, which will absorb the water vapor. Then, the collected water should be squeezed out of the wool and consumed when there is sufficient amount of it. Meanwhile, the salt and the minerals will remain in the pot.

In addition, one could dig a hole near the seashore to collect the water through several parallel tunnels that would make the water fresh at the end [when it passes through them repeatedly].

If one has to drink seawater, he should first mix it with apricot pips, burning coal, Armenian argil (type of earth), oak wood or fine wheat flour. This way, most of the minerals and mud will be collected in the bottom of the pot or the cup.

2. Misk (Musk)

Muslim narrated that Abu Sa'id Al-Khudri said that the Prophet b said:

"The best type of perfume is Musk."

In the Sahihain it is In addition narrated that A'esha said, "I used to anoint the Prophet s& with perfumed Musk before assuming Ihram, on the Day of the Sacrifice and before performing Tawaf around the (Sacred) House."

Musk is the king of all perfumes, it has the best aroma. Other types of perfumes are usually compared to Musk, but Misk is never compared to them. In addition, the hills and sands of Paradise are made of Musk.

Musk is a hot, dry substance of the second degree, and it brings comfort and joy to the hearts and strengthens the inner organs when it is drunk or smelled. Musk In addition brings strength and comfort to the external organs when anointed with it. Musk is profitable for old people and those who have excessive skin moistures, especially during winter, and In addition helps against fainting, shaking and the general weakness in the body as it excites the instinctive heat. Musk clears the white part in the eye and dries excess moisture in it, and In addition dissipates swelling in various organs. Musk In addition works as an antidote for some poisons, and helps against snakebite. It has many other benefits.

3. (Marjoram)

It is hot in the third degree and dry in the second degree, and when its aroma is smelled, it relieves cold headache caused by phlegm, colds, black bile and thick flatulence pressure. It In addition relieves the congestion, and clogs in the nose and head and dissipates most cold, wet swellings.

When Marjoram is used as suppository, it will increase the blood flow during menstruation and is favorable during pregnancies. When its dry leaves are crushed and used as a bandage, it will relieve blood traces that appear under the eye. It In addition helps relieve the pain of scorpion stings when it is mixed with vinegar [and then the affected area is bandaged with it].

Marjoram ointment In addition helps relieve backache, knee pain and fatigue. Those who are used to smelling Marjoram aroma will not suffer from water accumulation in the eye, cataract. When one administers its extract or water blended with the essence of bitter almonds in the nose, and helps against stuffiness that affects the nose and the head.

4. Malh (Salt)

Al-Bazzar narrated that the Prophet Marjoram said:

"You will soon be to the people just like what the salt represents to food, and the food's flavor doesn't become favorable unless there is salt in it."

Al-Baghawi said in his commentary on the Qura'an that Abdullah bin "Umar related from the Prophet Marjoram that he said, "There are four blessings that Allah has sent down to the earth from the heavens:

iron, fire, water and salt." This Hadith should only be related from Ibn 'Umar.

Salt is favorable for people's bodies and food. Further, salt is favorable and beneficial when blended with any substance, including gold and silver, as it makes gold more yellowish and whitens silver. Salt decomposes, cleanses, dries the thick humidity, strengthens and purifies the body and helps against open mangy sores.

When used as eyeliner salt, especially gem salt, will remove the excess fat or flesh "and the yellowish color from the eye. Salt In addition prevents malignant infections from spreading, works as a laxative and helps against pleurisy when the stomach is anointed with it. Salt cleanses the teeth, prevents them from decaying, and strengthens the gums and makes them firm. There are many other benefits for the salt.

The Letter Noon

1. The Nakhl (Date Palm)

The date palm is mentioned in the Qura'an in several places. In the Sahihain it is narrated that Ibn 'Umar said, "We were with the Prophet b and a spadix of date-palm was brought to him. On that he said, 'Among the trees, there is a tree which resembles the Muslim.' I wanted to say that it was the date-palm tree but as I was the youngest of all (of them) I kept quiet. And then the Prophet sg said, 'It is the date-palm tree.' I mentioned what happened to 'Umar and he said, 'Had you said it that would have been better to me than such and such."

This Hadith contains many benefits, such as the scholar training his students by asking them questions and testing their knowledge. It In addition contains parables and demonstrates the shyness of the Prophet's companions, the leaders and the commoners among them, as they all kept quite and were shy to answer the Prophet's question. The Hadith In addition demonstrates that the parent would be happy if his child does something right. The Hadith In addition demonstrates that it is allowed for the children to answer questions in the presence of their parents, even if the father did not know the answer, as this does not constitute misbehaving with the father. In addition, this Hadith compares the Muslim with the Nakhlah, the date palm, because of its tremendous benefit, constant shade and sweet fruit that it produces throughout the year.

Dates are eaten fresh, dried, ripe and unripe and are both a type of food and a cure. Dates are nutritious, a type of sweet, a drink and a fruit. The date-tree's trunk is used for building purposes, in making pots, and so forth and its leaves are used to make woven mats, baskets, vases and funnels, and so forth. Its fibers are used to make ropes and mattresses. In addition, its stones are used as fodder for camels and as ingredients in various medicinal remedies and in Ku'hl. In addition, the fruit of the date-tree is known for its beauty, refreshing shape, and the handsome way the fruits are arranged on their branches, which In addition brings comfort to the eye.

Merely looking at the fruits of the date tree reminds one of its Creator, Whose creation is both excellent and perfect, just as is His Wisdom. Therefore the date tree resembles the righteous believer, for he is pure goodness who brings about benefit both inwardly and outwardly.

In addition, the Nakhah was the tree trunk that

yearned and longed for the Messenger of Allah b when he no longer used it as a podium. The trunk yearned for the Prophet's closeness and for hearing his speech!

In addition, we should mention that the tree that Mary took refuge under when she gave birth to Jesus was the date palm.

There is a difference of opinion regarding which is better the date-tree or the (vine tree). Allah has mentioned both trees together in several Ayat (Verses) in His Book (the Qura'an), In addition, both trees are truly similar to each other, although each is at its prime in its natural habitat and the land that accepts it the most.

2. *Narjis* (Narcissus)

The Narjis is hot and dry in the second degree and its stems are used to relieve deep cankers that reach the nerves. In addition, Narjis cleanses and extracts septic substances. If the Narjis is cooked and one drinks its water, or boils it and eats it, it will cause vomiting and will extract the moistures that reside in the bottom of the stomach. When the Narjis is cooked with lentil plant and honey, it will cleanse the cankers from septic excretions and will cause the gastric ulcers to rupture.

Narjis blossoms are mild and beneficial against colds. They have a strong power of decomposition, open the nose and cerebral clogs, and help against headaches and black bile. Those who repeatedly smell Narjis during winter will have immunity form pleurisy during summer. In addition, Narjis helps relieve headaches caused by phlegm and black bile. Narjis aroma sharpens the mind and the heart and helps relieve many of their ailments. The author of At-Taysir once said, "Inhaling Narjis aroma heals against the epilepsy that attacks boys."

3. Noorah (slaked lime)

It is two parts lime and one part arsenic mixed with water and left to dry in the sun until it turns blue. Then one uses it as ointment and waits an hour until it starts its effect before touching water. Then one takes a bath and anoints himself with henna to remove the lime's hotness.

4. Nabq or Nabiq

It has several names: Nabq, Christ's thorn, lotus jujube, or rhamnus. Abu Nu'aym mentioned these in his book on Prophetic medicine, when he mentioned the Hadith,"When Adam was sent down to earth, the first of its fruits he ate was Nabiq."

In addition, the Messenger of Allah **b** mentioned the Nabq in a Hadith narrated by the Two Muhaddithain,

"On the night that I was token on the Night journey, I was shown Sidrat Al-Muntaha (a tree in the seventh heaven) and I saw its Nabq fruits which resembled the clay jugs of Hajr (a town in Arabia)"

Nabq is the fruit produced by the lote-tree. Nabq soothes the natural digestive process, helps against diarrhea, coats the stomach, relieves bile, provides nutrition for the body, taste to the food and causes phlegm. It In addition helps against inflammation caused by bile. Nobq is slowly digested while its flour strengthens the bowls and is favorable for bilious temperaments. The harm of the Nobq will be neutralized when eating honeycomb with it.

There is a conflict of opinion concerning if Nabq is wet or dry. The correct opinion is that wet Nabq is cold and wet while dry Nabq is cold and dry.

The Letter H'aa

Hindaba (Chicory)

Hindaba temperament changes according to the season. It is cold and wet in winter, hot and dry in summer and mild in spring and autumn. In general, Hindaba is cold and dry. Hindaba is beneficial and cools the stomach and causes constipation. When Hindaba, especially wild Hindaba, is cooked and eaten with vinegar, it constipates even more and is more favorable for the stomach and invigorating.

When Hindaba (chicory) is used as a bandage, it will relieve gastric inflammations, gout and hot ocular inflammations. In cases of scorpion stings, Hindaba helps when its leaves and stems are used as a bandage.

Hindaba In addition strengthens the stomach and opens the clogs in the kidneys, spleen, veins and intestines. It In addition clears and purifies the kidneys and helps them against the various hot and cold aches.

The sour Hindaba is the best for the liver, while its extract helps against icter (jaundice), especially when mixed with wet fennel extract. When Hindaba leaves are bruised and placed on hot swellings, it will cool and dissipate them. Hindaba In addition cleanses and clears the chest and dissipates the heat of irritated blood and bile.

The best way to eat Hindaba is without washing it so as to preserve

its effective ingredients. Hindaba works as an effective antidote against most poisons.

When Hindaba extract is used as eyeliner, it will clear and cleanse the eyes. Hindaba leaves are used in antidotes against scorpion stings, and against most poisons as we have stated. When the Hindaba is squeezed and its water is mixed with oil, it will help against all toxic substances in general. When Hindaba stems are squeezed and their water drunk, it will help against scorpion and hornet stings and against snakebite. Finally, the sap of its stems whitens the white area in the eye.

The Letter Waw

1. *Warss* (Ceylon Cornel tree)

Umm Salamah narrated, "The woman who has just delivered would remain for forty days afterwards [without praying or fasting]. One of us would then overlay Warss on her face to help against spots." Abu Hanifah, a linguist, said, "Warss does not grow in the wild.

Rather, it is cultivated. I think that it is only grown in the Arab lands, especially in Yemen."

Warss is dry and hot in the second degree. The best type of Warss is the red Warss, which is soft in the hand and does not have much bran. Warss is used as an ointment to treat spots, rashes and pimples that appear on the surface of the skin. Warss constipates, has a dyeing qual'ty and helps against leprosy when taken as a drink.

Warss has similar benefits to sea Qust, and if it is used as an ointment it relieves vitiligo (skin condition of unknown cause, characterized by patchy loss of pigment), rashes, pimples and ulcers. When the clothes are dyed with Warss, they strengthen the sexual drive.

2. Wasmah (Woad)

Wasmah is similar to the Nile's leaves and it is used to dye the hair black. We mentioned the subject of dying the hair black before.

The letter Yaa

Yaqtin (Gourd)

Yaqtin means gourd or pumpkin, although the word Yaqtin entails more meanings than these two. Yaqtin in Arabic entails every tree that does not have a stem, such as watermelon and cucumbers. Allah said:

﴿ وَأَنۢبَتۡنَا عَلَيۡهِ شَجَرَةٗ مِّن يَقۡطِينٖ ﴿١٤٦﴾ ﴾ (١٤٦) الصافات .

"And We caused a plant of gourd to grow over him." (37:146)

If someone says that the word tree means every plant that has a stem or a trunk and that which does not have a stem or a trunk is called Najm, not a tree. Hence, why did Allah say,

﴿ وَأَنۢبَتۡنَا عَلَيۡهِ شَجَرَةً مِّن يَقۡطِينٖ ﴾ (١٤٦) الصافات .

"A plant of gourd to grow over him." (37:146)

We answer this question by stating that the word 'tree' describes the plants that have stems in general. Yet sometimes, this word is meant to describe something specific [to describe Yaqtin for instance]. Understanding the areas where the texts speak in general terms and the areas where a specific meaning is meant is a great door to understanding the Arabic Language. The Yaqtin mentioned in the Qura'an is the pumpkin, which is In addition called Dubbaa, Qpr and Yaqtin.

In the Sahihain it is narrated by Anas bin Malik that a tailor once invited the Messenger of Allah **b**to eat from some food that he made. Anas went with the Messenger of Allah **b** and the tailor brought forth some bread made from barley and some soup that had Dubbaa and dried meat. I saw the Messenger of Allah **b** follow the traces of the Dubbaa all around the edge of the pot, which made me love Dubbaa ever since that day."

Abu Talut In addition said, "I entered upon Anas bin Malik while he was eating Dubbaa and saying [referring to the Yaqtin tree], 'You are a tree that is so dear to me because the Messenger of Allah b used to like eating you.'"

Yaqtin is a type of cold and wet plant and a light food that is easily digested. If the gourd was not spoiled in the stomach before being completely digested, it produces a good mixture in the stomach, especially when one eats similar or compatible types of food with it. For example, mixing mustard and pumpkin produces bitter humor, while eating it with salt makes it salty and with constrictive substances makes it constipate. When it is cooked with Safarjal (quince), it will provide good nutrition for the body.

Gourd is light on the stomach, especially for those who do not suffer from phlegm or cold condition. The wetness contained in this plant helps ease the thirst and headaches if one drinks its extract or washes his head with it. In addition, gourd soothes the stomach however one uses it, and is very beneficial for those who have hot temperaments.

In addition, when the Yaqtin is kneaded with dough and baked in the oven and then its extract is mixed with some light drinks, it helps cool down fever, quenches the thirst and constitutes a good, nutritious food. If it was mixed with quince jam and Manna, it eliminates bile.

When pumpkin is cooked and its juice is mixed

with some honey and Natron, it will cause phlegm and acid. If gourd was ground and then the head is bandaged with it, it will help ease the hot swellings in the cerebral,

When the gourd rinds are squeezed and the extract is mixed with rose oil and used as ear drops, it will help against hot tumors. In addition, its rind helps ease the swelling of hot eye infections and against gout.

In addition, gourd is very useful for those who have hot temperaments and those suffering from fever. When gourd finds some spoiled mixtures in the stomach it In addition gets spoiled causing harmful mixtures in the stomach. In this case, one should treat this condition with vinegar and sour substances.

In general, gourd is one of the lightest foods and the most easily digested. Anas ^ narrated that the Messenger of Allah **b** used to like eating it.

Conclusion

I thought that the best way to end this chapter is by mentioning a general advice concerning preventive measures so as to complete the book's benefit.

This is a chapter that Ibn Masawayh has collected in his book, Al-Mahathir. He said,

"Whoever eats onion for forty days and then his face becomes full of spots, has only himself to blame.

Those who want to economize and eat salted foods will have only themselves to blame if they catch mange or vitiligo.

Those who eat fish and eggs will have only themselves to blame if they catch hemiplegia (paralysis affecting only one side of the body) or facial paralysis."

Those who catch hemiplegia when they take a bath with their stomach full [of food], will have only themselves to blame.

Those who eat milk and fish will have only themselves to blame if they catch leprosy, gecko or gout.

* Whoever mixes milk and wine and then catches gecko or gout has only himself to blame,

Whoever has a wet dream but does not take a bath until he has sex with his wife and then if his wife gives birth to a retarded child, will have only himself to blame.

* Whoever eats his full of cold, boiled eggs and then catches Asthma will have only himself to blame.

* Whoever has sexual intercourse but did not wait until he ejaculates and then catches urinary calculus, (stone like mass that may form in the body under abnormal conditions), will have himself to blame. And

whoever looks at himself in the mirror at night and then catches facial paralysis or another disease will have only himself to blame."

In addition, Ibn Bukhtayshu' said, "Beware of eating eggs and fish together because they cause constipation, hemorrhoids and toothache. In addition, eating eggs excessively begets spots on the face. Further, eating salted foods and salted fish and having venesection (puncturing of a vein) after one takes a bath causes vitiligo and mange. Eating goat kidney on a regular basis will cause the prostate to be sterile, while taking a bath with cold water after eating soft-meat fish causes facial paralysis. In addition, having sex with a menstruating woman causes leprosy, and sexual intercourse that is not followed by taking a bath causes stones. Finally, spending too much time while answering the call of nature causes serious ailments."

Hippocrates said, "Less of a harmful substance is better than too much of a beneficial substance." He In addition said, "Preserve good health by preferring tiresome activity to laziness and abandoning having your fill of foods and drinks."

Further, a wise man once said, "Whoever wants to be healthy, let him eat good food, preserve cleanness and purity while eating, drink while thirsty, refrain from drinking excessive amounts of water and take a rest after lunch. In addition, let him walk after dinner and avoid going to sleep before first answering the call of nature or taking a bath after eating his fill. Further taking a bath once during summer is better than ten times during winter. Eating dried jerky meat at night helps bring about death. Having sex with old women brings the person closer to old age and sickens the healthy body." These words were falsely attributed to Ali. However, some of these words are from Al-Harith bin Kaladah the renowned Arab doctor.

Al-Harith said, "Whoever seeks longevity, although eternal living is not possible, should have lunch and dinner early, wear light clothes and refrain from excessive sexual activity."

He In addition said, "Four things weaken the body: sexual intercourse when one is hungry, taking a bath when one is full, eating dried meat and having sexual intercourse with an old woman."

When Al-Harith was dying, some people visited him and said, "Give us an advise that we could use after you." He said, "Only marry young women, eat ripe fruits when in season and refrain from seeking medications when you can bear the illness. Clean your stomachs once a month (i.e. vomit intentionally), so as to dissipate the phlegm and the bile and to allow the flesh to grow. When one of you eats lunch, let him lay down for an hour and when he eats dinner, let him walk at least forty steps."

A king once said to his doctor, "You might not remain with me for ever, so give me a prescription that I can use after you." He said, "Only marry young women, eat fresh meat and take medication when you are ill. Eat the fruit when ripe and in season and chew the food well. If you eat during the day, there is no harm if you lay down. If you eat at night, do not sleep until you walk even fifty steps. Do not eat except when hungry and do not force yourself to have sex or refrain from urinating. Cool hotness because it causes you tiredness. Do not eat food when your stomach already has food, nor eat what your teeth cannot chew, because your stomach will not be able to digest that food. Try to vomit once a week to cleanse your body. What a good treasure the blood in your body is, so do not cup it without necessity. Finally, take a bath, because it rids you of what the medication cannot rid you of."

In addition, Imam Shafiey said,

- "Four matters bring strength to the body:

  * eating meat, smelling perfume, taking baths without having sexual intercourse and wearing Kittan (linen).

- Four matters weaken the body:

  * excessive sexual intercourse, depression, drinking water repeatedly while the stomach is empty and consuming too much sour foods.

- Four matters strengthen the sight:

  * sitting next to the Ka'bah, using Kohl before going to sleep, looking at green things and cleaning up the sitting area [in the house].

- Four maters weaken the sight:

  * looking at dirt, crucified persons,' a woman's vagina and sitting while your back is to the

Qi'bloh (direction of the prayer).

- Four matters increase sexual power:

  * eating fowl-meat, the large Itreefal (a non-Arabic medication for constipation), pistachio and carob. - Four matters sharpen mind power:

  * avoiding unnecessary speech, using Siwak, and sitting with righteous people and with the scholars."

Plato said, "Five matters dissipate the strength of the body and might lead to death:

  * weakness, leaving loved ones behind, rage, rejecting good advice and the clever persons falling victim to deceit by ignorant people."

The doctor of Al-Ma'mun said, "Hold fast to five characteristics that whoever preserves them would never catch a disease other than death;

  * Do not eat food while there is still food in your stomach.

  * Do not eat a type of food that your teeth cannot chew, because then your stomach would not be able to digest it. Refrain from excessive sexual activity because it shortens life,

* Do not have sex with an old woman because it leads to sudden death.

* Do not revert to cupping without necessity. Vomit during the summer."

Hippocrates In addition said,

* "Everything that is excessive is unnatural." Galinus was once told:

* "Why do you not get sick that often?" He said, "I do not mix two types of unfavorable food together, nor eat food while not hungry, nor keep a food in my stomach which is bothering it."

* Excessiveness in four matters causes sickness:

* speech, sexual activity, sleep and eating habits.

* Excessive speech weakens the mind and hastens old age.

* Excessive sleep turns the face yellow, blinds the heart, irritates the eyes, makes one lazy to work and causes excess humidity in the body.

* Excessive eating habits spoil the orifice of the stomach, weaken the body, cause thick

flatulence and difficult ailments.

* Having sexual intercourse excessively depletes the strength, weakens the body, dries the moistures in the body, adversely relaxes the nerves, causes various clogs and harms the entire body, especially the brain because of the psychological effects it will have on it. Weakness in the brain, which will In addition weaken the soul, is worse than weakness in any other organ.

* The best time to have sex is when one feels a strong desire for a lawful partner (wife) who is beautiful, especially when the spouse is young, ready and excited. In addition, occasional legal sex makes it more desirable, especially when one does not have any concerns and does not use it excessively. In addition, legal sex is best when one is not full or hungry, not after conducting serious physical activity and not during extremely hot or cold weather. When one takes care of these ten matters we mentioned, sex will be most beneficial. Otherwise, if some of these matters were ignored, harm might be caused according to the seriousness of the matters that were ignored. If one does not take care of all these ten matters, he will be faced with a shorter

life span.

* Excessive diet is as dangerous to the healthy person as excessive eating habits when one is ill.

* Galinus said to some of his companions, "Beware of three matters and seek four matters, and you will not need a doctor.

* Avoid dust, smoke and foul odors. Seek nutritious foods, good scents (or aromas), sweets and take baths. Do not eat above your fill, nor pickle Batharuj (a plant) and basil, and do not eat walnuts at night. Whoever caught a cold should not sleep on his back nor should a depressed person eat sour foods.

* Whoever had venesection (puncturing of a vein), should not walk fast because this might cause death.

* Those who have an ache in the eye should not vomit.

* Do not eat too much meat during summer,

* Whoever is suffering from fever should not sleep in the sun. Do not eat old, seeded eggplant.

* Those who drink a cup of warm water every day

during winter will save themselves from illness.

* Those who rub their bodies with pomegranate rind while taking a bath will not catch a rash or mange.

* Whoever eats five flowers of iris with Greek mastic, roe aloes and Musk, will persevere the strength and health of his stomach the rest of his life.

* Eating watermelon seeds with sugar will cleanse the stomach from stones and will prevent burning sensation while urinating."

Four matters bring demise to the body:

* depression, sadness, hunger and staying up late at night Four matters bring joy:

* looking at greenery, running water, loved ones and fruits. Four matters bring darkness to the sight:

* walking bare footed, seeing hated faces mornings and afternoons or seeing the enemy, excessive crying and looking at thin lines for extended periods of time.

Four matters bring strength to the body:

* wearing soft clothes, taking a bath moderately, eating sweet and nutritious food and smelling good scents.

Four matters harden the face and rid it of its youth and health:

* lying, rudeness, asking too many questions without knowledge [or useful purpose] and sinning.

Four matters increase the youth of the face:

* chivalry, faithfulness, generosity and fear of Allah. Four matters bring about anger and hatred:

* arrogance, envy, lying and spreading calumnies. Four matters bring sustenance:

* standing up in prayer at night, seeking forgiveness [of Allah] often at night, giving away in charity and remembering Allah morning and evening.

Four matters prevent sustenance:

* sleeping in the morning, not praying often,

laziness and treachery. Four matters harm the mind and the intellect:

* eating sour foods and fruits excessively, sleeping on the back, depression and sadness. Four matters strengthen the intellect and the mind:

* when the heart is not busy [or concerned], consuming moderate amounts of food and drink, dieting on good combinations of sweets and nutritious foods and getting rid of the harmful substances in the body.

There are some matters that harm the mind:

* eating onions, beans, olives and eggplant excessively, having too much sexual intercourse, loneliness, worrying, intoxication, excessive laughing and depression.

Some wise men In addition said, "I became tired three times and could not find a reason for that except for three matters:

* I ate too much eggplant one day, olives another day and beans a third day."

We have mentioned several beneficial basics of the medicinal sciences that one might not be able to find except in this book. We In addition affirmed that the religion and medicinal science are close to each other. We In addition stated that Prophetic medicine cannot and should not be compared to the medicine of the doctors just as the medicine of the doctors cannot be compared to folk medicine.

This matter is deeper and more serious than we explained, but we mentioned what is sufficient for the reader to recognize its importance. Those whom Allah did not endow with sound comprehension in such matters let them know the difference between the power that is supported by divine intervention and knowledge, strong mind and sound comprehension that Allah has endowed the Prophets with, and between what all others have in this regard.

Someone might ask, "What does the guidance of the Prophet ^e have to do with the subject of medicines and cures and preserving the health?"

This question exposes the lack of understanding of such people, because this subject and many others are among what the Prophet **b** was sent with and what he has directed us to do. Sound understanding and knowledge of Allah and His Messenger are a bounty that Allah endows to whom He will among His creation.

We have explained the three principal basics of medicine in the Qura'an. How can anyone deny that the religion of he who was sent with the righteousness of this and the Next Life In addition contains what preserves the body? How can anyone deny that the religion In addition directs us to the best methods of staying healthy, just as it directs to the best methods of preserving the heart and preventing sicknesses that might attack them? These cures [that the religion contains] are mentioned in general terms and the specifics are left to those of correct minds and pure hearts to seek and implement, just as one does regarding matters of Fiqh. Do not be among those who reject something simply because they have no knowledge of it.*

When the slave is endowed with sufficient knowledge of Allah's Book and the Sunnah of His Messenger **b** along with sound comprehension of the Texts [of the Qura'an and Sunnah], he will rely on these sources and would not need anything else. In addition, he will be able to acquire all types of good knowledge from these sources.

All types of knowledge depends on knowing Allah, His Commands and creation. The Messengers of Allah **b** are the only source that we can acquire such knowledge from, because they have the best knowledge of Allah, His Commandments and creation. The Messengers In addition have the best knowledge of the wisdom behind Allah's creation and Commandments.

This is why the remedies provided by the followers of the Prophets are better and more efficient than the remedies of all others. In addition, the remedies provided by the followers of the best and the master of the Prophets, Muhammad bin Abdullah, are the best, most sufficient and beneficial remedies.

Only those who have true knowledge of the science of medicine and doctors and the medicine offered by the Prophets, can know the difference between them. The Prophets are those with the best minds, purest ways and deepest knowledge. They are the nearest to the truth among the creation. They are the best of mankind that Allah has chosen, just as the Messenger, Muhammad **b**, is the best among all the Messengers. The knowledge that Allah has endowed the Prophets and Messengers with and the wisdom and forbearing puts them in a category that does not permit comparison. Imam Ahmad narrated that the Messenger of Allah as said:

"You (mankind) are seventy nations (or distinct communities); you (Muslims) are the best and most honored among them to Allah."

This honor that Allah has endowed the Muslims with has appeared in their knowledge, minds, intellects and natural ways. The Muslims are the ones who searched through the knowledge of all other nations before them and In addition their wisdom, progress and their works, then added this knowledge to their own knowledge, forbearing and wisdom that Allah has endowed them with.

This is why the Christians are set aback by their silliness, lack of intelligence and apathy, while the Jews are set aback by their sadness, grief and anguish. Muslims, on the other hand, are endowed with sound minds, courage, understanding, joy, happiness and the tendency to help those in distress.

These are some secrets and facts that can only be comprehended by those who have sound minds, sharp intellect, deep knowledge and acquaintance with what the people have [of wisdom, knowledge, and so forth]. All success comes from Allah.

Index

www.ingramcontent.com/pod-product-compliance
Ingram Content Group UK Ltd.
Pitfield, Milton Keynes, MK11 3LW, UK
UKHW061539190726
13845UKWH00031B/1110